D0502437

MICHAEL OPPENHEIM, M.D.

T·H·E
MAN'S
HEALTH
BOOK

PRENTICE HALL
Englewood Cliffs, New Jersey 07632

Prentice-Hall International (UK) Limited, *London*
Prentice-Hall of Australia Pty. Limited, *Sydney*
Prentice-Hall Canada, Inc., *Toronto*
Prentice-Hall Hispanoamericana, S.A., *Mexico*
Prentice-Hall of India Private Limited, *New Delhi*
Prentice-Hall of Japan, Inc., *Tokyo*
Simon & Schuster Asia Pte. Ltd., *Singapore*
Editora Prentice-Hall do Brasil, Ltda., *Rio de Janeiro*

© 1994 by
Prentice-Hall, Inc.
Englewood Cliffs, NJ

All rights reserved. No part of this book may be reproduced in
any form or by any means without permission in writing from
the publisher.

10 9 8 7 6 5 4 3 2

This book is a reference work based on research by the author. The
opinions expressed herein are not necessarily those of or endorsed by
the publisher. The directions stated in this book are in no way to be
considered as a substitute for consultation with your physician.

Library of Congress Cataloging-in-Publication Data

Oppenheim, Michael
　　The man's health book / by Mike Oppenheim.
　　　　p.　cm.
　　Includes index.
　　ISBN 0-13-880550-4.--ISBN 0-13-880543-1
　　1. Men--Health.　I. Title.
RA777.8.066　1994
613'.04234--dc20
　　　　　　　　　　　　　　　　　　　　　　　　　94-4872
　　　　　　　　　　　　　　　　　　　　　　　　　CIP

ISBN　0-13-880543-1

ISBN　0-13-880550-4　(pbk.)

PRENTICE HALL
Career and Personal Development
Englewood Cliffs, NJ 07632

Simon & Schuster, A Paramount Communications Company

Printed in the United States of America

TABLE OF CONTENTS

INTRODUCTION

Men need to get healthier. Although women make 60 percent of office visits, men come in sicker. Being male, they often delay asking for help for too long. Of the ten leading causes of death, men lead in eight. Women suffer more high blood pressure than men but tolerate it better. Even obesity is less damaging to a woman's health. As in so many other male activities, ill health frequently leaves women holding the bag. When one of a married couple dies, the odds are six to one that it's the husband.

When I entered practice and began writing twenty years ago, almost no outlet existed to tell men about their health. Women's magazines devoted a fifth of their space to health-related articles. Men's magazines devoted zero space. When I wrote on something of intense male interest such as impotence, only a woman's magazine would publish it. When I mentioned a device, worn like a condom, to produce an erection, the avalanche of mail asking how to obtain one came from women. Men bought an occasional popular book on health, but most were written for women.

Yet even then men were starting to mend their ways. During the 1970s they began to exercise and quit smoking. During the 1980s they started worrying about their cholesterol. By the 1990s they grew concerned enough to give birth to the first men's health magazines (despite their unisex titles and fervent desire, older ones such as *American Health* and *Prevention* sell mostly to women).

Prevention was always a major concern of mine, so no matter what brought a patient in, if I discovered obesity, smoking, a high cholesterol, or no exercise, I warned about the consequences and laid out a program for reform. Few patients are willing to contradict their doctor, so almost everyone promised to shape up.

Practically no one did. Prevention is harder than enthusiasts claim. Some progress occurred, but I often lost patience with those who failed. Especially when it came to smoking in someone young, healthy, and reasonably intelligent, the sheer stupidity became too much to bear. "Don't you realize what's in store for you?" I thundered. "Don't tell me quitting is hard; it's nothing compared to the suffering and misery that's guaranteed if you don't."

During those early years, I noticed a pattern to the reactions: Men clenched their jaws and agreed to try harder; Women burst into tears.

That upset me as much as them, and I quickly learned gentler ways of keeping up the pressure. But I remain "harder" on men, and it works. Perhaps men are more accustomed to hearing orders: from bosses, drill sergeants, police officers, coaches, team captains. When my platoon sergeant or baseball coach threw a tantrum, I simply took the abuse and waited for it to pass. Men value bravado, and an important part is not letting other men see how much you hurt.

True bravery (in male terms) means going out of your way to endure pain. Men climb mountains, get into brawls, go to war, drive unsafely, play football, and fight bulls. Although unhealthy, these take bravado, and men like that.

Male behavior can be turned into an advantage. Being foolhardy, men smoke more than women; being rugged, they have better success at quitting. Women form 95 percent of the clientele at diet clinics, but men do better at losing weight.

Approached honestly, most men will take up a challenge. I will also challenge them to come to the office more often; it takes courage to give up control. In return they can expect benefits. They will keep those parts of their maleness that they hate to lose (potency, hair) and get rid of those present in excess (wrinkles, prostates).

Looking at the covers of women's magazines one sees women. Looking at the covers of men's magazines one sees . . . women again. Men must learn to share women's preoccupation with their bodies and their health.

CHAPTER ▪ 1

BLUEPRINTS

FOR

MANHOOD

TWO SEXES ARE BETTER THAN ONE

Although learning how you became an adult male has little practical value, it will help you understand why some problems are unique to your sex.

Why can't nature get along with a single sex? Don't assume that only simple bacteria and molds reproduce asexually. Many more complicated creatures do the same; others produce both sperm and egg and fertilize themselves. No natural law forbids even the most advanced animal from producing an egg that develops normally without male help. Some female lizards do this (all hatch into females).

A woman who generated a pregnancy alone would produce an exact copy of herself (a clone). Scientists know how to accomplish this with animals as complex as frogs. More progress must come before they can enable a woman to clone herself, but it should be possible within a century.

Two sexes make for variety, and nature seems to prefer this. An offspring who combines genes of two parents differs from both and from every individual that came before. All this variety means that species change more quickly, and evolution speeds up. This history of the earth bears this out. Life began over two billion years ago. Interesting things happened during most of this period, but the explosion of species began 500 million years ago when sexual reproduction appeared.

Although single-sex creatures such as germs reproduce by splitting into two copies, they evolve because their genes aren't perfectly stable. Genes rearrange themselves spontaneously and undergo chemical changes so that new traits appear (mutations). This happens very slowly, so even germs speed things up with a sort of sex life. Now and then two single-celled creatures press together, a hole appears in their walls, and they exchange some protoplasm. Although biology teachers joke about bacterial sex, this is not really intercourse, but it shows that nature is intensely interested in mixing genetic material. A separate sex, the male, provides this material most efficiently.

THE MALE OF THE SPECIES

You were destined to become a man as soon as the sperm containing half the genes you now possess entered the egg containing the other half (you might wonder what happens if more than one sperm enters; the answer is that the egg dies, but this is not a rule of nature; many higher plants do fine with double or quadruple their normal gene number).

During the first week after fertilization, nothing happens that foretells your sex or even that you'll end up as a human. The egg simply divides into other identical cells. During the earliest division—when there are two, four, eight, etc.—cells are so identical that each would grow into a complete person if separated. Although this occasionally happens, multiple births are not a good idea. The human womb is designed to handle one baby at a time; even twins have a higher incidence of miscarriages and birth defects.

After a week, you are a tiny ball of cells looking exactly like a cockroach or salmon at the same stage. Then cells begin to differentiate. In other words, each becomes destined to form part of the body and can no longer grow into a complete version of you. Differentiation occurs when some genes in a cell are permanently turned off while others continue to function. We don't know how this happens, but finding out is the leading wish of every researcher in genetics. The wonders we could perform by controlling gene expression are so dazzling that you should know a little about genes.

IT'S ALL IN YOUR GENES

Curled inside the nucleus of every cell lay long, stringy molecules called chromosomes. Human cells have forty-six (except eggs and sperm, which have twenty-three). Each chromosome is made up of thousands of genes. Each gene contains a single bit of information that controls the cell's operation, and *every cell in your body contains every gene!* After all, it's descended from the original fertilized egg, and each time a cell divides its chromosomes divide, too.

You should understand the implications. A cell in your brain contains the same genes as one in your finger, bone, liver, or thyroid. Almost all genes in a brain cell aren't functioning, only those that make it look and act like a brain cell. By turning these off and turning on others, the cell would change into something different—for example, a kidney cell.

In primitive animals, all genes in all cells continue to function. If you blow an adult sponge apart into a thousand separate cells, each grows into a complete sponge. More advanced animals lose this ability, but if you cut a large piece off a starfish or earthworm, nearby cells transform and replace it. Even a frog can grow a new leg under the proper conditions. The best a human can do is fill in an injured patch of skin or bone. Given the ability to manipulate gene expression, we could grow you a new stomach or arm, but I don't see that happening for a century or so.

When that week-old ball of cells begins to differentiate, the first changes are very basic: The cells become outer cells, middle cells, and inner cells—in scientific terms, ectoderm, mesoderm, and endoderm. The outer cells are destined to become skin, eyes, ears, and nervous system. Knowing embryology helps a doctor faced with a medical problem. Given a child born with a birthmark or other skin abnormality, the doctor looks closely for a neurological problem because a defect in the ectoderm can lead to both. He or she does not have to look so hard for a disorder of the digestive system, which is derived from endoderm.

The Origin of Genitals

The mesoderm gives rise to sex organs. After three weeks a clump of cells appears that's destined to become both the urinary and genital system. Very primitive animals have neither. More advanced ones have a single system that combines both. Even birds use a single opening for excretion and reproduction.

Around week six, certain cells form a pair of primitive gonads, which become ovaries or testes. Others make up a genital eminence, which develops into external sex organs. At this point boy and girl fetuses look identical. Within the next two weeks the gonads begin to look like testes or ovaries, but the external genitals still appear indifferent.

The Male Shape

At eight weeks the fetal testes begin secreting male hormones, which gradually produce features we recognize as masculine—the penis and scrotum as well as internal structures such as prostate and spermatic duct. Soon after the testes come to life, they begin to descend down the abdominal cavity, settling into the scrotum by the end of the eighth month.

You might conclude that a girl results when the fetal ovary secretes estrogens, but you'd be wrong. The fetus already has plenty of female hormones: its mother's. The growing ovary doesn't have to do anything to encourage a female fetus to grow into a girl. Furthermore, if a male's fetal testes fail to make male hormones, that baby comes into the world looking like a normal girl (the testes don't descend, so they're not visible). The parents will raise the child as a girl; no one will notice anything disturbing until puberty doesn't occur.

This means that the female is the basic body design for a human. Making a male requires major alterations. Since nature isn't perfect, extra design changes increase the chance of error, and this helps explain the greater frailty of men.

Being born gets you over the first hurdle.

BECOMING A MAN

The Second Hurdle

Being born male marks the initial step toward manhood but not the most important. Socialization is essential during the first decade of life, puberty during the second.

By socialization I mean how your parents and other people treat you. Children learn an amazing amount during their first few years. They learn a language with more facility than you or I. Given the opportunity, they can learn two at the same time.

Parents quickly teach a child that it is either a boy or a girl. Although they may know nothing about sexual intercourse, children develop strong feelings about gender and become terribly offended if anyone puts them in the wrong category.

In the preceding section I mentioned that a fetus whose testes fail to produce male hormone is born looking like a girl. The truth will not come out until a doctor investigates why puberty didn't occur. Then no doctor in his or her right mind informs the child. Telling a teenage girl that she's a boy is too devastating. It's unlikely that even the parents will learn the truth; they would be almost as devastated. Most likely the doctor will explain that the child has defects in her sex organs that make childbearing impossible but that she can otherwise lead a normal life. Then a surgeon will remove the testes (undescended testes occasionally become malignant) and the doctor will prescribe estrogens so that she develops an adult female appearance.

Although you know that you're a man because of your upbringing, it's critical for your mental health that your body matches your expectations. This is accomplished by ingenious changes that occur beginning around age ten.

Having formed a boy, male hormone production decreases late in pregnancy. At birth, boys have about the same level of male hormone as girls. Then it rises to a peak at three months of age before dropping again. No one knows what this spurt accomplishes; it may be essential to your development or a meaningless remnant of a past evolutionary process. By age three most children know which sex they belong to, but despite rapid growth during the first nine or ten years, little happens to make boy bodies look different from girls.

Then comes puberty, which enlarges and matures the sex organs but also changes body shape (women's hips and men's shoulders widen), tissue distribution (men become more muscular, women fatter), and hair distribution (hair recedes along the forehead and temple to form an adult pattern). Both sexes grow more hair.

STAGES OF PUBERTY

Early Adolescence

A close examination reveals several curly hairs at the base of the penis. The scrotum appears slightly darker than other skin and shows a few wrinkles.

Soon after a boy's tenth birthday (although it can happen as late as fifteen), puberty officially begins with the period known as early adolescence, which lasts from six months to two years. The penis lengthens, and the testes grow more rapidly, settling into their adult configuration with the left lower than the right. Patients regularly ask why one testicle hangs lower than the other. My answer is a lesson in survival of the fittest.

Used by politicians and businesspeople, the phrase *survival of the fittest* means that one must be ruthless to prosper. Many people believe, incorrectly, that this is how nature works. In fact, organisms evolve and change because some parents have more offspring than others. These parents are more "fit," because they have some useful quality (better eyesight, bigger antlers, more colorful feathers) that yields greater success with the opposite sex, resulting in more children. Naturally these children resemble their parents. Unfit parents have fewer children, so eventually everyone resembles the fit parents, and the unfit die out.

But they die out quietly—not because someone has killed them. Survival of the fittest in evolutionary terms means survival of the most fertile, not of the biggest bully. Remember this when someone claims that being nasty is nature's way.

Long ago men had testicles of varying length. When they hung equally, a man could not bring his legs together without great pain, so he walked with feet spread apart. Women laughed at this waddle. Since they did not find it sexy, women preferred not to mate with such men. Those with unequal testicles walked with a handsome, manly gait that women found more attractive. Eventually equal testicles disappeared because so few children were born with them.

During this period pubic hair remains fine and silky and confined to the base of the penis. The first ejaculation occurs about a year after testicular growth accelerates, at the time that a small clump of pubic hair is in place. This may occur at night or during masturbation. Although not as well publicized as the first menstruation, it comes as a big surprise.

A few hairs appear at the corners of the upper lip. Hair around the anus appears before facial hair, but no one regards this as a milestone.

Middle and Late Adolescence

Middle adolescence in boys begins at age twelve (or as late as fifteen; plenty of overlap occurs) and lasts six months to three years. Here boys finally escape the humiliation of being shorter than girls by entering a growth spurt during which they may shoot up six inches per year. Four inches is the average. Girls begin their spurt around age twelve, boys at fourteen, so there is an uncomfortable gap. Growth stops after the spurt, so the longer it's delayed, the taller the individual. When a girl threatens to grow "too tall," doctors can administer estrogens to bring on puberty earlier.

The adult shape appears during this period. Male hormones increase muscle mass, and their greatest effect occurs on upper chest and shoulder muscles. Male hormones also lengthen bones, giving men thicker, broader shoulders as well as longer arms and legs relative to their body. Female hormones widen the pelvis, so women have broader hips.

When a boy reaches thirteen, parents notice that his former indifference to dirt has reversed dramatically. He may take several showers a day, seek out clean clothes without being asked, and express an interest in deodorants. Adults smile and tell each other that the boy is aware of girls. In fact, the boy is aware that he smells. Body odor and armpit hair appear at this time. Odor is another affect of male hormone; women normally have some male hormone; those who have none remain odorless.

Women lacking male hormone also don't get acne, another disturbing event of this period. Parents are too willing to tolerate a little acne in their teenage children. It's more upsetting than they realize and easy to treat.

During middle adolescence pubic hair grows darker and coarser, starts to curl, and spreads widely over the pubis. The penis grows thicker and longer, the scrotum darker and more wrinkled. Male hormone enlarges the cartilage and muscles of the larynx to give the voice a whining quality and make it crack; the satisfying male baritone takes a few years to appear.

Boys become fertile around age 14, girls a year or so earlier. Curious about sex, they look intently for information and find plenty in movies, television, and among their friends. It's the wrong information and often results in pregnancies and venereal disease (VD), in these adolescents.

Late adolescence marks the end of the line. Beginning between ages 14 and 16, it may continue into the early 20's. Nothing new appears, but everything reaches the adult pattern. Hair spreads to the chest, chin, and inner thighs. A fringe of pubic hair grows up toward the belly button to give a diamond shape. This requires a male level of male hormone. Women normally don't grow this fringe; they keep a triangular pattern. The larynx reaches adult size so the voice deepens and stops breaking. Growth slows and stops.

TEACHING ABOUT SEX

You can teach a child something if he considers you an authority. When a boy looks to his father as the last word on baseball, cars, and algebra, it's because the father acts like he knows what he's talking about—and talks freely. A decade of silence on sex ruins your credibility.

Good sex education begins a few months after a child is born. Children play with their genitals as soon as they acquire enough manual dexterity, usually at five or six months. Despite Freudian teaching, this is normal infantile curiosity and exploration, although manipulation here brings more pleasure than most other areas of the body even in an infant, so he may devote an unnerving amount of attention to his penis. Needless to say it's a bad idea to slap his hands away or even (as more progressive writers suggest) distract him with toys and play. This behavior almost always fades around one year of age as he becomes able to explore the rest of the world.

Children chatter about their genitals as soon as they can talk. In most cases they quickly learn that parents don't share their interest, so they drop the subject and save their talk and experimentation for times when you're not around. Both same-sex and opposite-sex play is a normal part of growing up. You can't prevent it, and it does no harm.

Your first active step in sex education is to stay away from infantile euphemisms; use the correct names for the genitals. Answer the child's questions as they come; don't put them off till later because he'll get the answers elsewhere, and you'll never hear the question again. Answer questions during the first few years, but don't give more information than the child is ready to absorb. If he wonders where babies come from, it's all right to say they come out of the mother's belly and leave it at that. Later he'll want more details, and if he doesn't ask by the age of five or six, you should provide the information before his friends enlighten him. If you've been straightforward all along, this will be easy. Of course, he'll get the usual lurid version from friends and the media, but since he considers you the authority, you'll have a chance to straighten him out. Children who learn about sex from their parents stand a better chance of avoiding later disasters. Unfortunately, to most adults "sex education" means the traditional discussion of the birds and the bees with a preadolescent.

I still remember the embarrassment of listening to my father explaining the facts of life. Although obviously as uncomfortable as I, he knew that he had a duty to perform. At the time I looked on intercourse as one of the mysterious activities adults seemed to enjoy—like watching movies with no action or drinking foul-tasting liquids like coffee and whiskey. I knew sex had something to do with childbirth, but it wasn't clear why adults liked it. Of course, it seemed a wildly grotesque and forbidden activity which, to a ten-year old, was reason enough. When my father explained that a man put his penis inside a woman's vagina, he was not providing new information, and his solemn manner implied that intercourse was some sort of religious act. That increased my confusion, since I and my contemporaries assumed that it was exactly the opposite. I was relieved when he wandered away from the subject of genitals, but it was no more enlightening to hear him talk about women who "sell themselves." I'd never heard of that. What did that have to do with intercourse, I thought. What did they sell themselves for? This was not an educational experience.

If talking about sex with your boy makes you uncomfortable, don't do it. The child will be equally uncomfortable and won't learn a thing. Give him a good book on the subject. Your pediatrician has favorites. Two good ones for beginning readers are *How You Were Born,* by Joanna Cole, Mulberry, 1984 and *Where do Babies Come From?* by Margaret Sheffield, Knopf, 1991. Excellent introductions for older readers include *Growing Up Feeling Good,* by Ellen Rosenberg, Puffin, 1987, and *The What's Happening to My Body? Book for Boys,* by Lynda Madaras, Newmarket Press, 1988. Although aimed readers age ten or older, your boy is better off reading it earlier—before his friends give him the wrong information. The subject holds enough interest for a seven- or eight-year-old so that he'll struggle through.

Please don't send the boy to your doctor for a talk. It will embarrass the doctor as much as it would you. Schools could do the job if allowed to teach about sex from kindergarten on. That's not possible in this country (some European countries do it; all have a lower teenage V.D. and pregnancy rate). When it exists, U.S. sex education consists of a bland discussion of hormones and what happens after sperm meets egg. Some mention sexually transmitted diseases—unfortunately emphasizing AIDS which is not a risk for most middle-class students but legally required in some states.

Teenage Sex

I believe that teenage sex is stupid, but many Americans believe that it's sinful—an important difference. No one is obligated to take action against stupidity, but sin is terrible, like crime. No good person allows it to happen.

Teaching teenagers about birth control and avoiding disease infuriates many parents. This is teaching how to sin without suffering the consequences, they believe. They are certain that this knowledge encourages students to have more sex than they would otherwise. Parents who make a big fuss are a minority, but this is enough to convince school boards that it's not worth the trouble. The end result is no sex classes or classes that offend no one but also don't help students to behave sensibly.

Fortunately, most teens grow into adulthood without suffering great harm from sexual activity provided they avoid catastrophes. The greatest is not disease or even teenage pregnancy; it's early marriage. Even if the bride isn't pregnant, this is a terrible start to adult life.

Finally, sex is not as universal as many believe. By age 19, forty percent of American women and twenty percent of men remain virgins.

CHAPTER ▪ 2

THE ROLE

OF

NUTRITION

THE NUMBER ONE FACTOR FOR HEALTH

Although America was a rich country 150 years ago, a working man and his family lived on bread, cheese, beer, and an occasional piece of meat. Everyone except a few eccentrics considered meat the most desirable food, so the middle and wealthy classes consumed enormous quantities—often half a dozen meat courses per meal—as well as much alcohol and sweets. Fruit was interesting but exotic (you might find an orange in your Christmas stocking). Nobody admired vegetables or grains, because that's what poor people lived on.

Men of their times, nineteenth-century physicians regarded meat as the basis of a healthy diet as well as an important adjunct in treating illness. High-quality meat was essential and poor quality was harmful, and no one objected to fat. In fact, experts disapproved of lean cuts because everyone knew that healthy animals were fat. Sick people required meat even more; a patient too weak for solid food received the healthiest possible liquid: an infusion of fatty beef in salt water. We still call it bouillon. Someone too sick to eat might receive his or her bouillon by enema.

Today a forty-year-old American, European, or Japanese enjoys a better than even chance of living past eighty. One hundred and fifty years ago he was approaching the end of his life expectancy, and this remains true in poor nations today. Medical science contributed modestly to this spectacular increase in longevity—mostly through childhood immunization. Improvements in diet and sanitary engineering played the greatest role. By sanitary engineering, I mean a clean water supply, sewers, and garbage collection: measures that have reduced the deadly infections of past centuries to such a minor threat today that doctors routinely misdiagnose them.

Enormous increases in farm production as well as advances in food preservation and transportation have given everyone access to a much greater variety, but as usual, technology has been a mixed blessing. Modern men enjoy a rich variety of good food along with an avalanche of fast food, nonfood, and processed-to-death food, which too many men make the mainstay of their diet.

Food has become so cheap that even the poorest in wealthy countries can afford an adequate diet (in the United States the poorest must live on the street to accomplish this; since the 1980s general relief buys food or shelter, but not both). Anyone who doubts this abundance should notice the incidence of two diseases of overconsumption among the poor. Unheard of before the industrial revolution, obesity and tooth decay are now more common among the poor than among wealthier classes.

Improvements in nutrition have literally redesigned our bodies. We are several inches taller than in previous centuries. Our ancestors would be shocked at the sight of today's teenagers; they are sexually mature because puberty now occurs three years earlier.

What a Nutritious Diet Can Accomplish

Attention to diet is, without a doubt, the most important positive action a man can take to improve his health. Not only is eating right vital for the growth, development and optimal functioning of a man's body, but current scientific findings indicate that it can offer substantial protection from several chronic degenerative diseases as well.

Over the last two decades we have been bombarded with an onslaught of dietary advice. On a regular basis we are given new dietary guidelines and recommendations which inevitably cause a certain amount of confusion for health conscious Americans.

Eating right isn't as difficult as some people think. As long as you are able to maintain an overall diet that is low in fat and high in complex carbohydrates, you're starting down the right track. Don't worry about making radical changes in what you eat or giving up all of your favorite foods. I will help you achieve an optimal diet—one that gives you all of the nutrients you need for an active lifestyle and enhances your longevity by including natural, whole foods.

In the section on nutrients found on page 21–23 I cover all of the elements of good nutrition and on pages 38–43 you will find my six simple rules for achieving the best diet. Immediately following is an important discussion on the relationship between diet and five of the leading causes of death in this country.

Diet and atherosclerosis (hardening of the arteries). The cause of heart attacks, heart failure, and strokes, atherosclerosis is entirely a nutritional disorder and 100 percent preventable by diet alone—an enormous benefit because atherosclerosis leads the mortality list in the U.S. and most advanced nations. For

American men in their forties, heart disease causes one sixth of all deaths. This rises to thirty-three percent after fifty, to forty percent after seventy, nearing fifty percent at eighty-five.

Although atherosclerotic arteries are "hard," hardness is not a major concern. The problem, as most men know, is that atherosclerotic arteries become clogged. The clogging material is cholesterol which begins piling up on the inner surface of arteries at a shockingly early age. The classic studies occurred during the 1950's when autopsies on soldiers killed in Korea revealed extensive cholesterol deposits in men in their teens and twenties.

Atherosclerosis affects all arteries, but large vessels have room for a great deal of buildup, so the weak links are smaller arteries. When obstruction reduces blood flow to the coronary arteries, the oxygen starved heart muscle hurts (producing chest pain or angina) or pumps too weakly (heart failure). When lack of blood kills a piece of heart muscle, we call it a heart attack. Temporary plugging of a small artery in the brain produces transient neurological defects (local weakness, dizziness, confusion). A stroke occurs when obstruction kills a piece of brain.

It turns out that the heart attack rate in the U.S. has drifted down thirty percent since 1960 and continues to decline. The stroke rate had dropped by half. An improving diet deserves some credit although other actions (less smoking, more exercise) have played a role. Despite this decline, heart attacks and strokes remain the greatest health risk for most men but a risk that a perfect diet can reduce to zero. You'll learn specifics in pages 41–43, but you've probably guessed that it's the sort of high fiber, high plant food, low fat, low meat diet that experts have touted for decades. To achieve zero atherosclerosis you must begin early, but it's never too late because evidence is growing that a man who dramatically improves his diet can dissolve cholesterol buildup.

Although efficacy varies, the best diet also protects against a host of other diseases and chronic disorders. Here are the facts plus some speculation that seems on the right track.

Diet and cancer. For the nonsmoking man, prostate and colon/rectum make up the leading cancer sites with bladder cancer a distant third.

What's In Your Food
(Average Chemical Composition By Per Cent)

Food	% Water	% Protein	% Fat	% Carbo-hydrate	% Mineral
Almonds	5.1	21	54	16	2.2
Apples	85	0.4	0.5	13	0.5
Artichokes	79	2.0	0.1	17	1.0
Avocado	70	2.2	20	6	1.0
Banana	75	1.1	.6	22	1.0
Blackberry	86	1.0	1.1	11	0.5
Butter	11	1.2	85	0	3
Cabbage	90	1.9	.20	5	1.0
Cheese	39	24	30	1.5	4.5
Cream	74	2.5	18	4.5	0.5
Dates	20	2.1	2.8	70	1.60
Eggs	73	12	12	0.5	1.1
Garlic	65	6.8	0.1	27	1.5
Grapes	78	1.3	1.2	19	0.6
Grapefruit	86	0.5	0.0	7.3	0.4
Hickory Nuts	3.7	15	67	11	2.4
Horseradish	77	2.7	0.3	16	1.5
Huckleberries	78	0.8	0.6	17	1.0
Jerusalem Artichoke	79	1.5	0.1	17	1.1
Kale	93	5.1	0.2	8.2	1.2
Leek	87	2.8	0.3	6.5	1.2
Lentils	12	25	2	53	3.5
Lima Beans	68	7.1	0.7	22	1.7
Milk (skim)	90	3.2	0.3	5.2	0.7

What's In Your Food (*continued*)
(Average Chemical Composition By Per Cent)

Food	% Water	% Protein	% Fat	% Carbo-hydrate	% Mineral
Millet	11	9.1	3.8	70	1.9
Mushrooms	89	2.6	0.3	6.1	0.7
Nectarines	83	0.6	0.0	16	0.6
Oatmeal	7.3	16	7.2	68	1.9
Olives	30	5.2	51	10	2.3
Peaches	88	0.7	0.1	9.4	0.5
Pears	84	0.6	0.5	14	0.4
Potatoes	75	2.1	0.2	21	1.1
Pumpernickel	42	4.2	0.7	43	1.3
Rhubarb	94	.60	.70	3.6	.70
Rice	13	7.8	0.9	76	1.0
Rye	16	11	1.8	67	1.8
Spinach	88	3.5	.60	4.4	2.1
Strawberries	88	1.0	0.6	77	0.8
Stringbeans	84	3.9	0.2	8.3	1.2
Soy Beans	10	34	17	34	4.7
Tapioca	11	0.4	0.1	88	0.1
Tomatoes	94	.90	.20	3.7	1.0
Truffles	77	7.7	0.5	6.6	1.9
Turnips	89	3.5	.10	11	1.2
Walnuts	2.5	28	56	11	1.9
Water Cress	92	1.9	0.1	1.3	1.5
Watermelon	93	0.5	0.2	6.0	0.3
Wheat (whole)	36	8.9	1.8	52	1.5
Yams	72	1.8	0.2	23	0.9

Prostate cancer. With 165,000 new cases in 1993, this is the leading male malignancy. Incidence rates have risen slowly for several decades, probably because of better detection and an aging population. The best diet seems to provide some protection. As a strictly male medical problem, I devote a large section to prostate cancer later on.

Colon and rectal cancer. About half as common as prostate cancer, bowel cancer incidence has been declining slowly for white men but increasing in blacks for the past forty years, possibly because of changes in fat consumption.

Obesity increases the risk, and a low fat diet decreases it. Consuming a great deal of fiber protects against colon and rectal cancer, perhaps by speeding passage of waste and carcinogens through the bowel, perhaps by altering the mix of bacteria that normally live in the bowel and produce carcinogens.

Bladder cancer. As a filtrate of body fluids, urine concentrates any toxin in the body, so environmental carcinogens are the major cause of bladder cancer. Furthermore, since men make up eighty percent of victims, something related to maleness increases our risk. Men smoke more than women, and smoking doubles the risk of bladder cancer. Men tend to work around chemicals more than women, and workers in the dye, rubber, paint, and leather industry suffer more bladder cancer. No specific dietary factor increases the risk; a flurry of stories about coffee and artificial sweeteners lit up the tabloids a decade ago, but subsequent studies haven't backed the initial reports. Vitamins and minerals discussed later on may provide protection.

Pancreatic cancer. Although much less common than the above three, it's a particularly unpleasant malignancy, almost invariably fatal, occupying fourth place in mortality behind lung, prostate, and bowel cancer. Located deep inside the abdomen, the pancreas is difficult to examine, so pancreatic diseases tend to be silent during early stages.

After rising for most of the century, the rate has remained steady since 1970—most likely a balance between declining smoking (which doubles or triples the risk) and the increasing number of the elderly. Men suffer 30 percent more pancreatic cancer than women. Most cases occur after age 65 with black men suffering forty percent more than white men.

Aside from not smoking, following a low fat diet provides the best protection.

Distinct nutritional factors in cancer prevention. Studies suggest that cruciferous vegetables (cauliflower, cabbage, broccoli, and brussels sprouts) protect especially well. Consumption of large quantities of allium plants (onions, garlic) greatly lowers the risk of stomach cancer although this is not a major threat in the U.S. The same chemicals that give these vegetables their distinct odor and lower the risk of stomach cancer also have a cholesterol lowering and anti-inflammatory action, and we may hear more about them in the future.

Advocates of natural living denounce additives and modern food processing. Given a choice I'd eat only fresh, organically grown food, but no one in an urban society except the rich have this choice, so we all consume foods prepared by one or another chemical or industrial process. While modern additives don't make food better, they are a vast improvement over traditional methods, and you must look with deep skepticism on anyone urging a return to preservation by old techniques, some of which are still found in markets today. They cause cancer. Areas of the world (some quite advanced such as Japan) which enjoy salt-cured, smoked, and nitrite-cured food suffer an enormous rate of upper digestive tract cancer—esophageal and stomach. Stick to modern chemicals.

Evidence exists that vitamins A, C, E, and selenium offer significant cancer protection, and I discuss the specifics in the next chapter.

Unlike the case with atherosclerosis, diet is only one of many factors causing cancer, so the best diet can't eliminate all risk, but a thirty to fifty percent reduction is to be taken seriously.

Diet and high blood pressure. This is almost a purely dietary disorder. In industrialized countries, blood pressure rises with age, reaching dangerous levels in many individuals. This elevation doesn't occur in members of primitive societies who consume little salt, and where hypertension is unknown.

Humans have always yearned for whatever food is in short supply, and primitive (or simply poor) societies have trouble acquiring meat, sugar, alcohol, and salt. Once people become prosperous enough to eat whatever they want, they go overboard with formerly scarce food. Americans have a passion for salt, consuming at least ten times more than their bodies require.

All countries have their junk food—easily prepared, intensely tasty, cheap, and often not very nutritious. French fries are a variation.

American junk foods contain enormous amounts of salt, not because preparation requires it but because we like saltiness. History provides part of the explanation. Before the development of refrigeration and canning, salting was the easiest way to preserve food because germs can't grow in an extremely salty environment. When canning appeared early in the nineteenth century, canners canned heavily salted foods. Salting wasn't required, but considering the defects of early canning technology this wasn't a bad idea. Unfortunately it preserved our bad habit. Food canned without salt seems tasteless.

As you'll learn further on when I give the details on salt avoidance, a person who never added salt to food, never cooked with salt, and never bought food prepared or canned with salt would still consume more than enough.

Not everyone on a western diet develops dangerously high blood pressure, but we have no easy way of determining who among us is "salt sensitive." However, most high blood pressure makes itself known by middle-age, so if you've passed fifty with a normal pressure, the odds favor that it will stay normal no matter how much salt you consume.

Diet and diabetes. Affecting perhaps two percent of the population, diabetes comes in two forms. Childhood (i.e. insulin dependent) diabetes appears suddenly, usually affects children but occasionally adults, and requires insulin from the beginning. According to the most popular theory, the disease develops when a virus provokes a misguided immune reaction to destroy insulin producing cells in the pancreas.

Diet may play a role in provoking childhood diabetes. Prevention comes too late for readers of this book, but they should take notice when planning a family. In the U.S., exclusively breast fed infants have one-third the risk of diabetes. Around the world its incidence parallels cow's milk consumption. The country with the highest consumption, Finland, suffers five times as much diabetes as the U.S. In Japan where milk is not part of the diet, childhood diabetes is rare.

Researchers suspect that the immature infant's intestine absorbs some cow's milk protein (mature intestines don't absorb large molecules) and that this foreign protein stimulates their immune system. This causes no problem until something happens to incite an attack on the insulin producing cells. Then their sensitized immune systems mount a more vigorous attack. Human milk contains no foreign proteins, and infants who receive no other food during the first six months of life grow up with a more sensible immune system.

More common than the childhood form (three quarters of cases), adult-onset diabetes is probably an unrelated disorder. Heredity plays a major role; your risk is about thirty percent if a parent or sibling is affected (it's ten percent for insulin dependent diabetes). Diet provokes adult onset diabetes, and the major offender is not the popular villain, sugar, but calories. Almost all adult-onset diabetics are overweight, and the best treatment is not pills, insulin, avoiding sweets, or even a diabetic diet but simple weight loss. Staying thin prevents adult-onset diabetes with over ninety percent efficiency. Losing weight often returns an overweight diabetic's blood sugar to normal and allows him to discontinue medication or insulin.

Diet and gastronintestinal disease. Although it sounds paradoxical, the digestive tract requires large amounts of indigestible food to function properly. The small intestine digests refined sugar, meat and dairy products with such efficiency that almost no residue remains to enter the colon. When mills developed machinery to remove the dark bran from wheat and produce beautiful white flour, bread also became too digestible. White bread appeared late in the nineteenth century just as increasing prosperity in western countries enabled almost everyone to eat as much meat, milk, and sweets as the rich in previous centuries. Western colons, accustomed for thousands of years to masses of indigestible plant fiber, hardly noticed the small remnants that entered now and then. Unfortunately, an important colonic function is water absorption, and the longer stool remained, the drier it became. A century has been too little time for evolution to adapt colons to much smaller volumes of much harder stool. The bowel muscle pushes too slowly, generates more pressure than its weak tissue can handle, and often appears to grow frustrated and irritable.

Almost everyone blames his last meal for an attack of vomiting, bloating, dyspepsia, diarrhea, or abdominal cramps, but no patient of mine has denounced the local restaurant after I've diagnosed his appendicitis, diverticulitis, hiatal hernia, hemorrhoids, or irritable colon. Yet all are common where people eat the usual high fat, low fiber western diet, rare where they don't. All seem the consequence of long-term abuse of the digestive tract described above, so the earlier one begins the best diet, the greater the benefits (ironically, men quickly blame food when I diagnose an ulcer, but ulcers are the one gastrointestinal disease not related to diet).

WHY YOU NEED NUTRIENTS

Men suffer plenty of diseases they could prevent with a better diet. Even men in good health endure a food-related disorder (obesity) as they age because muscle mass (which generates a great deal of heat) diminishes and fat (which generates much less) increase. By the sixties, calorie needs have dropped by about 30 percent.

All living creatures burn food to obtain energy. Once again, this is not an analogy but literally what happens. Complex food molecules are torn apart and reduced to carbon dioxide and water, generating the same amount of heat whether this occurs in a flame or a living cell. In a cell, as you'd expect, burning occurs more slowly. Any food that you can digest (i.e., burn) contains calories. Indigestible substances (some types of fiber) and foods that are basically extracts or chemicals (coffee, tea) contain none.

Cold-blooded animals require as much energy for activity as mammals and birds, but almost none when resting motionless. Warm-blooded animals have an insatiable appetite for energy; humans consume two-thirds of their daily calories just to maintain their body temperature at rest. This explains why it takes a frustratingly large amount of exercise to burn off calories.

Protein

Proteins are huge, complex molecules that serve for structure (muscle, skin, nerve) and metabolism (hormones, enzymes, blood). Although flesh is a rich source, proteins occur widely in nature, so anyone who eats a varied diet need not pay special attention to meat.

A man needs 45 to 60 grams per day—3 to 4 ounces. Laypeople find it hard to believe that the equivalent of one lamb chop per day provides our protein needs, but this is not controversial. Americans, like humans in most wealthy countries, consume too much protein—two to four times more than necessary in the United States. Although a healthy person can consume a great excess without harm, this accomplishes nothing useful because the body doesn't store protein. Using as much as it needs, it converts the rest to carbohydrate or fat.

Men who exercise believe that protein builds muscle. Although true, even the most vigorous body builder adds only a fraction of an ounce of muscle per day, so that's all the extra protein he needs.

Fat

A fat molecule consists of glycerin attached to three fatty acids: chains containing four to twenty-four carbon atoms and their accompanying hydrogens and oxygens. Triglyceride is the medical term, so a test for triglycerides measures the fat in your blood. Besides meat, eggs, and dairy products, nuts and vegetable oils make up the richest sources.

Except for a small amount of stored carbohydrate, the body converts excess calories from food into fat, a concentrated source of energy. Burning a gram of fat produces nine calories; a gram of carbohydrate or protein produces four. Even the thinnest person requires fat, because we store very little carbohydrate (the average man carries around 150,000 calories of fat, 2,000 of carbohydrate). Less than a day of fasting uses up stored carbohydrates.

Besides storing energy, fat covers blood vessels, nerves, and organs to protect from physical damage and insulate against heat loss. It also contributes to your body structure, especially to the membranes that cover cells and cell nuclei, and it provides chemical building blocks for important body substances such as prostaglandins.

Dietary fat requirements are small because your body makes glycerin and fatty acids from simple molecules. The exceptions are two fatty acids, linoleic acid and arachidonic acid. Both are widely distributed in the food supply, so no special effort is required to consume your daily requirement. No minimum fat requirement exists, but a tasty diet is difficult without at least 10 percent of the calories from fat.

Carbohydrates and Fiber

The most familiar carbohydrates are sugars: small molecules that plants manufacture by combining carbon dioxide and water during photosynthesis. Glucose, the most important, has the formula $C_6 H_{12} O_6$—meaning it's made from six carbon dioxides and six water molecules. Animals (as well as plants) obtain energy by burning carbohydrates, returning them to carbon dioxide and water. Our cells burn only glucose; we consume other sugars such as fructose, maltose, or sucrose as well as other carbohydrates, but we convert them to glucose before use.

Plants make their tissue by stringing sugars together to form large molecules called complex carbohydrates. Some, such as starches, taste good and form part of our diet. Others (cellulose, gums, lignin) are entirely indigestible by higher animals. Called roughage or fiber, indigestible plant matter provides no nutrients but plays an essential role in our diet. Those who consume too little suffer from chronic constipation; generous amounts provide the sheer bulk that our intestines require to move food along smoothly; they also serve the protective functions discussed earlier.

We burn dietary glucose so quickly that none remains a few hours after a meal. Fortunately humans and other animals convert some sugar into a complex carbohydrate called glycogen, storing it in the liver and muscle. Although we store less than a day's supply, this enables us to avoid depending entirely on other sources of glucose—fat and protein. In the absence of glycogen, the body manufactures glucose from both fat and protein. This produces a condition called starvation ketosis, in which tissue breakdown products make the blood too acid, leading to a queasy feeling and slowdown of normal metabolic activity. Provided that you consume a minimum of carbohydrates (at least 15 percent of your calories), you can burn fat without ketosis. The best diet is at least 50 percent carbohydrate.

Don't FORGET VITAMINS AND MINERALS

Vitamins are small organic compounds required in tiny amounts for the chemical reactions that support life. Minerals are basic elements (iron, copper, calcium, etc.).

While essential for your nutrition, vitamins, minerals, and trace elements exert a fascination out of proportion to their importance in organizing your diet, but they are important, so here are the basics.

Vitamin A plays a vital role in the function of your retina and skin. Common in the poorest countries, blindness from lack of vitamin A almost never occurs elsewhere because so many foods contain it: green and yellow vegetables, yellow fruits, dairy products, eggs, and liver. I have never heard of a case of deficiency in the United States or read a case report in a medical journal, but now and then I read about vitamin A poisoning, usually in someone who consumes large amounts in an effort to improve his or her vision or complexion. Remember that vitamins participate in chemical reactions essential for your body's operation, but consuming more than these reactions require won't make you supernormal any more than feeding extra voltage into your television will improve the picture. In fact, when doctors use Retin-A, Accutane, and other vitamin A derivatives to treat skin disorders, they are taking advantage of their toxicity, not their normal action.

No one is certain how vitamin A protects against cancer of the digestive system, bladder, and lung, but this effect is most obvious when we compare people who consume plenty of vitamin-rich foods with those who don't. Evidence that vitamin A supplements reduce cancer risk is modest but growing. I have participated in such a study for almost ten years. During this time, over 20,000 doctors have consumed pills containing either aspirin, vitamin A, or a placebo to determine the effect on their health—mostly the incidence of heart attack and cancer. After five years it was obvious that aspirin protected against heart attacks, so researchers discontinued that leg of the experiment. The vitamin A results should be out by the time you read this.

The recommended daily allowance (RDA) of vitamin A is 5,000 units daily. Recommended dietary allowances include enough to perform the strictly chemical functions of the vitamin with a generous margin of error.

B vitamins, originally isolated from the same source (liver and yeast), are grouped together for that reason alone. Their actions are unrelated, and no reason exists for considering B complex more useful than any other combination. Experts recognize eleven B vitamins, but several don't seem necessary for humans.

Vitamin B_1, or thiamine, is part of an enzyme system that breaks down glucose to provide energy. Obviously a fundamental process in all living creatures, glucose breakdown is a complex reaction requiring dozens of steps. Many vitamins take part, a fact responsible for their reputation as a source of energy. The true source of energy, of course, is glucose. Lack of glucose produces fatigue; ironically, vitamin deficiency leads to many symptoms, but lack of energy is not prominent.

Every doctor learns about beriberi in medical school, but traditional thiamine deficiency is almost unknown in the United States because the vitamin is so widely available in meat, whole grains, dairy products, legumes, and nuts. However, interns and residents at city hospitals see a peculiar form in men who consume almost all their calories in the form of alcoholic beverages. Called Wernicke's encephalopathy, it's a neurological disorder producing muscle weakness, numbness, difficulty walking, and delirium. A single thiamine injection produces dramatic improvement provided that the deficiency is not too chronic. The RDA of vitamin B_1 is 1.5 milligrams daily.

Vitamin B_2 or riboflavin, is another trace chemical important in energy metabolism as well as visual function. Deficiency is so uncommon that no name exists, and it almost never occurs except in severe malnutrition when other deficiencies are also prominent. Meat and fish, especially organ meats, as well as dairy products, grains, green leafy vegetables, and eggs contain riboflavin. The RDA of vitamin B_2 is 1.7 milligrams daily.

Vitamin B_6, or pyridoxine, plays a role in glucose metabolism but is more strongly involved in buildup and breakdown of proteins—so much so that the body's need varies with protein intake: The daily requirement is 1.5 milligrams of pyridoxine for every 100 grams of protein. Meats, liver, whole grains, cereals, and vegetables contain pyridoxine.

Like vitamins B_1 and B_2, deficiency of B_6 is rare; unlike them B_6 has important medical uses as well as many risky interactions with drugs.

Isoniazid, the most important antituberculosis drug, causes an unpleasant neuritis in a small percentage of patients. Pyridoxine prevents this, so everyone taking isoniazid should take extra pyridoxine. Some drugs antagonize the action of pyridoxine, so doctors prescribe extra B_6 for patients on penicillamine, cycloserine, and hydralazine, among others. On the other hand, patients taking L-dopa to treat Parkinson's disease must religiously avoid B_6 because it breaks down L-dopa, a drug that resembles natural chemicals that pyridoxine acts on. Women who become depressed taking oral contraceptives often feel better when they take 50 milligrams of pyridoxine per day. This also cures an uncommon anemia called pyridoxine-responsive anemia, a disease probably not caused by a simple deficiency, so this is a case where pyridoxine works as a drug, not a nutrient.) The RDA of vitamin B_6 is 2 milligrams daily.

Vitamin B_{12}, the first vitamin to perform a miracle cure, is essential for growth and reproduction of all animal cells, but most critically in humans for maturation of red blood cells and metabolism of nervous tissue. A deficiency leads to a relentlessly progressive, fatal anemia (pernicious anemia) accompanied by profound weakness and paralysis. Not rare, pernicious anemia is not the result of dietary B_{12} deficiency but of a stomach defect. The stomach secretes a substance called intrinsic factor, which combines with B_{12} and enables the small bowel to absorb it. For unclear reasons, the stomach sometimes loses the ability to secrete intrinsic factor, so B_{12} (formerly called extrinsic factor) passes through and out of the digestive tract.

During the 1920s researchers discovered that feeding patients enormous amounts of liver relieved their anemia. Although life-saving, this was an unappetizing diet; fortunately scientists soon isolated a liver extract and later the pure vitamin. Nowadays victims of pernicious anemia (and of stomach and bowel diseases that prevent B_{12} absorption) do fine on a monthly injection.

The B_{12} story is an exhilarating milestone in medical history. As late as the 1920s medical doctors performed precious few dramatic cures. Surgeons did so routinely (untreated appendicitis leads to an agonizing death, so a simple appendectomy is a real miracle). A doctor feeding liver extract to a miserable, bedridden patient could watch him or her perk up within days, arise and walk in a week, and return to normal life in a few months.

The news of B_{12} spread like wildfire through the general public as well as the medical profession, and seventy years have hardly dimmed its reputation as the premier energizer. Doctors prescribe it liberally as a placebo, although I know more than a few who are convinced that it works, and many patients request B_{12} when they feel they need a boost. Actors and singers who can afford it have a nurse on hand to give an injection before every performance.

Good research shows that B_{12} energizes only those enfeebled by B_{12} deficiency, but I carry a vial on my rounds for patients who ask for it; I never suggest B_{12}, but I don't object to requests. It's a safe drug, and much useful magic surrounds B_{12} besides its history. Laypeople (but not doctors) consider an injection superior to a pill. Even more impressive, vitamin B_{12} is the only colored drug in common use. When I fill a syringe with vivid red liquid, patients know that strong medicine is coming.

Liver is the richest source, but all parts of an animal contain B_{12}, including eggs and dairy products. Dietary deficiency is almost unheard of, except in pure vegetarians who eat no eggs or milk products. They should take supplements, but injections aren't necessary. The RDA for vitamin B_{12} is 2 micrograms daily.

Folic acid and B_{12} invariably appear together in textbooks because both participate in cell growth and reproduction, and the anemia from a deficiency of either produces identical, abnormally large (megaloblastic) red cells. Despite this similarity, the two are not chemically related. Virtually all foods are rich in folates, especially green vegetables, liver, yeast, nuts, and cereals. Deficiency occurs rarely, except in chronic alcoholics and those with intestinal disease that prevents absorption. Long-term therapy with several antiseizure drugs and oral contraceptives occasionally interferes with folic acid's action, producing a megaloblastic anemia.

Unlike B_{12}, folic acid has value as a preventive. Pregnant women take supplements to lower the incidence of several neural birth defects. Given to women with suspicious, precancerous cells on their cervix, 10 milligrams of folic acid a day for three months seems to normalize the cells. Although not in the front ranks of the anticancer vitamins, folic acid shows tantalizing possibilities. The RDA for folic acid is 200 micrograms daily.

Niacin's scientific names are nicotinic acid or nicotinamide. Another B vitamin, it's unrelated to the nicotine in tobacco, so researchers invented a different name to avoid confusion. Niacin is another factor in the chemical reactions that allow cells to make energy. All meats and fish, as well as whole grains, green vegetables, nuts, and legumes, are rich sources.

Lack of niacin leads to pellagra, known to medical students as the disease of the three D's: dermatitis, diarrhea, and dementia. In severe cases victims suffer a sunburn-like rash, and vomiting accompanies diarrhea along with delirium and hallucinations. Pellagra was endemic in the American south for centuries, and doctors noticed that the poor suffered most, but occasionally the prosperous fell victim. Some families included many cases; others were spared. Using common sense, doctors concluded that pellagra was a contagious disease aggravated by poor hygiene.

It was well into the twentieth century before researchers corrected this impression. Pellagra appeared where people ate a great deal of corn and almost no meat, a characteristic of the old south. To synthesize niacin, the body uses tryptophan, one of the twenty amino acids that make up protein. Meat, fish, poultry, nuts, and legumes contain plenty of tryptophan, but the protein in corn contains little. It takes only a little meat and a modest variety in the diet to achieve an adequate intake, so niacin deficiency is no longer a problem.

Massive doses—several hundred times the RDA—lower blood cholesterol and reduce the risk of a heart attack. Despite the high dose, niacin is easily the cheapest treatment for a high cholesterol—a tenth the cost of newer drugs. Despite this advantage, doctors don't prescribe it much because of the side effects. Almost everyone taking an effective dose (2 to 6 grams a day) feels an uncomfortable flushing; the skin turns red and often itches. A large minority also suffer stomach irritation. One can minimize these reactions by dividing the dose, taking it after meals, and taking aspirin before each dose, but most patients remain at least mildly inconvenienced, so doctors prefer newer drugs that rarely cause discomfort. I encourage patients to try niacin, but your doctor may not mention it, so you may have to. The RDA of niacin is 20 milligrams daily.

Pantothenic acid participates in reactions that break down carbohydrates and fats and synthesize hormones and many other substances. Volunteers fed a diet low in pantothenic acid for several months develop headaches, vomiting, muscle cramps, weakness, and numbness in the extremities. This proves that pantothenic acid is essential, but medical science hasn't identified a deficiency disease in people consuming their regular diet, probably because pantothenic acid occurs so widely. There is not even an official RDA, but experts estimate an adult requirement of 4 to 10 milligrams per day.

Biotin also takes part in the buildup and breakdown of fats and carbohydrates. This is another essential vitamin that hardly ever presents a nutritional problem because so many foods contain it: meats, eggs, dairy products, yeast, and nuts. It's also synthesized by colon bacteria. Almost all cases of deficiency occurred in patients on long-term intravenous feeding with an artificial diet. They suffered inflamed, peeling skin and hair loss that resolved as soon as doctors added biotin. No one knows how much biotin your diet should contain; 30 to 100 micrograms is the current estimate.

Vitamin C, also known as ascorbic acid (ascorbic = antiscorbutic = antiscurvy), is essential for synthesis and maintenance of connective tissue—the tough, rubbery tissue that holds everything together and fills in the spaces between organs. Connective tissue lines your blood vessels, forms tendons and ligaments that attach muscle to bone and bone to bone, and make up almost all your skin except for the thin layer of epidermis on the surface.

The oldest known deficiency disease, scurvy devastated ship crews during the age of sailing ships when fresh food was unavailable and sailors consumed only preserved meat, dried beans, bread, and alcoholic beverages for months. Symptoms were what you'd expect of deteriorating connective tissue: bleeding first into the skin, bleeding gums and eventual loss of teeth, fragile skin, poor wound healing, swollen, painful joints and muscles. Death usually occurred from internal bleeding.

Most men know that citrus fruits are rich in vitamin C, but many foods contain it, including other fruits, milk, organ meats, and vegetables. Nowadays scurvy occasionally turns up, almost invariably in a old man living alone on a diet limited to hamburgers, snack foods, sweets, and alcohol.

Among fashionable vitamins, B_{12} leads in the older generation, C in the younger. More evidence exists for the virtue of taking extra C, but it's a complicated, confused matter. Everything began, of course, with Linus Pauling, probably the greatest chemist of the twentieth century, who became an apostle of vitamin C during the 1960s and praised its action in preventing colds and cancer, boosting immunity, and prolonging life.

Aged 92 as I write, Pauling continues to consume a staggering 18 grams per day (300 times the RDA) and urges us all to do the same. To a certain extent there is less here than meets the eye because he began dosing himself at sixty-five, and a healthy 65-year-old stands a good chance of living into his nineties. On the other hand, Pauling provides a living example of vitamin C's safety. Taking 18 grams would terrify me, but his claims for its good qualities seem less outrageous now than twenty-five years ago, when I was younger and unconcerned about my own health and the possibility of growing old.

Besides its function in building connective tissue, vitamin C strengthens the immune system in ways we are beginning to understand. Scientists have long studied those parts of our defenses that neutralize bacteria and viruses. Until recently they paid less attention to defenses against equally destructive toxins that we swallow or breathe in from our environment, as well as toxins normally produced within the body. No animal is perfect, and normal metabolic activity generates highly reactive chemicals, with names like free radicals and oxidants, that damage tissues, make normal cells malignant, and may produce the steady deterioration that we call aging.

Just as white cells and antibodies fight off most infections, other substances neutralize damaging free radicals, oxidants, and similar toxins. Since we know that an infection may overwhelm the best immune system, it comes as no surprise that some toxins escape, at least long enough to do damage. Boosting our supply of toxin neutralizers with extra vitamin C seems a sensible preventive measure. To a surprising extent, the food industry accepts this. Thus, bacteria in our intestine act on nitrates and nitrates used in processed meats to produce nitrosamines, a potential carcinogen. Vitamin C blocks this conversion, so it's routinely added to processed meats (I include this strictly as an example; processed meats form no part of my recommended diet).

Vitamin C appears to lower the risk of colon, rectal, bladder, stomach, and lung cancer. Because the best evidence comes from comparing subjects who ate varying amounts in their diet, the benefits of taking extra vitamin C are not so clear, although this may change in the future. I take 1 gram (1,000 milligrams) per day, despite Pauling's heroics. The RDA of vitamin C is 60 milligrams daily.

Vitamin D, although called a vitamin, is really a hormone. It's synthesized in the skin and under ideal conditions isn't required in the diet. Like a hormone, vitamin D then travels in the blood to distant sites and attaches to cell receptors to act. In combination with other hormones, vitamin D regulates the calcium level in blood and bones; in the intestine it permits absorption of dietary calcium and phosphorus. Fish oils, eggs, and liver are rich sources, but nowadays so many foods are fortified with vitamin D that attaining enough is easy.

When it's lacking, calcium and phosphorus aren't absorbed, their blood level drops, and the body makes up the deficit by extracting calcium from bone, which becomes soft and deformed. Called rickets in children and osteomalacia in adults, Vitamin D deficiency rarely occurs in tropical climates even among the poor because solar radiation converts substances in the skin to the vitamin (irradiating food does the same). Not much sun is required, so vitamin D deficiency shouldn't occur in temperate countries except in extreme circumstances. During the 1950s and 1960s British doctors began seeing rickets in children of dark-skinned Indian and Pakistani immigrants who lived in sunless British cities, but this declined as more food was fortified.

Doctors prescribe massive doses of vitamin D to treat several uncommon hormonal or kidney diseases in which blood calcium is low. No common disorder (such as osteoporosis) benefits from this, and healthy people who consume excess vitamin D absorb more calcium than their body can handle. As a result, calcium precipitates in the kidney (causing kidney damage and stones); produces calcification in other tissues such as heart, lung, and skin; and leads to fatigue, headaches, diarrhea, and vomiting. Poisoning yourself requires supplements of pure vitamin D; you can't take in too much from excessive sunlight, fortified food, or the usual multivitamin. The RDA for vitamin D is 400 units daily.

Vitamin E, alpha tocopherol, seems to act as a general anti-oxidant, preventing formation of harmful oxidation products within the body and scavenging those that appear. Premature infants receive extra vitamin E to prevent damage from the pure oxygen that they require.

Alpha tocopherol is widely available in whole grains, vegetable oils, eggs, nuts, and legumes. Experimental volunteers remain frustratingly healthy for month after month on a diet lacking vitamin E, so it may serve no specific metabolic function in humans. On the other hand, a host of symptoms quickly appear when animals become deficient, including sterility, muscle deterioration, heart disease, and anemia. As a result, enthusiasts promote vitamin E to improve human sexual performance, cure muscle cramps, prevent atherosclerosis, and boost energy. No evidence exists that this works, but its antioxidant action provides reason enough to pay attention.

Unlike the case with A and D, vitamin E supplements are reasonably safe, so although no one knows if taking a few hundred units per day prevents cancer better than the RDA, there's probably no danger in doing so. The RDA of vitamin E is 30 units daily.

Vitamin K participates in the complex series of reactions necessary to make blood clot. Bleeding, often catastrophic, happens in its absence. Leafy vegetables, as well as liver and other meats, contain vitamin K. Almost all deficiency bleeding in adults occurs as the result of blood-thinning drugs (Warfarin, Coumadin) that block vitamin K action and prevent clots in disorders like pulmonary emboli, abnormal cardiac rhythms, and in people with artificial heart valves. Bacteria in your colon make vitamin K, perhaps all that you require, but this is not certain, so an RDA exists. The RDA of vitamin K is 80 micrograms daily.

Minerals Are Also Important

Dozens of elements are essential for life, but a lesser number should concern you in day-to-day nutrition and as disease preventives.

Calcium, the major mineral in bone and teeth, also occurs throughout blood, body fluid, cells, and tissues. It's essential for muscle contraction, cardiac function, nerve conduction, cell structure, blood clotting, and many other functions that we haven't discovered. Calcium is so central to life that three hormones (vitamin D, parathyroid hormone, and calcitonin) precisely regulate its action as well as its entry to the body (the intestine), exit (kidneys), and storage (in bone).

Dairy products, green leafy vegetables, shellfish, and fish eaten whole (such as sardines) are good sources, but calcium is one nutrient that's marginal in the American diet. Experts encourage those who don't drink a quart of milk a day (skim milk is fine) to take a gram of calcium. Because calcium seems to protect against colon cancer, probably by binding toxins in the intestine, I suggest that everyone follow this advice. Plain calcium carbonate (chalk) is the cheapest. You can buy large bottles, but antacid tablets such as Tums taste better.

When blood calcium drops, muscles and nerves become irritable, producing painful cramps, tingling, and muscle twitching that progresses to convulsions and death. In reality the body regulates calcium so efficiently that these symptoms occur only in advanced deficiency or when the hormonal system can't function (such as after surgical removal of the parathyroid glands). During most cases of calcium deficiency, blood levels are kept near normal by calcium removed from bone, eventually producing rickets and osteomalacia.

An elevated calcium leads to weakness, depression, vomiting, constipation, cardiac irregularities, and abnormal calcium deposits in tissue and bone. Again, diet or even supplements are rarely responsible. Most serious elevated calcium occurs during advanced cancer, and almost all the remainder from hormone disorders due to overactive glands or excessive vitamin D intake. The RDA of calcium is 1.2 grams daily.

A single *iron* atom rests at the center of each of four units of hemoglobin, the red molecule filling your red blood cells that transports oxygen from lungs to tissue. A single iron atom also anchors the similar, smaller myoglobin molecule that stores oxygen in muscles and gives them their red color.

Meat, egg yolks, yeast, whole grains, green vegetables, legumes, and nuts contain iron, but the body absorbs meat and egg iron more efficiently than vegetable iron. Although rarely a problem in healthy men, iron deficiency anemia is the leading nutritional disorder in young women, who can lose more iron in menstrual bleeding than a normal diet provides. Every woman with heavier than average periods should take iron supplements, but men should not. Here's why.

Unlike calcium, which pours into and out of the body with abandon, humans hold onto iron with ferocious stinginess. In fact, we have no way to excrete it; urine, bile, and sweat contain almost none. A tiny amount leaves each day in cells normally shed from our skin and intestinal lining. This conservation appears more extraordinary when you realize that adults have two quarts of red cells, and these cells live only four months. They are then removed from the circulation, broken down, and converted into bile by the liver, which excretes bile into the small intestine to help digest fats—all except the iron, which is extracted and sent back to the bone marrow to make more hemoglobin. As a result, we require only 1 percent as much iron as calcium. Many experts classify iron with the trace elements.

Besides iron in active use, we store only about 1 gram, mostly in the liver and spleen. When more enters the body, it settles out in various tissues, and pure iron is as toxic as other metals. Long-term excess damages the heart (leading to heart failure), liver (cirrhosis), and pancreas (diabetes). Multivitamins contain too little iron to worry about, and even those who consume a few iron pills rarely get into trouble, but no good comes of it. A woman with iron deficiency anemia can usually blame it on menstruation, but men don't have this excuse. A man who needs iron is bleeding from somewhere that shouldn't bleed, almost always in his digestive tract, usually from an ulcer or tumor. Iron will cure the anemia, but the bleeding will continue. The RDA for iron in man is 12 milligrams daily.

Zinc participates in many areas of tissue growth and reproduction, so children and pregnant women need more, but men need some. Skin, gastrointestinal lining, immune cells, and the testes reproduce the most rapidly, so zinc deficiency causes skin inflammation, poor wound healing, hair loss, diarrhea, depressed immunity, and sterility. These symptoms are most obvious in a rare genetic disease called acrodermatitis enteropathica, in which zinc absorption is defective; large doses of zinc produce dramatic improvement.

Dietary deficiency is largely confined to poor areas of the world because meat, dairy products, grains, and nuts contain plenty of zinc. Its miraculous effect on acrodermatitis enteropathica (like that of B_{12} on pernicious anemia) has encouraged zinc's use to improve fertility, immunity, and wound healing and to grow hair and improve the complexion. Although evidence for this is unimpressive, taking a few times the RDA is probably safe, but—as I've mentioned—metals quickly become toxic. The RDA of zinc is 15 milligrams daily.

Selenium plays an important role in oxygen metabolism and breakdown of peroxides as well as cell growth. Because it occurs widely in meat and vegetables, deficiency doesn't occur—except perhaps in the Keshan province in China, where the soil lacks selenium. Seen only in this province, Keshan disease leads to a degeneration of the heart and other muscles that selenium cures.

Selenium protects animals against viruses and chemicals that cause cancer. Evidence for protection in humans is less clear, but studies show a higher rate of lung, stomach, rectal, and esophageal cancer in areas where soil has a low selenium content.

Selenium is also toxic to animals; farm runoff water high in selenium has eliminated the wildlife from some wildlife refuges. Poisoning in humans has occurred from industrial exposure but not diet, although this may change if more evidence appears of its anticancer properties and taking supplements becomes more popular. The RDA of selenium is 70 micrograms daily.

Magnesium, a close relative of calcium, shares many actions. Besides forming part of the structure of teeth and bones, magnesium is essential for nerve transmission as well as muscle and heart activity. Deficiency causes weakness, irritability, confusion, increased muscle tension and spasm, and eventually seizures. Magnesium excess suppresses nerve and muscle activity so well that doctors give large doses to control seizures in certain conditions such as toxemia of pregnancy.

Grains, nuts, and legumes are rich sources, but meat and fruit also contain modest amounts, so dietary deficiency in healthy men rarely appears outside the laboratory. Despite the prominence of weakness as a symptom, Americans mostly ignore magnesium, remaining loyal to the traditional energizers: B vitamins, especially B_{12}, and iron. In contrast, Germans consider subtle magnesium deficiency a significant cause of chronic fatigue, anxiety, and generalized aches and pains. German patients consume a great deal on their own, and doctors prescribe it liberally. People with healthy kidneys can consume a great deal of magnesium safely, so there's no harm in imitating the Germans, just as anyone can consume the minced animal genitals with which the Chinese treat similar symptoms. However, folk medicine doesn't work well outside its own culture, so Americans achieve better results from the B's. The RDA of magnesium is 400 milligrams daily.

Iodine is among the few elements with a single function. The thyroid gland requires iodine to make its hormone, which regulates the rate at which the body uses energy. Ocean seafood is the only significant natural source of iodine, so a mild deficiency was once extremely common. When intake becomes inadequate, thyroid tissue swells, enabling it to extract iodine more efficiently from the blood. A visibly swollen thyroid is called a goiter, and in past centuries goiters were so common that women considered them a mark of beauty.

Only in severe deficiency does thyroid hormone secretion drop, producing lethargy, mental dullness, loss of appetite, constipation, chilliness, and increasingly puffy and swollen skin (but not obesity; you have to be healthy to get fat).

Adding iodine to salt was the first great public health triumph of the twentieth century. Ironically, today iodine occurs almost everywhere in the environment—in dough conditioners, food additives, and even automobile exhaust—so iodized salt is no longer necessary. Fortunately, a modest excess is not dangerous; in fact iodine solutions are the best expectorant, loosening tenacious sputum. Doctors prescribe them to treat bronchitis and asthma. The RDA for iodine is 150 micrograms daily.

Fluoride accumulates in teeth, making the surface enamel harder and resistant to decay. Although present in almost all foods, water is the major effective source, along with oral supplements and direct application of fluoride to newly erupted teeth. Since fluoride enters developing teeth, it probably does little good once permanent teeth are fully formed after age fourteen.

Excess dietary fluoride produces white mottled patches on the teeth, which do no harm; much heavier intake, generally through industrial exposure, causes abnormal, painful calcification in the bone, ligaments, and muscles. Despite warnings that fluoride causes cancer, this doesn't happen.

In a high school health science class in 1955, I learned that 5 percent of Americans reached adulthood with no cavities. That number had stood for a century, but today over 50 percent have no cavities, and this figure continues to rise. Although epidemic over most of the world, tooth decay is declining in the United States; this is one of our great unsung public health triumphs. Fluoridation is responsible.

Thirty years ago, water fluoridation opponents portrayed fluoridation as an evil conspiracy by dentists. This is ironic because the spread of fluoridation has devastated the dental profession. Income has dropped, dental schools across the country are closing their doors, and I no longer read editorials warning of a shortage of dentists.

Only half the water supply is fluoridated, although dietary supplements and topical applications help more of the population. Everyone should make sure his or her family—especially children—receives the benefit. A reasonable daily dose is 1.5 to 4.0 milligrams. Drinking water should contain 1 part per million.

A dozen other elements, including manganese, copper, silicon, chromium, cobalt, and molybdenum, are probably or definitely essential but don't represent a significant health concern. Lack of nickel, tin, vanadium, and even arsenic produces disease in some animals and plants, but no one has discovered their role in humans.

Who Needs Vitamins and Minerals?

Everyone needs them. People who don't consume enough get sick. Americans tend to believe that "not eating right" produces vitamin deficiency, but this is only true in places like East Africa or Bangladesh. The consequences of a bad American diet (fast foods, processed foods, sweets, beverages, and high salt, fatty, and fried foods) are mostly disorders of excess: obesity, heart attacks, high blood pressure, and tooth decay. Nutrient deficiencies exist, but they are more subtle. Preventing cancer, for example, may require more than the bare minimum that prevents scurvy, beriberi, rickets, etc.

Some circumstances increase the chance for a distinct deficiency in otherwise healthy people.

Reducing Diets. A diet can contain enough vitamins and minerals until it drops below 1,000 calories daily. At that point, supplements become necessary. An ordinary multivitamin is probably enough, but you shouldn't follow such a diet without a doctor's supervision.

Vitamins and Vegetarians. A balanced meatless diet contains enough vitamins unless it also lacks milk and eggs. Vitamin B_{12} only occurs in animal products, so anyone on such a strict vegetarian diet must take extra B_{12}.

Vitamins and Infants. Breast-fed babies don't need vitamins for the first three months. After that, dark-skinned infants and those who get little sun exposure should have extra vitamin D. Formula-fed babies need extra C and D unless the formula itself contains them.

Vitamins and Drugs. So many interactions occur that entire books exist to warn doctors. I've mentioned some important ones earlier, and your doctor will use his or her judgment on others at the time of your prescription. Most interactions have the same significance as the warning on the label of common over-the-counter cold remedies ("Do not take this product if you have heart disease, high blood pressure, thyroid disease, diabetes, or enlargement of the prostate unless directed by a doctor"). Reading this always makes me nervous, but I can't remember the last patient who suffered a reaction, so I allow everyone to take them.

Most drug–nutrient interactions are uncommon, but the risk increases with the length of time you take the drug and its toxicity. Antibiotics, seizure medications, blood thinners, and cancer chemotherapy cause the largest number of reactions. Most doctors don't know whether their patients are taking supplements; make sure you provide that information when you receive a new prescription.

Vitamins and Stress. Physical stress reduces the blood level of certain vitamins, especially C. Common sense tells us that reversing this drop will help, and many health educators urge those under physical as well as emotional strain to take supplements. Some vitamin products are advertised as specific for stress.

Vitamins and Illness. Vitamin C has a modest effect on cold symptoms, but if you feel bad enough to think about seeing a doctor, it's wrong to temporize with vitamins.

Minerals. Men should take a passing interest in calcium. Everyone slowly loses calcium from bone beginning in the mid-thirties. By middle age, many women suffer collapsed vertebrae, hunchbacks, and broken hips. Men get into trouble later because their bones are larger to begin with, but everyone should consume a quart of milk a day or take a gram of calcium.

As mentioned, young women often need extra iron, but giving iron to a man with iron deficiency anemia without finding the cause is clear malpractice.

Vitamin and Mineral Supplements. Should you take them "just to be safe"? Yes, if it makes you feel better. Some doctors go overboard warning of the dangers of taking too much. While you can poison yourself with vitamins, it takes a very large amount to do so. Other experts stress how unnecessary they are. That's true, but most human activities are unnecessary, including most things we enjoy. Everything is relative. A vitamin pill is better for you than a stick of gum, not as good as a carrot.

A Sensible Rule. Taking multivitamin and mineral supplements is OK provided that you're otherwise in good health. If you really need something, a supplement probably won't help. For example, there's too little iron in a typical multivitamin with iron to cure iron deficiency. If you truly need the vitamin A or D or folic acid, something serious is wrong, and you must see a doctor to find out. It may turn out that some extra A, C, E, or selenium lowers your risk of cancer; for the moment I advise against taking more than a gram of vitamin C per day or more of the others than you can get in a multivitamin.

Your Dietary Goals

When in doubt, remember that the healthiest diet must accomplish four goals:

1. Prevent disease caused by a poor diet. In America and most of Europe, atherosclerosis is the leading nutritional disorder; although well behind, high blood pressure and cancer remain significant.
2. Travel comfortably through your digestive tract. You should think about other things between meals instead of the constipation, cramps, bloating, hemorrhoids, and other symptoms produced by food that is difficult for the human intestine to handle.
3. Taste good. A dull diet is depressing, and I mean this in a medical sense. A feeling that food has lost its taste is one of the first signs of severe depression. Plenty of healthy activities contain an element of discomfort (medical procedures), deprivation (losing weight, breaking habits), or tedium (daily exercise). As one of the joys of life, eating must always be a pleasure.
4. Provide essential nutrients. I place this last because it's the easiest to achieve.

Quick Reference Chart for Vitamins and Minerals

Vitamin	USRDA	What It Does	Food Sources
A	5,000 IU	Helps maintain skin; engenders good vision	dark green leafy vegetables, yellow vegetables
B$_1$ (thiamine)	1.5 mg	Helps break down glucose to provide energy; aids nervous system functions	pork, milk, eggs, green peas, wheat germ
B$_2$ (riboflavin)	1.7 mg	Assists in energy release from foods; participates in protein metabolism	milk, poultry, organ meats, cereals
B$_3$ (niacin)	20 mg	Helps body release energy from foods	poultry, fish, peanuts, milk, potatoes
B$_5$	10 mg	Helps body process nutrients	dark green leafy vegetables, milk, eggs
B$_6$ (pyridoxine)	2 mg	Helps regulate brain functions; involved in protein processing	beans, nuts, eggs
B$_{12}$	6 mcg	Assists in normal functioning of the nervous system; involved in maturation of red blood cells	eggs, beef, liver, milk
Biotin	300 mcg	Plays key role in formation of fatty acids	liver, milk, eggs
Folacin	200 mcg	Aids in formation of red blood cells	dark green leafy vegetables, cereals, orange juice
C	60 mg	Aids in healing wounds; essential for synthesis of connective tissue	tomatoes, strawberries, citrus
D	400 IU	Required for normal bone growth; regulates calcium level	salmon, tuna, milk, fish livers
E	30 IU	Helps maintain normal red blood cells; acts as general anti-oxidant	whole grains, lettuce, wheat germ
K	80 mcg	Assists in clotting of blood	cabbage, broccoli, soybeans, leafy vegetables

Mineral

Mineral	USRDA	Function	Sources
Calcium	1–2 grams	Required for formation of bones and teeth	milk, sardines, dark green leafy vegetables
Iodine	150 mg	Helps manufacture hormones	seafood, iodized salt, dairy, vegetables
Iron	12 mg	Required in transport of oxygen in blood	eggs, meat, liver, cereals
Magnesium	400 mcg	Helps body release energy and grow bones and teeth	legumes, milk, whole grains, seeds
Phosphorus	800–1,000 mg	necessary for bone growth	eggs, poultry, fish, meat, legumes
Selenium	70 mcg	Plays major role in oxygen metabolism and cell growth	meat, seafood, liver
Zinc	15 mg	Plays major role in healing wounds and repairing tissue	meat, eggs, poultry, fish, cereals

Key: USRDA = Recommended Dietary Allowance
    IU = International Unit
    mg = milligrams
    mcg = micrograms

Good NUTRITION: SIX BASIC RULES TO USE

Plenty of writers devote entire books to nutrition, explaining how subtle changes in your diet will fine-tune your health. I teach that achieving good nutrition is easy. A sensible man should follow a few rules and get on with his life.

Rule 1:

Eat a variety of food.

By consuming a mixture of fresh fruits and vegetables, breads, cereals, proteins, and dairy products, you'll get everything you need. If you want more specifics, the Department of Agriculture adds that you need the following daily:

> Six to eleven servings of breads and cereals
> Three to five servings of vegetables
> Two to four servings of fruits
> Two to three servings of proteins
> Two to three servings of dairy products.

Although the Department can define a serving, it's not worth learning. A serving is a reasonable portion.

Rule 1 is all you need to fulfill your nutritional requirements. You don't need to learn which foods are rich in, say, riboflavin. I don't know myself. I looked it up to write this chapter; before that I never had a reason. As far as nutrients are concerned, variety matters most.

Since the important dietary diseases in this country are the consequence of excess, most of the remaining rules tell you what to avoid.

Rule 2:

Reduce your protein intake.

I suggested this earlier. Excess protein itself won't harm someone in good health, but high-protein foods tend to be high in calories and (in the case of meat) accompanied by fat.

Rule 3:

Avoid fat, especially animal fat.

Dietary cholesterol and (to a greater extent) animal fat, which the body turns into cholesterol, end up as rock-hard deposits on your arteries: atherosclerosis. As decades pass, deposits build up and can eventually cut off the blood supply. When this occurs in the heart, it's a heart attack, in the brain it's a stroke.

Rule 4:

Think about sugar.

Although we consume 130 pounds of sugar per person per year, health-conscious Americans view sugar with the same disapproval that fundamentalist Christians reserve for sin. Like sin, sugar is probably not good for you, and it certainly contributes to obesity and tooth decay. Despite the common belief, it does not cause serious diseases such as diabetes, atherosclerosis, or heart attacks.

Children (who are most susceptible to tooth decay) and adults with a weight problem should stay away from sugar. Everyone else should not take it so seriously. Remember that three elements that improve the taste of food most intensely are fat, sugar, and salt. Of these, the first is by far the greatest source of disease in our society, so an ideal diet is very low in fat. You can attain some benefits by cutting out the other two (giving salt priority), but a diet lacking all three becomes more spartan than most people will tolerate.

Everyone worried about their teeth and weight must stay away from sugar; otherwise I don't greatly disapprove of sweets except for those made with fatty dairy products such as cream and milk—read the labels. Simple sugar turns up in a surprising number of products and under many names.

Brown sugar, raw sugar, syrups, and honey are all plain sugar. Some enthusiasts object to including honey, but it is not superior. Honey is essentially sugar plus bee droppings plus dirt and debris from the hive.

Read labels. Simple sugars under other names include sucrose, glucose, maltose, dextrose, lactose, fructose, and corn syrup. Canned vegetables, breads, and breakfast cereals often contain sugar as the first or second ingredient, but many don't.

My own researches have turned up a reliable rule for evaluating fast food, snack foods, and other heavily advertised products: If it's low in fat, it's high in sugar and vice versa. For example, low-fat frozen yogurt is heavily sweetened. Granolas that boast of their absence of sugar contain plenty of fats and oils. Neither is necessarily unhealthy, but you should realize that "low fat" or "low sugar" don't mean "low calorie."

Plenty of intensely sweet foods contain little sugar: fresh fruit, dried fruit, and fruit canned in its own juice or without sugar are prime examples.

Rule 5:

Develop a taste for complex carbohydrates.

When I was a child, experts frowned on "starch," and only the constipated showed any enthusiasm for roughage. Today we treat complex carbohydrates with more respect. This is partly because nothing remains after you've listened to experts denounce protein, fat, salt, and sugar, but the truth is that a mixture of fruits, vegetables, nuts, and whole grain (not whole wheat) cereals and bread is the healthiest diet a human can follow. Primitive cultures who eat nothing else suffer no atherosclerosis, high blood pressure, or heart attacks and almost no hemorrhoids, constipation, irritable bowels, appendicitis, ulcers, gallstones, and tooth decay. They would suffer less cancer if they lived long enough, but most die early of violence, starvation, parasitic diseases, and bacterial infections.

Rule 6:

Think about salt.

Excess salt causes high blood pressure. In the single culture that loves salt even more than we do (Japan), strokes from high blood pressure are the leading cause of death. Seventeen percent of American adults have hypertension; strokes are third on the list, of the most frequent causes of death in the United States.

If you never added salt to food, cooked with salt, or ate canned, baked, processed, preserved, restaurant, or snack food with salt, you'd still consume more than enough sodium for your body's needs. Unfortunately, we grow up with a taste for salt, so simply withdrawing it from a familiar food is a disaster (try no-salt canned soup!). On the other hand, substituting spices makes food taste better. Wealthy countries neglected spices once they could afford to eat all the fat, salt, and sugar they wanted.

Learn to enjoy the unsalted flavors of foods. Despite this cheerful advice, much unsalted food is uninteresting, but experimenting will teach you what tastes good. I enjoy unsalted potato chips and nuts as much as the salted variety. Most breakfast cereals contain salt (and sugar); exceptions are shredded wheat, puffed wheat, rice, and corn as well as a few others, and they taste as good. Read labels.

Remember items extremely high in salt: condiments (soy sauce, steak sauce), pickled foods, cheese, cured meats, soup, and almost any popular snack or fast food.

Cholesterol and Good Nutrition

The immediate benefits of the best diet include elimination of constipation, cramps, bloating, and other symptoms of irritable bowels, a condition caused by lack of dietary fiber that probably affects 20 percent of the population. Nothing is perfect, so another immediate consequence is flatulence. A high-fiber diet is gassy, an annoyance that may or may not diminish with time.

Although far more substantial, the long-term benefits are hard to appreciate—and it's important that you appreciate them, because the best diet requires that you give up some food that you wouldn't give up without a good reason. I haven't eaten sausages or ice cream in thirty years, and I enjoy everything I eat now. But I still remember how good they tasted.

You monitor long-term benefits by knowing your blood cholesterol. A low level in someone in good health and following a good diet not only demonstrates low risk of atherosclerosis but of chronic gastrointestinal disorders and malignancy. If you can bear sticking your finger with a lancet, buy the home testing kit and measure your cholesterol monthly until it reaches a healthy level; then measure yearly. Don't test more often; cholesterol levels change slowly, and a single meal has no measurable effect.

A skilled technician can draw blood painlessly from a vein, so you may prefer this. Talk to your doctor about visiting the office or a neighborhood clinical lab to have the test *without* paying for an office visit. Performing the test costs a few dollars, so you shouldn't pay more than $15 to $20 for the service.

The Ideal Cholesterol. An average blood cholesterol in the United States is 220 mg per 100 cc, but this is almost certainly not a natural average for a healthy human. Healthy members of primitive cultures average well under 150. Although this is undoubtedly a better level, a primitive man probably leads a strenuous life, goes hungry now and then, and shares his food with a number of intestinal parasites.

American doctors treat a cholesterol under 200 as good news; since it's below average, the man's risk of heart attacks and other consequences of atherosclerosis also drops. Although it's nothing to sneeze at, a below-average risk of the leading killer of American men leaves some remaining risk. With more effort, you can do better.

At a cholesterol below 180, heart attacks are rare; at 150 they probably don't occur, and you can achieve this by diet alone. I keep my level in the 170s despite coming from a high-cholesterol family (levels over 240; my father had his first heart attack at forty-six). Yet food is one of my great pleasures; I snack continually, eat out several times a week, and have a taste for sweets. I love my diet, although friends have long since stopped inviting me to dinner because I refuse so many foods. I could drop my cholesterol still more, but that would involve more cutbacks than I could tolerate. You might feel different, but don't make a decision until you reach 180.

Aspects of an Effective Low-Fat Diet. You can eat the following:

- All vegetables except coconuts and avocados.
- All fruits.
- All grains, cereals, and nuts.
- Fish; chicken and turkey without the skin.
- Alcoholic beverages. I rarely touch alcohol because I don't like the taste, but modest amounts do no harm, and the other ingredients in alcoholic beverages are probably good for you. Every few years someone publishes a survey showing that people who consume small amounts of alcohol are much healthier than those

who consume large amounts and slightly healthier than those consuming none at all. No one has explained the last finding; perhaps people who drink modestly enjoy life more than teetotalers.

■ Egg whites; oils that are liquid at room temperature except for coconut and palm oil.

The following are best avoided:

■ Animal meat. Fat, not protein, is the problem here, so some health writers urge you to trim off fat or to boil rather than fry your steak. Although this eliminates a good deal of fat, plenty remains because much fat is interlaced with the meat. It's all right to broil and trim as a first step, but in my experience few men achieve a cholesterol below 180 without a big drop in animal meat consumption.

■ Dairy products except for skim milk, cottage cheese, and fat-free frozen yogurt.

■ Anything hydrogenated or partially hydrogenated, including hydrogenated vegetable oils, peanut butter, and margarine. Hydrogenation is a chemical process that hardens liquid fats, making food look better (i.e., peanut butter no longer appears oily), but it converts good fats into bad ones.

■ Oil that's solid at room temperature.

■ Egg yolks, pastries, cakes, pies, and any dessert with a crust or made with milk or cream.

If you eat out a great deal, take an interest in how the food is prepared. Foods cooked immersed in fat, such as french fries and egg rolls, are hopeless. It doesn't help your cholesterol to order fish or vegetables in a restaurant that covers them in butter. Although Mexican food is generally one of the healthiest, traditional Mexican cookery uses lard, but some restaurants advertise the fact that they don't.

Salt—a Lower Priority

Compared to what the average American eats, the healthiest diet is very low in fat, lower in protein, and higher in fruits, vegetables, and fiber. It's also far lower in salt. In the real world, a man makes choices and the blunt fact is that the consequences of a high-fat diet (such as heart attacks) are irreversible; atherosclerosis itself may be reversible, but only slowly and with a very rigorous diet. The consequence of chronic high salt intake, high blood pressure, is quickly reversible. Cutting out salt can accomplish this with mild hypertension, but drugs control almost all elevated pressures. A lifetime on drugs may not be ideal, but once pressure returns to normal, the man doesn't have hypertension or any risk of its consequences—an impressive benefit.

The healthiest diet avoids both salt and fat; many men make the change with little difficulty, but it's a big, big change. If you must make a choice, give fat priority.

Sugar—Still Lower

Although complex carbohydrates are better, simple sugars are not forbidden. Candy is OK provided that it's made without milk or fats. So are soft drinks. Puddings and mousses are acceptable for the same reasons, although you're not likely to find a cook that makes them this way.

This Diet Works

Your cholesterol must drop on this diet. The more strictly you follow it, the more it drops. If you drop below 150, not only will you never get atherosclerosis, but any cholesterol plaques in place will probably dissolve (doctors debate this, but many experts, including me, believe it).

This is not a reducing diet. Low-cholesterol or low-fat food is not necessarily low in calories. You can eat as much as you want, so don't expect to lose weight unless you're trying.

If you're having trouble, don't blame your metabolism. Your body may sabotage a reducing diet by slowing its metabolism as you lower your calorie intake, but this doesn't happen here. If your cholesterol isn't dropping, you're eating too many bad foods. I indulge now and then, but not enough to raise my cholesterol. You shouldn't feel deprived on this diet. If you do, you'll slack off. Do your best. If you reach 200, that's pretty good.

CHAPTER ■ 3

THE IMPORTANCE
OF
EXERCISE

The Benefits

Although never more important than good nutrition, regular exercise helps maintain health, guards against disease and, as increasing evidence indicates, slows the aging process. Exercise is of value to all men at all stages of life. This is especially true since daily activity alone rarely provides sufficient physical impetus to maintain fitness. Except for men in careers that include intense training (ballet, professional athletics), any man who wants to enjoy the benefits of exercise must make a special effort.

Specifics. Since 1962, in one of the most famous and extensive empirical studies ever undertaken, researchers have monitored the health of 17,000 Harvard alumni who entered college from 1916 to 1950. Although many findings were no surprise—smokers and those with high blood pressure fared poorly—analyzing physical activity turned up some intriguing results.

At first glance, one can poke holes in the results. After all, active men tend to eat better, weigh less, and smoke and drink less. These are all qualities geared to keep them healthier. However, the researchers were well aware of this, so they factored out these beneficial aspects, and let their results reveal the benefits of exercise alone.

Men who consistently burned 2,000 calories per week enjoyed notably better health than those who burned less than 500. Their rate of coronary heart disease dropped by one third. They suffered approximately 20 percent less incidence of cancer. They even showed a slight decrease in deaths by accident and suicide.

Varsity athletes who settled into a sedentary lifestyle upon graduation fared as poorly as those who were inactive throughout their college years. Students who avoided athletics during school but became active later in life reaped appreciable health benefits.

Men who exercise are found to sleep better. They also experience less stress, depression, and constipation, fewer headaches, and exhibit more self-confidence. Exercise intensity strengthens bone as well as muscle, so active men suffer less osteoporosis, as well as less muscle atrophy, as they grow older.

A man who exercises regularly lowers his blood pressure; whether he lowers his cholesterol level remains a matter of debate, but he certainly doesn't raise it. We do know that exercise will not dissolve atherosclerotic build-up. That requires proper diet. But the exercising man suffers less of the consequences of coronary artery disease, including heart attacks. He also enjoys a lower risk of adult-onset diabetes, colon cancer, and psychiatric disease.

In regard to stress, a study at the University of Southern California compared a tranquilized, non-exercising group to a group that exercised but did not take a tranquilizer. The latter group was more relaxed and exhibited fewer psychiatric problems. One of the leading theories behind the stress-reducing effects of exercise is the increased level of the hormone norepinephrine in brain of those who exercise regularly. This hormone is reputed to have a calming, contenting effect.

ENDURANCE VS. STRENGTH

Exercise is a means of increasing either endurance or strength. Aerobic (endurance) exercise strengthens the cardiovascular system. A stronger heart pumps more blood per beat and pumps longer before tiring. Conditioned vessels supply more blood to muscles and carry away waste products more efficiently. Many consider cardiovascular endurance to be the key component of good health.

Endurance exercises work by expending calories. You burn calories fastest through the vigorous, rhythmic movement of large muscle groups, producing a continuous blood flow throughout the muscles. Good aerobic exercises include walking, jogging, jumping rope, bicycling, swimming, cross-country skiing, and such interactive sports as tennis, basketball, and racquetball.

Strength training (anaerobic, i.e., "without air") builds muscle and helps create a desirable body composition. Instead of rhythmically contracting and relaxing, muscles act with intensity against resistance. Tension builds, impeding blood flow rather than increasing it. Fatigue occurs quickly, so you cannot perform strength exercise for too long. When circulation is impeded, a reflex response rapidly increases blood pressure. This is why doctors discourage patients with hypertension and cardiac disorders from even moderate free weight or isometric regimens.

Strength improves the ability to perform myriad actions, many of which add to life's pleasure. A generation ago, athletes involved primarily in aerobic sports religiously avoided strength training on the theory that muscle building decreased performance. We now know that the opposite is true: Sensible weight training plays an important role in all athletics, often in the development of lean muscle mass.

WHAT HAPPENS WHEN YOU EXERCISE

In the Muscles. Working muscles utilize more glycogen (stored glucose in the mitochondria of the cells), take up more glucose from the blood, and burn fat transported in the blood from storage sites. The increased metabolic effort requires extra oxygen and greater blood flow; in their absence, muscle fatigue occurs very quickly. Our brain triggers the changes to meet these demands. The glycogen comes initially from carbohydrate sources but, in the presence of continued activity, eventually derives from stored fat.

In the Lungs. The depth and rate of breathing increases immediately. The normal adult ventilation of 10 to 12 liters per minute can increase ten times during strenuous exercise. A healthy nonsmoker's lungs can easily take in enough oxygen for any amount of reasonable exertion. Feeling "out of breath" really has nothing to do with your lung capacity: It means that your heart and blood vessels aren't transporting sufficient oxygen to the muscles. This becomes clear when you remember that endurance exercise strengthens your cardiovascular system, not your lungs.

In the Blood Vessels. Soon after muscles begin working harder, waste products diffuse into nearby tissues, causing a massive dilatation of blood vessels, which allows increased blood flow. These same waste products stimulate the brain to direct a massive flow of circulation to the working muscles. During vigorous exercise, muscles may receive 20 times their normal circulation.

In the Heart. The heart rate increases to provide this circulatory flow. A nonathlete in his forties has a resting heart rate of about 70 beats per minute; during moderate exercise, the rate may double and reach 180 beats during utmost exertion. The average man ejects 75 milliliters (five ounces) of blood at his resting heart rate; exercise can increase the volume of flow over 50 percent. This resting cardiac output of about five liters per minute (70 beats multiplies by 75 milliliters) can quadruple during exercise.

Blood Pressure. Two components make up a pressure measurement; Systolic (the maximum pressure generated as the heart contracts) and diastolic (the minimum pressure when it relaxes). A level of 120/80 millimeters of mercury is considered the traditional normal reading, but no one's blood pressure remains constant—just as no one has an absolutely fixed heart or breathing rate. Therefore, readings between 100-140/60-90 are considered acceptable.

Systolic pressure rises with exercise, reaching as high as 180/190, but diastolic pressure shouldn't change. The increased *pulse pressure* enables the heart to expel blood quickly, then relax in order to accept its next load. A rise in diastolic pressure due to exertion is a sign of heart disease—an indication that the heart can't respond properly to an increased work load. When doctors perform an exercise electrocardiogram (ECG), rising diastolic pressure—and not an abnormality on the ECG—can be the first signal of cardiac weakness. An abnormal result makes an exercise program *more* rather than less important, since it will have the effect of strengthening the heart, the most important muscle of all. But close medical supervision will be necessary to avoid too strenuous a program.

PLAN AHEAD AND BE REASONABLE

Regular exercise takes time and discipline. Men who develop the workout habit in school can easily continue it even as their life fills up with job and familial responsibilities, and becomes increasingly more complicated. For older men unused to an exercise regimen, adding several hours of activity per week takes planning. They must give the matter considerable thought. This doesn't mean getting bogged down in a Hamlet-like "should I or shouldn't I?" syndrome. It just means that exercise is not to be entered into lightly or casually.

Obviously, exercise is only one of many valuable options for the man who chooses to stay as healthy as possible. Too crowded an agenda may result in failure on all fronts. Only realistic, applicable goals will lead to lasting success. Don't overstate your goals, or expect your regimen to produce a series of instant successes. And don't get frustrated and chuck your whole program just because things don't seem to be going your way. Remember Lao Tse's dictum, "The longest journey begins with one step." Then again, a less-revered, anonymous sage once said, "Watch that first step, it's a bitch."

Nevertheless, persistence and positive thinking will get you just as far in your exercise program as it will in the other elements of your life. Find the positive element in every situation and build upon it.

Oddly, one of the most common mistakes a novice makes is to overtrain, which can lead to serious overuse injury. But don't feel bad. Many a bodybuilding pro is guilty of the same overzealous behavior. Over-exercising is counterproductive: After all, muscle growth (hypertrophy) occurs during rest, not while working out. "Less is more" is the watchphrase here. Also beware of overdoing such aerobic activities and sports as running, swimming and skiing. All three can lead to joint and other injuries. They're all such fun, the natural tendency is to hit the track, pool, or slope to excess.

Make Sure It's Fun

Now, there's a key word—*fun*. Make exercise fun, like watching a favorite movie, or delving into a good book. Don't be put off by the fact that you're the flabbiest guy in the gym, that your exercise form needs a lot of work, or that you have no idea what purpose the various exotic cardiovascular machines serve. Don't get defensive or feel like a jerk. Instead, take the exercise learning process with good grace, and don't be afraid to laugh at yourself a little bit. Relax and enjoy your exercise time.

And, in order to approach exercise with a mature attitude, share in the secret that most exercise mavens hate to acknowledge. Genetics play a big role in the tendency towards obesity, in body type and shape, and in the ability to make training gains. Physically, all men are not created equal. Accept who you are, and do the best with what you have. Exercise experts who urge every man to achieve physical perfection and meet unrealistic dietary demands are doing great harm to the fitness movement. In other words, a little exercise is better than no exercise at all.

Ideally, a good regimen consists of three non-consecutive workout days a week. Don't feel overly guilty if you're forced to skip a session or just get lazy. Your life is pretty dull if there are no emergencies or special occasions that disrupt your schedule. Visiting a sick friend or going on a romantic date is sometimes simply more important than flexing your pecs. But don't make a habit of slacking off; it's only a prelude to giving up your regimen altogether.

Giving sports activity plenty of priority is a fine idea, but remember that all sports are not created equal. An aerobically effective sport raises the pulse and keeps it high for the duration. So bowling, golf, baseball, leisurely hikes, and sightseeing bicycle jaunts should not be central to your aerobics program.

Exercising with a friend is an excellent way to keep your workout sessions fresh, but don't depend on him (or her) too much. His lackluster exercise habits might rub off on you. Then again, he could be a shining inspiration. Other ways to keep the zing in your workouts is to bring a little music along via your Walkman, switch gyms if you're getting tired of the same old scene, add new exercises to your program, get some attractive workout clothes, and vary the weight and/or repetitions in your routine.

Choices Are Important

Read a lot. There are a number of good exercise magazines featuring detailed body part routines. There are at least as many others that seem to consist mainly of supplement ads and redundant "inspirational" articles. By the same token, there are plenty of good exercise books out there—and plenty of bad ones. Avoid books that are ill-disguised promos for specific products or celebrities (same difference); or quick-fix tomes with little scientific validity (*Twenty Minutes to a Better You*). Anything under the aegis of the American College of Sports Medicine is worth a read, especially in regard to pre-program screening techniques and program preparation. This organization tends to be on the cutting edge, although some of their material is decidedly for advanced trainees.

Choose your health club very carefully. Steer clear of those "lifetime" memberships and places that look more like discos than gyms. If you yearn for a disco fix, put on an old Donna Summer record. Remember, the dropout rate at health clubs equals that of diet clinics. Don't be a statistic.

Never buy a home exercise machine as a first step. It's inevitably going to gather dust, and serve only to line the pockets of the manufacturer. Durable home equipment costs a fortune, but you'll probably want to purchase a stationary cycle, rowing machine, treadmill, cross-country ski machine, or stair-climber somewhere down the line.

An extremely important consideration is to consult a physician before beginning your exercise program. Even if you're under forty, thin and in ostensibly perfect health, some hidden cardiac or other problem can be lurking in the background. We've all heard stories of young athletes collapsing and dying on the running track or sports field. If you're planning to include anaerobic exercise and crosstraining sports that push your cardiovascular system to its limits in your regimen—as well you should—a check-up becomes all the more vital. Here is what you might expect:

Screening for Young Men

Prior to any assessment, a fully completed medical history should be provided by the would-be trainee—this holds true for any age group. Major health problems include cardiorespiratory disease, diabetes, epilepsy and asthma, as well as conditions of a musculoskeletal and neurological nature. The doctor will be listening carefully to your heart. Those rare athletes who drop dead during a game often suffer from subtle congenital heart abnormalities like hypertrophic cardiomyopathy and subaortic stenosis. Simple tests such as an electrocardiogram and ultrasound exam (echocardiogram) can confirm such problems. You don't need an exercise electrocardiogram or other sophisticated test unless the doctor suspects coronary artery disease, or you suffer from alarming symptoms such as excessive shortness of breath, fainting spells, or chest pain. A normal blood test is also usually sufficient. An assiduous physician will determine your percentage of body fat; relative flexibility and strength levels; blood pressure; and possible genetic predeterminants nestled in your family tree.

Screening for Middle-Aged Men

A healthy fifty-year-old doesn't require more screening than a man half his age. In most respects, middle-age is the prime of life. Although many experts agree on this, in the real world when you suddenly announce the intention to exercise, your doctor will be unable to resist the urge to carefully test your heart.

Although a resting electrocardiogram almost never detects coronary artery disease in someone who feels quite well and is not complaining of problems, you'll probably receive one anyway. Stressing the heart with exercise reveals much more; when narrowed arteries become unable to supply the heart's increasing blood requirements, the electrocardiogram usually becomes abnormal. Stress ECGs are virtually *de rigeur* for middle-aged trainees. Provided the outcome is normal, you might actually enjoy the experience of marching on a treadmill until you're exhausted, while a bank of instruments records your cardiogram and blood pressure. Then again, high-impact aerobics night with the Marquis DeSade might not have been without its pleasures for some guys.

For every man in this age group with risk factors, such as high cholesterol or a history of smoking, the stress ECG becomes even more essential. Although accurate, it is wrong about five percent of the time (no test is perfect; 95 percent accuracy is considered good). Determining that the results are in error requires expensive and sometimes potentially hazardous procedures.

Screening for Older Men

Exercising is one of those things it's never too late to do. Fitness gains tend to reverse themselves depressingly quickly if a consistent, ongoing program isn't adhered to. Therefore, the older man who has never worked out is on a near-equal footing with the older man who worked out in his youth, but lost the habit over the course of time.

You'll require an exercise ECG not only to detect heart disease, but to measure your functional capacity—how vigorously you can exercise, how much weight you can safely lift. Your doctor will make sure your arteries, bones and joints can handle the extra stress. Chances are they probably can. More and more older men who have no exercise background have begun an aerobics program, and can be seen hoisting free weights at gyms throughout the country.

DESIGNING AN EFFECTIVE AEROBICS PROGRAM

Building your cardiovascular system requires exercise at 60 to 75 percent of your maximum heart rate. Less exercise puts too little stress on the system to produce the desired training effect. More makes you too tired before doing you very much good. Although physiologists use increasingly complex techniques to monitor aerobic intensity, measuring your pulse rate will work just fine. Count your resting (normal) pulse rate for 15 seconds and multiply the number of beats by four. This will give you the number of beats per minute, which varies from 60 to 100, depending on such factors as age, weight, and sex. Then check your pulse again during a vigorous aerobic workout and multiply by four. The number of beats should equal what is called your target heart rate, i.e., the level of intensity you want to reach. After your session is over, and you've rested for three minutes, monitor your pulse rate again. It should have returned approximately to your resting rate.

Your maximum heart rate is 220 minus your age. At age forty, this equals 180 beats per minute. To obtain your target heart rate, take the percentage of the maximum heart rate at which you plan to exercise: 70 to 85 percent of 180 equals 126 to 153 beats per minute. Eighty or more percent of your maximum heart rate would represent an advanced training level. The trick, of course, is to sustain the intensity.

And your heart rate is only a guideline. Getting healthier requires persistent increased energy production. Exercise scientists who measure the difference in energy expenditure between sedentary and active men find a difference of only 300 calories a day, so that's all you should initially burn. It takes 100 calories to jog or walk a mile on a flat surface, to bicycle two miles, or to swim 400 yards.

Keep Your Heart Level Up

But whatever the aerobic activity, the essence is to maintain a continuous elevated heart rate. Good breathing technique is also important, allowing a consistent flow of oxygen for sustained energy. To strengthen your cardiovascular system effectively, you should try to exercise four times a week, for at least 20 minutes but no more than an hour. As a beginner, start out modestly at five to ten minutes, and gradually work up to 30 minutes.

Ideally, aerobics and anaerobics go hand-in hand. A strong cardiovascular system helps you to manage a strenuous weight training regimen. Don't try to "combine" your strength and endurance training: The time frame and extent of physical adaptation needed for aerobic versus anaerobic activity is quite different. By keeping strength and endurance goals separate, you'll avoid extraordinary strenuous and injurious activity.

Besides doing wonders for cardiovascular, respiratory and pulmonary health, aerobic activity is great for general as well as specific muscle toning and increasing fat-burning capability. Naturally, with all the activities to choose from, it only makes sense to ask which ones are best for you. They'll all work your heart and lungs, so that's not the determinant. You have to ask yourself two questions: What activities do you enjoy doing? And what body parts would you like to tone while you're getting all those cardiovascular benefits? It's as easy as that. Now let's look at some of the great aerobic alternatives available to you.

Benefit by Jogging and Walking

Jogging makes few demands in terms of time, equipment and expense. If you lead a very full life, it is a practical choice. Walking is without doubt the most universal exercise, a good option for men of all ages and in all states of health.

The 1970's was the prime time for the jogging craze and for best sellers on the subject with exotic names like *The Royal Canadian Air Force Exercise Plan*. Although the Canadian Air Force still collects royalties from this fine book, jogging is no longer the rage, and yet it continues to enjoy modest popularity.

About two hours per week is all the jogging time you'll need. Jogging is a steady trot about twice as fast as a brisk stroll. Put on some old clothes and running shoes, and be sure to carry a watch. Jog up the street for 5 minutes and back. Check your pulse as soon as you stop. If it's below seventy percent of your maximum heart rate, add a minute each day until it reaches the desired level. Cut back a bit if the rate is too high.

Four minutes of jogging is surprisingly tiring if you're out of condition, but don't be discouraged. It may take a few weeks to get where you want to be. Once you reach that goal, add a minute here or a block there or any distance that seems convenient. It should take another week or so until you're ready to advance again.

A pleasant change will occur somewhere between reaching the 15 and 25 minute interval. You'll notice that you're no more tired at the end of your jog than you were a few minutes after beginning. That means you've gotten yourself in condition, and can probably jog an hour without running out of gas.

Now you can set up a regular jogging schedule. Thirty minutes, four days a week will keep you in trim even if you skip a day now and then. This means you can't confine jogging—or any exercise—to weekends and holidays. You'll develop the habit best by jogging at the same time each day, which often means the first thing in the morning.

Some exercise experts denounce running on concrete. Although dirt is more low-impact and probably better, concrete shouldn't lead to major problems. Remember to do a warm-up before jogging, since this is more important than your choice of running surface.

A half-hour's jog takes you about three miles, so you can explore an extended area of your neighborhood. Lay out different routes, trying not to run on the same path too often. Skip jogging in the rain, and never jog on an icy surface without wearing cleats. But jogging in a drizzle is tolerable, provided the weather is fairly warm.

If You Can't Jog, Walk

Walking is a fine aerobic exercise with the lowest dropout rate. No matter how inactive you are, you'll notice improvement after a month of a good walking regimen: Stronger legs, greater endurance, a slower resting pulse.

Make sure you have a pair of comfortable shoes. Despite grim warnings in the sports journals, there's no harm in using ordinary sneakers or running shoes, especially during the early months. Wear cotton or wool socks; as they absorb sweat better.

Forget the funny waddle you saw in the Olympics. If someone tells you to walk with toes pointed straight ahead, ignore that too. Walk naturally with your toes pointed slightly outward. If you think you have a foot or gait problem, see a podiatrist. When you walk, move at a brisk pace, as if you were hurrying to an appointment. For an average-size man, 120 steps per minute is reasonable. Swing your arms, but don't exaggerate the motion. Do five to ten minutes of stretching exercises before every walk and a similar workout afterwards to cool down.

You should walk an hour a day, four days a week. At first, your pulse should reach 60 percent of its maximum rate after about 15 minutes. As you progress, you'll walk faster, elevating it higher. If you have trouble raising your pulse to that level, try carrying weights or wearing leg weights or a weighted backpack. Walk 20 minutes per day the first week; 30 minutes the second week; 40 minutes per day by the third week; 50 by the fourth; and 60 by the fifth week. After that, don't increase your actual time, but try walking a little faster each week. Don't increase your active pulse rate on a weekly basis by more than six to ten beats per minute. It's reasonable to take two months or more to reach 80 percent of your maximum rate.

Jot down your maximum heart rate for each walk. Calculate the average for every week. Record your resting pulse before getting out of bed on days that you walk. A gradual lowering of the rate demonstrates a healthy training effect.

Eventually, you might want to think about competing in a racewalk. Most large urban areas have a club that sponsors competitions. To find the one in your area, write The Walkers' Club of America, 445 East 86th Street, New York, N.Y. 10028. Or, you can walk for fun. These same clubs sponsor noncompetitive walks—health walks, historical walks, and walks for charity. You should also consider joining a group that sponsors hikes, such as The Sierra Club.

Jumping Rope, Not Just For Kids

Next to walking, jumping rope is about the most cost-efficient activity of all. Incidentally, it's also one of the best. You'll increase agility, improve your reflexes, tone your waist, hips and legs—and few activities are as relaxing as jumping rope. Get yourself a sturdy leather rope with wooden handles and try to jump on a hard surface. Jump for three minutes, rest one minute, then jump for another three. This is nowhere as easy as it sounds; you'll have to work your way up to that level. Not counting your warm-up and cooldown, you'll have yourself a great seven minute aerobic workout.

Keep your arms straightened at your sides, and swing the rope over your head using an easy wrist motion, with your knees flexed a bit, and a light spring in your toes. You can vary your jumprope regimen to great effect. Jump on the left foot, then the right, and keep on alternating; jump with your feet wider apart; jump with one foot positioned behind the other, etc.

Other Choices

Aerobic dance. No, it's not for ladies only, although you may feel a little silly at first. Think of it as striking a blow against sexual stereotyping. Find out what your instructor's credentials are, and make sure the routine is low impact and high intensity.

Cardio-Circuit Training. Give all your body parts some benefit with a rigorous gym workout. That is, if you can get close to all these popular machines. Try a combined 30 to 45 minute routine, four days a week, on the treadmill, the air and/or turbo cycle, stair climber, air rower, cross-country ski machine, and upper body ergometer. This is for the ambitious trainee looking to cram some serious body toning into his aerobics time.

Cross-Country Skiing. This may not be practical as a regular alternative for many men, but it makes for a fabulous winter vacation workout, or a weekend break from your standard aerobics regimen. For sheer conditioning—and sheer fun—it can't be beat.

Bicycling. Another great choice, but only provided you pedal steadily against a high gear to maintain a rapid pulse. This is difficult in a city environment, because you must move rapidly over level ground without stopping too often.

Swimming. A wonderful year-round aerobics activity, especially if there's a heated pool at your health club or YMCA. You can even design an innovative swimming regimen of your own, alternately emphasizing the upper body and the legs. If you already love to swim, make it one of your aerobic mainstays.

Calisthenics. This old high school gym class stand-by is a budget-minded way to combine aerobic and anaerobic benefits. Try jumping jacks, squat thrusts, toe touches, leg raises, and push-ups. It also makes a great warm-up.

A TOTAL BODY WORKOUT FOR BEGINNERS

Now that you've got a handle on your endurance program, you'll want to try some strength (progressive resistance) training. There tends to be a certain amount of pretentiousness and ego connected with working out, although far from universal on the part of everyone. Stick to the basics, learn to accept good advice, and you're sure to be okay.

Since this is not an exercise book per se, remember that there's always much more for you to learn. Pick up knowledge as you go along, keeping your mind open and your attitude light. Join a friendly gym where the well-trained staff will help you set up a program geared to your specific needs and wants. No two bodies are alike.

How often should you work out? Initially, it's best to stick to a fundamental full body regimen, performed three non-consecutive days per week (say on Mondays, Wednesdays and Fridays). Don't forget your warm-up: A good warm-up routine can consist of about three to five minutes of cardiovascular exercise, and five to ten minutes of stretching. Assuring flexibility not only helps prevent injury, it allows your muscles to be more effectively stimulated. Stretch slowly and deliberately, never forcing the stretches. Follow the American College of Sports Medicine guidelines when choosing an effective stretching routine. Many widely used stretches aren't all that effective.

Try to be fairly rested when you exercise: It's not a good idea to hit the gym after a hard day at work. Never choose a program that is too strenuous for you—you'll be an exercise dropout in record time. Start very light in terms of weight, duration, and intensity. As little as twenty minutes of training per session can be extremely salubrious. Three sets per exercise consisting of ten repetitions (reps) per set is perfect for the novice. Gradually increase the weight until you can do those ten reps comfortably, but somewhat challengingly. It can't be said often enough. *Don't strain and don't overtrain.* Keep an exercise log to record the date of the workout, the body parts worked, the names of the various exercises, your number of sets and reps, the amount of weight used, and the nature and degree of your progress. Combine realistic goals with intelligent motivation and relevant exercises, and progress should be considerable.

A newcomer should be careful to rest about one minute between each set of repetitions. It's a no-no to hold your breath when exercising; you should try to breathe as naturally as possible. But it is important to coordinate your movement with your breathing: Inhale on the lowering phase and exhale during the exertive phase. For pulling motions, exhale as you bring your hands towards your body, and inhale as you push them away. Exhale when you bend forward at the waist, and inhale as you raise the torso up.

Weights or Not?

You may be asking, should I use free weights, exercise machines, or both? The easy answer is to use both. However, there are advantages and disadvantages in each case. Machines get the nod for fostering pure toning effect, whereas weights are better for adding sheer mass and bulk. You'll have to jump from machine to machine to accommodate different muscle groups, but changing the resistance is a lot easier than changing weight plates. Tendons and ligaments are worked heavily when weights are involved, but machines are designed to move the resistance in an ergonomic pattern. To develop joint strength specifically, free weights are a must. For elderly exercisers or those suffering from an injury or extremely weak individuals, machines are numero uno. The incidence of injury while working out seems to be fairly evenly divided between weights and machines, although the machine manufacturers would have you believe otherwise.

Key among strength training variables is intensity—the amount of stress, energy, and the degree of difficulty needed to perform a given exercise. Intensity can be raised or lowered by altering the number of reps and sets, speeding up or moderating your exercise motion, and adopting a positive or negative training emphasis. A positive or *concentric* contraction occurs in the lifting phase and a negative or *eccentric* contraction in the lowering phase of an exercise. For those starting out, low reps are recommended to decrease muscle discomfort and soreness. A slower speed is recommended to discourage injury, reduce gravitational pull, and to encourage adherence to proper exercise form. Negative training emphasis is encouraged to better match muscle movement with resistance forces.

A Sample Daily Routine

Now here's a sample total body resistance training routine, to be performed on three non-consecutive days, in conjunction with aerobic activity. As a beginner, you should concentrate on the following major muscles groups: Shoulders, arms, chest, back, abdominals and legs.

- Shoulders:
  Dumbbell Military Press (3 sets per arm x 8-10 reps);
- Biceps:
  Alternating Dumbbell Curls (3 sets per arm x 8-10 reps);
- Triceps:
  Lying Triceps Extensions (3 sets x 8-10 reps);
- Chest:
  Incline Bench Press (3 sets x 8-10 reps);
- Back:
  Bent-Over Rows (3 sets x 8-10 reps);

■ Abdominals:
  Crunches (3 sets x 10-12 reps);

■ Legs:
  Standing Calf Raises (3 sets x 10-15 reps);
  Squats (3 sets x 8-10 reps).

Start with one or two sets of each exercise if you can't do three sets right away. Keep the weights light. Feel free to include machine as well as free weight activity.

An Intermediate Total Body Program

As your routines become more strenuous and complex, pay even more attention to the role of proper nutrition, and be sure to eat or drink some form of carbohydrates approximately one hour before working out. This intake can be in the form of popular carb-loading drinks, which contain glucose, fructose, or glucose polymers. Even as you get past the basics, never sacrifice form and good technique just to add weight. Form and technique must always be foremost in your mind.

Become familiar with the three types of muscular contraction:

■ *Concentric:* the muscle shortens in length as it overcomes resistance

■ *Eccentric:* the muscle increases in length to accommodate resistance

■ *Isometric:* the muscle resists outside stress without actually exhibiting motion.

It's probably time for you to move on to supersetted routines. A superset is an extended exercise set, in which an exercise is immediately followed by one or more other exercises, with no rest in between. With superset routines, available carbohydrate stores in the body are quickly diminished, leading to the breakdown of stored fats as a back-up energy source. A concentration superset focuses on a single muscle or muscle group with one intense exercise followed by another. Opposing muscle groups supersets focus on distinctly disparate groups.

Completing the Circuit

Circuit training is another workout variation, one which can offer very rapid and dramatic training results. The trainee performs one set of his initial exercise, then moves on to another or several other exercises, before performing a second set of the original exercise, thus completing one *circuit*. With this kind of training, all muscles groups are exercised in a proportional manner, resulting in parallel strength gains. We usually think of circuit training in terms of machine workouts, where resistance can be changed efficiently and quickly, thereby allowing for rapid change from one exercise to another, and back. While circuit training generally consists of back-to-back exercises for the same body part, it can also be used to train antagonistic muscle groups.

A split system workout is when you work on only certain body parts on given days; e.g., chest on one day and arms and legs on another. This is great for intense, productive, time-efficient workouts. Most intermediate training programs discourage working on a given body part more than two days a week. This is because your muscles need more rest to recuperate as you employ progressively heavier resistance.

Periodization—long-term, scientific program planning—is another process you should get acquainted with. Here you become acutely aware of training goals, how one phase or aspect of training leads to another and influences it. Training variables are foremost in consideration: You learn to manipulate them in a sophisticated fashion, resulting in an infinite variety of exercise possibilities. You become knowledgeable about the relationship between volume training and intensity, and how volume can be estimated by the total number of sets times repetitions. Also how training intensity can be determined by the percentage of maximal strength manifested in a particular exercise (the one-repetition maximum, or 1 RM).

You may now be at the stage where a personal trainer will be of considerable advantage to you, if you're willing to invest the time and money. If not, you can successfully go your own way, adding acumen as well as muscle growth. At times, you will definitely have to shake up your regimen to overcome *sticking points* or *plateaus*—that's when you're no longer making any discernible progress with your existing program. You'll also have to make changes simply to keep yourself motivated.

A Full Body Superset Routine

Here's an example of a full body superset routine you might want to try:

- Legs:
  Start with the Leg Press, completing 1 set of 10 reps; then immediately reposition yourself to do the Leg Press Calf Raise, again 1 set x 10 reps. Then do another set of Leg Press. Alternate and complete a total of 3 sets of both.
- Back:
  Pull-Ups (1 set x 10 reps), followed by Bent-Over Rows (1 set x 10 reps); return to the Pull-Ups. Alternate for 3 sets x 10 reps.

- Chest:
  Alternate 3 sets x 10 reps of Flat Dumbbell Press and Flat Dumb-bell Flyes.
- Abdominals:
  Alternate 3 sets x 10 reps of Sit-Ups and Leg Lifts.
- Shoulders:
  Alternate 3 sets x 10 reps of Barbell Military Press and Trap Lifts.
- Triceps:
  Alternate 3 sets x 10 reps of One-Arm Extensions and Kickbacks.
- Biceps:
  Alternate 3 sets by 10 reps of Concentration Curls and Seated Alternating Curls.

The minimal equipment necessary for this workout shouldn't result in undue access delays.

CHAPTER ■ 4

MENTAL AND EMOTIONAL HEALTH ISSUES

Seventy percent of patients seeking help from psychologists and psychiatrists are women. Men are not "saner" than women; women are simply more likely to admit to themselves that they need assistance and more readily seek help. Perhaps to compensate, men turn to other ways of dealing with stress and emotional pain. Men abuse alcohol and drugs three times as much as women do, and commit over 90 percent of violent crime.

Testosterone is traditionally blamed for men's "bad" behavior, but while male hormones make males more aggressive and irritable, they do not make them more stupid, impair their judgment, encourage them to repress their emotions, or make them respond poorly to stress. Two factors other than testosterone are responsible for most of the unnecessary pain in a man's emotional life.

First is temperament. *Temperament* refers to an inborn pattern of behavior that tends to remain constant throughout life. Some individuals are high-spirited and sociable, others withdrawn, still others touchy and critical. Parents notice these characteristics almost from the cradle, so they are probably inherited.

Second is *learning*. Mostly from his parents, but also from friends, the media and his culture, a boy learns how a man should behave. Everyone understands the enormous effect of family on a man's coping tactics, but we fail to appreciate how much American society contributes. For example, the Confucian culture, which still influences China and Japan, teaches that a man owes absolute, unquestioning loyalty to his superiors. Although it sounds outrageous to us, this philosophy keeps stress at a minimum in a rigid social system. Our democratic society encourages us to give loyalty where loyalty is due, and to refuse to accept injustice. American men feel they must not tolerate unfair treatment—an agonizing source of stress in many jobs and relationships where alternatives are limited.

EMOTIONS AND HEALTH

Unfortunately, the stress men face doesn't just make them unhappy or more likely to drink. It also harms their health. There's obviously some link between your thoughts and what happens inside your body. Just thinking about your favorite foods makes you salivate, even if there's no food in sight. But salivating is a single, very simple response. Is there more to the mind/body relationship?

Researching the Mind and Body

Researchers began to accumulate evidence of a mind/body connection in the mid-1970s with the discovery of the endorphins, the "good" hormones that seemed to block chronic kinds of pain and lift certain types of depression. A few years after the discovery, scientists at the University of Tennessee looked into whether or not a person's thoughts could affect their endorphin levels. The Tennessee researchers worked with a group of patients suffering from "incurable" back pain. They began by measuring the endorphin levels in the patients' spinal fluid, then giving them placebos ("sugar pills"). About 30 percent of the patients responded to the placebo; that is, they felt better. But it wasn't the placebos that eased their pain, it was the fact that their endorphin levels had gone up. What made the endorphins rise? It was not the placebos, but the patients' thoughts. Somehow, the belief that they would soon feel better was "translated" into increased production of endorphins and possibly other substances that killed their pain.

Many other studies have confirmed and expanded upon these early findings. For example, researchers at U.C.L.A. measured the effect of emotions on the immune system. They used "method" actors who were trained to "feel" the emotions of the characters they portrayed, to really become angry or happy or whatever the script dictated.

The actors were instructed to play out "happy" and "sad" scenes, while the researchers took various measurements from the actors' bodies, including the secretory IgA (immunoglobulin A). IgA, an antibody found in the mouth and other parts of the body, is an important part of the immune system. When the actors acted out the happy scenes, their IgA went up but when they played through the sad scenes, it went down. Here was strong evidence that emotions could influence your immune system and your health.

Just how strong the mind-body connection might be is suggested by a 1990 article in the *Journal of the American Medical Association*. It seems that the death rate for elderly Jewish men falls right before Passover. Passover is an important Jewish holiday, especially for fathers and grandfathers, who head the family celebrations. As soon as the holiday is over, the death rate for the men jumps up, then falls back down to average. A University of California study found the same phenomenon, this time with elderly Chinese women whose death rate falls shortly before the Harvest Moon Festival, an especially important holiday for elderly women. The numbers suggest that somehow the joyful, eager anticipation of the Jewish men and elderly Chinese women helps keep them alive until the party's over.

There are two sides to every coin, of course. If good thoughts strengthen your health, than bad thoughts can do the opposite.

FEAR, UNCERTAINTY, AND DEATH

The first strong evidence that unhappy thoughts can harm you accidently came out of our space program. Back in the 1960's and 1970's, the young engineers and Ph.D's at Cape Kennedy who were putting men on the moon began dying of heart attacks at an alarming rate. Drinking, drug abuse, and divorce were also suspiciously high. When people die of heart disease, you normally look at the standard risk factors: high cholesterol, high blood pressure, obesity, diabetes, and cigarette smoking. These were not out of line at Cape Kennedy; they weren't to blame for the deaths. Neither did the scientists have blocked coronary arteries, the usual cause of heart attacks.

Some in the government wondered if the Russians weren't to blame, but soon found that the real culprit was fear. Thanks to budgetary problems, the work force at Cape Kennedy was steadily cut back. One day the men were rocket scientists, among our best and brightest, the next day they were on unemployment. Instead of exalting at our space program's success, the scientists had unusually high levels of depression and anxiety. Their fearful agitation prompted massive outpourings of adrenaline and other substances that destroyed their heart muscles. They were literally frightened to death.

Effects on Your Heart

These findings are supported by various laboratory studies showing that fear, uncertainty, agitation and similar feelings can harm the heart. In one early study, a group of caged rats were forced to listen to a recording of "cat noises" at regular intervals. The rats didn't know it was only a recording; they thought the cat was really there, about to pounce. Pretty soon, the rats began dying. Autopsies showed that their heart muscles had been destroyed, just like the scientists'. But it's not just rats and scientists. If you let an aggressive tree shrew attack a submissive shrew, than separate them but let them see each other, the submissive one will die within a few weeks. If you keep moving rabbits back and forth between cages, never allowing them to adjust, they'll start dying in about six months.

Not every encounter with fear is deadly, but it can effect you. A 1988 article in the *New England Journal of Medicine* describes how stress can harm the heart in more subtle ways. Patients who already had coronary artery disease ("clogged arteries") were asked to do mental arithmetic, speak in public, and perform other potentially stressful tasks. The researchers found that when certain patients were nervous, several things happened. Less oxygen flowed to their heart muscles, the amount of blood pumped by the heart with each beat fell, and/or the heart wall itself moved in abnormal ways.

WHAT IS STRESS?

There are many definitions of stress, all revolving around the "fight or flight" response to danger. The idea behind fight or flight is simple. The human body only wants to expend as much energy as must in order to handle ordinary activities. But when danger arises, your body goes into high gear. Your heart beats harder and faster, extra sugar is pumped into the bloodstream for energy, muscle tone increases, your vision becomes sharper, your breathe heavier. These and other changes instantly prepare you to either fight or run for your life.

When You Should Use the Fight or Flight Response

The fight or flight response is a wonderful mechanism for saving your life, but it must be used carefully and sparingly. The powerful chemicals released by the body to kick off "fight or flight" can damage the body if you trigger the response too often, or for the wrong reasons. The right reason for using fight or flight is imminent, serious danger. A car is about to run you over, someone is going to punch you, an angry dog is running toward you. The wrong reason is, well, there are no wrong reasons, simply times when it's inappropriate to trigger the response. Why is it inappropriate? Because although you correctly perceive a danger, you can't fight and you can't flee. Your body is shoved into high gear, but you have to stand there and take it.

People didn't have to deal with rude clerks and traffic tickets during their days as cave dwellers. Life was simpler, and the distinction between danger and non-danger was clearer. Today, however, most situations we face are irritating, not life-threatening. Nonetheless, we keep triggering off the "fight or flight" response. We can't punch our bosses or wives, or run away when they give us a rough time. Neither can we fight or flee when the kids get on our nerves, when we get a traffic ticket we don't deserve, or when the stock market falls. At times like these, we need a "stand tall and respond with reason" response. Unfortunately, we tend to jump right to "fight and flight" with relatively slight provocation. We unleash the harsh chemicals within our bodies, but don't use them up fighting or running. Instead, we stew in our own juices.

The Modern Meaning of Stress

This brings us to a modern definition of stress: *Stress is our response to what happens to us.* Setting aside physical trauma, most of life's events are not stressful. It's our response that makes them so. An argument with your wife does not have to be stressful but often is—because we allow ourselves to become angry and resentful. Even things that would scare most people silly need not be stressful to us. For example, returning to Earth from the moon in a space craft is not inherently stressful, not if you have full confidence in the craft, not if you believe that what you're doing is no more dangerous than a Sunday morning stroll through the neighborhood. If, however, you keep thinking about what will happen to you if a few little computer chips fail, you will be stressed. The event—riding a spaceship home—is the same. Your perception—it's safe or it's not safe—makes it stressful or stress-free.

Hearing a noise in the middle of the night can be tremendously stressful—if you think it's a burglar. But if you know it's just the cat scratching at the door, it's not stressful at all. Perception is the key to stress.

WHAT ANXIETY DOES TO YOU

Anxiety is a feeling of uneasiness, uncertainty, fear, and agitation related to stress. People become anxious because they fear some danger, although they may not know the shape that danger will take, or from where it will come. Anxiety is often prompted by critical situations such as taking a test, being called in for an I.R.S. audit, or by a general concern about life in general.

Telltale Symptoms of Anxiety Attacks

When you're anxious, your muscles become tense, you perspire, your heart rate increases, and you breathe more rapidly and deeply. You feel restless. Your attention span and ability to follow directions drop. You may feel an increased need to urinate or defecate. If you're with other people, you may ask lots of questions, keep changing the topic of conversation, and constantly look for reassurance. Severe cases may lead to anxiety attacks, complete with dizziness, profuse sweating, rapid heart action, fainting, gastrointestinal upset, and feelings of imminent disaster or death. The symptoms of anxiety and anxiety attacks are similar to those of stress.

Stress and Blood Pressure

Hypertension (high blood pressure) is a major modern killer. Although the mechanisms of high blood pressure are complex, the basic equation is simple: *Flow* times *resistance* equals *pressure*. Flow is the cardiac output, how much blood the heart pumps out with every beat. Resistance is how easy or hard it is for the blood to flow through the arteries. If either the flow or resistance rises, blood pressure goes up. When flow or resistance drops, blood pressure falls.

When you're stressed, when you think you're in danger, a part of the brain called the hypothalamus sets off a chain of events that prepare you to run or fight for your life. As part of this stress reaction, the heart beats faster and harder, pushing up the blood pressure. And with chronic, continual stress, the blood vessels "clamp down" and get smaller. This increases the resistance, raising the blood pressure even more. Indeed, studies have shown an increased incidence of high blood pressure among people living in high-crime areas.

High blood pressure is just one side effect of stress. Long-term or repeated stress can lead to depression, increased risk of diabetes and/or peptic ulcer disease, a decrease in sex hormones, and a general drop in the immune system's ability to fight off disease. The platelets may become more "sticky" then they should be, putting you at greater risk of heart disease. Body chemistry usually returns to normal when the stress is over. But with too much stress, body chemistry may become "stuck" in the stress gear, leaving you with permanently high blood pressure and an increased risk of heart disease, ulcers and other problems.

Stress Can Affect Your Immune System

It's difficult for some to imagine how thoughts can strengthen or weaken the immune system. After all, the immune system isn't a single, stationary "target" for your thoughts; there are millions of immune system cells spread throughout the body. However, in the 1970's researchers found nerve connections linking the brain and the nervous system to the bone marrow, the thymus, the spleen, the lymph tissue, and other parts of the body where immune system cells cluster. The mind may not be in direct connection with the individual, far-flung cell of the immune system, but it does have direct links to various places where young immune system cells are "schooled," and where mature cells "check in."

Researching Effects on the Immune System. An interesting study involving hundreds of West Point cadets showed how emotions can influence the immune system. The cadets had their blood checked to make sure they had no EB-virus antibody (no indication of infectious mononucleosis). During their rigorous, stressful, academically, and emotionally demanding stays at West Point, some of the cadets developed mononucleosis, others did not. The ones who came down with the disease were the ones who felt more pressured and who had poorer grades. In other words, the ones who felt more stressed got sick.

Despite their smiling pictures in space ships, astronauts are also under a great deal of stress. If you check them before and after a space flight, you'll find that their T-cell response is reduced during the first four days after returning to earth. The stress of hurtling out to space in a little metal crate and then risking being burned up as they crash through the Earth's atmosphere to (hopefully) land intact is quite enough to weaken their immune systems.

You needn't blast off into space to be stressed. Your immune system can be thrown for a loop when a spouse dies, when you're taking care of a severely ill loved one, when you're going through a difficult divorce, or when you're preparing for and taking important tests. A substance called *cortisol* is one of the culprits. Cortisol goes up when you're stressed, helping you deal with short-term danger. But chronic stress leads to a long-term elevation of cortisol, which can break down the body's muscles, weaken the bones, and harm the immune system. Elevated cortisol levels have been associated with diabetes, depression, cancer, heart attacks, stroke, high blood pressure, and other diseases. We doctors have known for years that you can cause certain diseases just by giving patients large doses of cortisol.

What About Silent Sizzlers?

"Well," some people say, "that's certainly too bad about stress, but it doesn't effect me. I'm the calm type." It would be nice if you could judge a package by its wrapping, but the truth is that some of the calmest people I've ever met were burning up on the inside, burning with stress. You can check for these "silent sizzlers" by hooking them up to special monitors in the doctor's office and having them play a video game. They don't know that the game is rigged; they can't win. If you watch these "silent sizzlers" you think they're taking it all in stride, not caring if they win or lose. But the monitors tell the real story of stress being played out inside their bodies, complete with the outpouring of powerful stress chemicals that make their hearts beat harder and faster, blood vessels constrict, sugar pour into their bloodstream, and otherwise keep their internal alarm bells ringing.

ARE YOU STRESSED?

There is no perfect profile of the stressed person, for everyone responds to life's events differently. Losing a girlfriend, for example, may be a disaster for one man, but just an inconvenience for another. To get a rough idea of how you react to life's everyday and extraordinary events, check off the items below that apply to you. Do you:

_____ Hate to waste time?
_____ Drive fast, even if you're on time?
_____ Tend to over-schedule your days?
_____ Get impatient if other people speak too slowly?

_____ Race through meals, bathing, house-cleaning, gardening and other chores?

_____ Hate losing, even if the game's just for fun?

_____ Feel like intimate relationships are taking you away from work or other more important things?

_____ Often do more than one thing at once?

_____ Neglect hobbies because there isn't any time?

_____ Feel like you should be in charge of everything, because other people don't do it right or take too long?

_____ Tend to get upset when someone else does well, and you don't?

_____ *Have* to be on time for everything?

_____ Speak rapidly, forcefully, and use obscenities?

_____ Use numbers to measure success (how much money made, how many units produced, how many acres owned)?

The more items you checked, the greater the odds are that you are under stress. Many physical ailments, such as ulcers and back aches, may also signal stress.

How to Handle Stress

There is no all-encompassing cure for stress, and there are some stressful things you can't do anything about. For example, you might not be able to quit your job, even if the boss gives you a rough time. But there are some things you can do to counteract at least some of your stress:

1. Don't try to do more than one thing at once.
2. Don't stuff your schedule too full. Only plan to do what you can comfortably accomplish in one day. Save the rest for another day.
3. Drive slower. Even if the traffic is terrible, take it easy.
4. Leave a little early.
5. Set aside a little time every day for exercise and relaxation. A casual stroll in the early morning or evening is an excellent way to relax.
6. Spend some time with family and friends, even if you have to take time away from work or hobbies.
7. Don't automatically volunteer to take on more responsibility or work just to get ahead. Carefully consider whether or not you can do so without eliminating your leisure time.
8. Wherever you're going, make it a point to look at one nice thing on the way—a flower, the sunset, an interesting building, some hot cars.

9. Next time you chat with someone at a party or gathering, don't talk much. Just sit back and listen, asking just enough questions or making just enough statements to keep the conversation going.

10. If someone's doing something slower than you would do it, don't interfere.

11. Before taking on a new task, ask yourself if you really need to do it, if it must be done right now, and if someone else couldn't do it instead.

12. Devote a little time every day to a hobby such as reading, gardening, woodworking, or stamp collecting. Don't try to become a great reader or gardener; don't try to make money from your hobby, just have fun.

13. Unless your boss objects, take a five- or ten-minute break every couple of hours while you're working.

14. Look for a reason to compliment someone (co-worker, family member, friend) every day.

15. Unless you absolutely need it for work, leave your watch at home.

16. Deliberately lose the next time you play a game with children, your spouse or a friend. Take pride in how cleverly you disguise the fact that you're losing on purpose.

Remember, stress has more to do with how you respond than what actually happens to you. You don't always have much power over what's happening, but you can change the way you respond.

Dealing with Your Anger and Guilt

Anger seems to be epidemic today. Whether it's people fighting over a parking space or entire communities rioting because they're dissatisfied with a court verdict, anger is a major social problem. It's a terrible health problem, as well. Judiciously used, anger is a tool used to spur you on when you're in danger. Overused, anger leads to the release of tremendous amounts of adrenaline, cortisone and other powerful substances that can lead to neck pain, tension headaches, ulcers, and other problems.

Anger leads to a lot of pain for nothing, for anger doesn't work. You can intimidate some people by screaming at them, but anger won't get you the things that really count in life—self-esteem, a feeling of contentment, love and respect, and the ability to love others. Most of the time it won't even get you the parking space, because the other guy will probably yell right back at you. These days, who knows, he may even shoot you!

Tips for Dealing with Your Anger

If you find yourself getting angry too often:

1. Understand that you're usually angry for a different reason than you think. You're not angry because someone beat you to the parking space; you're mad because you feel he's slighted you, or you're frustrated because you're in a big hurry. When spouses argue, the real issues are generally money, power, or child-rearing philosophies, not who should wash the dishes. If you feel yourself getting mad, ask yourself why. Are you fighting the wrong battle?

2. Let go of your anger. You might be surprised at how easy it is to tell yourself, "Forget it, it's not worth it." With a little practice, many people report that they're able to switch off anger. They do so by reminding themselves that anger stands in the way of their real goals in life. If you're dealing with old angers, e.g., if you're mad at your father because he was anything from a bad Little League coach to an alcoholic wife-beater, remember that your anger is not hurting him. Your anger has given you that ten-year ulcer, not him. And that third grade school teacher who humiliated you in front of the entire class? That was thirty years ago; she's forgotten all about you. Your anger is hurting you, not her.

3. Forgive the person you're angry at. Often, people don't know they've done something wrong. There's a good chance that the guy who cut in front of you on the freeway didn't even see you. He wasn't out to hurt you; he's just a bad driver. Forgive him. And even if someone is out to get you, even if they deliberately sabotaged your presentation so you wouldn't get the promotion, forgive him. Don't *forget* what happened; protect yourself against future attack and work to expose that rotten apple before he destroys the company—but forgive him. The immediate danger is over. Now it's time for careful planning, and anger only gets in your way.

Overcome Your Guilt

Although guilt is less talked about than anger, many men carry a heavy load of guilt. They feel guilty because they aren't caring enough as husbands or they aren't great fathers. They don't make enough money. They put their mothers in rest homes instead of taking her in. There are many reasons to feel guilty, but ask yourself if what you've done was really so bad. Were you wrong to say "no" to your friend's request, or has he been taking advantage of your generosity? Have you really been a poor father, or are you trying to live up to some ridiculous "perfect father" standard?

Tips to Overcome That Guilt

If you really have done something wrong, or failed in some way:

1. Admit your error to yourself. Drop your defenses and excuses—admit it.

2. Apologize to the person/people you've harmed (unless doing so would harm them even more). Tell your wife you've been a bad husband, tell your co-worker you've been bad-mouthing him to the boss. If your confession leads to punishment, accept it.

3. Make amends to the person/people you've harmed. Do something special for your wife. Tell the boss that the guy you've been bad-mouthing is really terrific. If that's not practical, do something for society (such as donating money to charity).

4. Make a plan for doing better. Ask your wife what you can do to be a better husband. See a marriage counselor. Make a point to either speak well of your co-workers, or keep your mouth shut.

5. If you are a religious person, participate in your religion's forgiveness rituals.

6. While always striving to do your best and never excusing your misdeeds, accept yourself for who you are. Movie stars and quarterbacks get a lot of money and adulation, but the "average Joes" are the backbone of this country. We could do quite well without another seven-foot basketball player, but we need all the accountants and janitors and factory workers and farmers and doctors and clerks and managers and everyone else who puts his or her nose to the grindstone. It's fine to delight in the achievements of others, but be sure to look with pride at your accomplishments, no matter how small you think they may be.

CONFRONTING YOUR GRIEF

Grief is a powerful emotion that can weaken your defense against disease. Studies have shown that following the death of a spouse, the survivor's immune system may weaken, dropping dangerously low in about six months. It takes another six months for the immune system to fully recover. During that one year period, the survivor has a greater chance of contacting all kinds of diseases.

Grief can strike from many quarters. You may lose a parent, a sibling, a friend, a spouse, or perhaps worst of all, a child. Some may grieve the loss of a limb following an accident or the loss of health after developing a serious, lingering disease or disorder. Others grieve the loss of money and prestige following a career setback.

With grief, joy and enthusiasm seem to vanish as the mind's eye focuses on what's been lost. The good things in life are still there, along with the hopes and dreams, but the inner eye doesn't notice. Every pain is magnified, every joy diminished.

Grief is an absolutely natural human response to life's unfortunate events. There is no shame in grieving, but it should not be prolonged unnaturally. To help us through the grieving period, and to keep grief in perspective, many cultures and religions have devised grieving rituals. Many have various "levels" of grief, during which one may almost completely withdraw from society for a brief period of time, then partially return, and finally completely take up his role in the family, workplace, and society.

How to Cope with Grief (There's No Cure)

There is no cure for grief. Indeed, grief should not be "cured" but allowed to run its natural course. There are steps to take to help ensure that grief does not linger unnaturally, including:

1. Do good for others, for doing so helps you feel good about yourself and about life. It can be as simple as paying someone an unexpected compliment.

2. Give yourself a goal. Decide that you're going to perform a certain number of good deeds, read so many books, or finally paint the spare room. In other words, give yourself something to do and something to look forward to.

3. Participate in your religion's or culture's grieving rituals, even if you're not a firm believer. The rituals give you something to do and help keep you in society by instructing others to comfort you.

4. Continue looking for joy just as you normally did once the initial, intense period of grief has passed. Don't force yourself to be happy, but be receptive to all the things that made you happy before. Don't drop out of society. Keep visiting friends and participating in your hobbies. Stay on the bowling or softball team.

5. Remember that while no one can replace the people you've lost, your heart always has more room for another loved one. Let them in—when you're ready.

6. Know that your grief will fade with time, if you let it. The pain of losing a loved one may never totally disappear, but it will fade with time—if you allow it.

LOOK ON THE BRIGHT SIDE: OVERCOMING DEPRESSION

Depression is booming in these troubled days, with millions of people feeling helpless to improve their situations. They have little hope for the future, either their own or society's. Depressed people often feel that nothing is worth much of an effort. Besides, they're usually fatigued and worn out and lack interest in life.

Psychologists and psychiatrists have identified many types or depression, such as agitated depression, anaclitic depression, bipolar depression, endogenous depression, involutional melancholia, reactive depression and retarded depression. We've probably all suffered from the very common reactive depression, which is a normal response to loss or tragedy (such as the death of a loved one). The person suffering reactive depression is sad, despairing, and discouraged, usually in proportion to the loss he has suffered. Given time, reactive depression clears up by itself. Others types of depression, such as endogenous depression, seem to be related to chemical imbalances in the body. With these forms, there may be exaggerated feelings of sadness, dejection, emptiness, hopelessness, and worthlessness, all out of proportion to whatever unpleasant things have happened. Indeed, there may be no obvious connection between the person's life and his depression.

The diagnosis of depression can be complex, but there are some general signs to look for, including: Vague, unfocused feelings of dissatisfaction; feeling helpless to change things you don't like; wishing that people would listen to you once in awhile; putting up with things rather than changing them because you're sure that trying to change them would only make things worse; feeling that you're unimportant, and will remain that way; having trouble imagining yourself successful, popular, powerful; having trouble expressing your feelings to people; thinking that nobody would notice if you just disappeared one day; and occasionally feeling that suicide might be a simple way out.

Ideas to Help Overcome Depression

Although counseling and medication are required for more severe forms of depression, men suffering from milder forms can take steps to improve their energy and interest in life:

1. Don't dwell on what's wrong—think and talk about what's good in your life. If you can't think of any good things in your life, ask a friend or relative to tell you.

2. Schedule as many "happy" things as possible into your day. Set aside time to go to the movies and read the funny papers. Watch little kids playing in the park. Go to birthday parties, Christmas

parties, graduations, anniversaries, and other joyous occasions. Don't force yourself to be happy; just be there.

3. Help others. Doing so will help you feel good about yourself.

4. Go to individual or group counseling. Talk things out, listen to the others. Find a counselor or group interested in hearing you out and helping you move on. Avoid those that want to spend ten years rehashing all the bad things that ever happened to you.

5. Give yourself a goal and work toward it every day, a little at a time.

6. No matter how you feel, stand tall and walk proud. Act as if you're a success, and some of your acting will rub off on you.

7. If you have been struck by loss or tragedy, allow yourself to grieve. Accept your reactive depression as a natural process that will run its course.

8. While focusing on the good things in life, beware of people who demand that you *always* be happy. Your emotions belong to you, not them.

NEW DRUGS THAT AFFECT EMOTIONAL HEALTH

In times past, psychiatrists were sure that severe mental illnesses such as depression, mania and schizophrenia were caused by actual brain disease, with disordered nerve transmission and even visible anatomic abnormalities. The normal range of human character traits (pessimism, optimism, shyness, gregariousness, fear of novelty, etc.) were considered to be the result of early childhood experiences.

Today, we are beginning to wonder if mental illnesses and normal traits aren't all ranges of temperament. One might place profound depression at one extreme, then move to chronic pessimism, moodiness, a normal temperament, general cheerfulness, intense optimism, and, finally, mania. Disease is at either end of the spectrum. What's in between isn't disease, but some of it can be the source of intense stress.

Research into both animal and human brain function over the past twenty years has supported this biological approach to personality, but doctors paid little attention until recently, when it became unnervingly clear that drugs could change temperament. Safe drugs, that is. Humans have used alcohol, opiates, and cocaine to relieve stress for thousands of years, and they work—for a time. Shy people become more gregarious after a few drinks. Amphetamines make the world appear more hopeful. Unfortunately, these drugs also damage the brain. Modern psychoactive medications, such as lithium, older antidepressants, and tranquilizers push people with extreme mood disorders toward the middle of the spectrum without damaging healthy brain tissue, but they have a fair number of unpleasant side effects

The New Wonder Drugs

New psychoactive drugs with fewer side effects appeared at the end of the 1980's, and psychiatrists began prescribing them for less severe illnesses. Newer antidepressants such as Prozac and Zoloft worked no better than the older ones for typical depression, but some patients began reporting improvements in areas other then mood. Uncertain individuals became self-confident. Wallflowers found themselves socializing comfortably. Pessimists felt that the future looked exciting. Not only were some patients becoming well; the doctors found that they were "better than well."

The patients themselves quickly passed the word. Prozac exploded into popular consciousness in 1989. It was even featured on the cover of news magazines. After a period of enthusiasm, the media began denouncing Prozac. Stories of Prozac's deranged victims replaced tales of miraculous transformations. The Prozac's Survivor's Group was organized. Lawsuits were filed. Moralists warned against chemically tampering with the human spirit.

The media lost interest in Prozac after a year. Stories of catastrophic side effects didn't pan out, but the drug's good effects remained. Most doctors prescribe Prozac and its relatives for depression, mania, and a few other serious psychiatric disorders. As I write, your chance of receiving Prozac or a similar medication to relieve stress remains slight, but the subject remains full of debate and controversy. (I've noticed a number of otherwise healthy doctors taking it themselves.)

Your Goal: A Healthy Mind

Life contains plenty of pain and frustration. Luckily, the good outweighs the bad for most people. Anger, guilt, grief, and feelings of failure harm our emotional and physical health; joy, optimism, and confidence strengthen us. Your goal is mental and emotional health, which has been defined in countless ways. If we can work at what we enjoy, have someone to love and something to look forward to, emotional difficulties will fade to a minimum, and we will be healthy and content.

CHAPTER ■ 5

A MAN'S HEALTH PRIORITIES

Uncontrollable influences on health include age, heredity, and gender (males are worse off). Experts also include race, but this is misleading because the overwhelming influence is not race itself but social factors like income, educational level, and dietary preferences. While there's nothing you can do about the aforementioned four influences, five others are well within your control: habits, medical care, exercise, diet, and mental attitude.

This chapter describes the best strategy for staying healthy. It's simpler than you think, and four short sections are plenty. Each discusses the five influences in order of their importance during four periods from youth to old age. No one is perfect; I don't expect you to do everything, but you'll benefit most by following my advice in order. Thus, a smoker who wonders if he should have an annual physical has his priorities deranged.

Each section begins with a checklist that measures how well you're taking care of yourself. I spent a good deal of time deciding what to include as well as the weight to give each element, and I left out everything over which you or your doctor have no control. As a result, you can improve your score. Sixteen is perfect. Consider yourself fairly responsible if you score fourteen or more. Ten or below is very bad. Take this checklist seriously; anyone can score fourteen with a modest effort. Perfection takes work, but (unlike in many areas of life) it's attainable.

HEALTH PRIORITIES IF YOU'RE UNDER 40

A man who wants to reach forty should use his seat belt, practice safe sex, and keep his temper. To enjoy life after forty he should stay thin and not smoke. It's traditional to tell smokers and the obese that they'll die young; this is an exag-

CHECKLIST FOR
THE YOUNG MAN

_____ Check three times if you've never smoked more than a rare cigarette.

_____ Check if you've smoked more but quit permanently.

_____ Check if you practice safe sex with everyone except long-term relationships. Don't check if you occasionally slip up.

_____ Check if you drink lightly. Consider this a weekly consumption of no more than four cans of beer or four wine glasses of wine or two cocktails.

_____ Check if you avoid the sun; wearing a sunscreen and a hat counts.

_____ Check if you brush and floss daily and have regular dental checkups.

_____ Check if you've lost your temper enough to have a fistfight no more than once as an adult _and_ you don't have a handgun in the house.

_____ Check if you exercise as much as I recommend.

_____ Check twice if your weight is near normal.

_____ Check three times if your cholesterol is under 180.

_____ Check twice if it's between 180 and 200.

_____ Check twice if you consider yourself a conservative, safe driver and always wear your seat belt. Considering yourself a skillful driver doesn't count. Don't check if you regularly ride a motorcycle. Nondrivers can check twice.

If you wonder why I include measures like dental hygiene on the same list as avoiding a heart attack, you should remember the purpose of good health. It's not a laudable accomplishment like balancing your budget, but a positive pleasure. Healthy people have more fun. Unfortunately, except for a general sense of well-being, much of the benefit of a healthy young man's life lies in the future. Below age forty, a man scoring a perfect sixteen may not seem notably happier than a flat zero. In fact, the zero probably leads a more colorful life.

Things change as years pass. You might think that a fifty-year-old man who has recovered from a heart attack feels worse than his neighbor who has lost all his teeth, but this is not necessarily so. The heart attack certainly came as a blow, but people adapt. The man most likely went on with his life, sometimes depressed by his disease but mostly not thinking about it. The man wearing false teeth is never unaware that they are less convenient than the real thing. No one can say which man feels more burdened by his disability, but no one can deny that the man with neither leads a more pleasant life. Take your teeth seriously.

geration. Although their lives are shorter, many live to a good age, but it's a life of chronic illness.

PRIORITIES

1. Habits   4. Exercise
2. Diet   5. Medical Care
3. Attitude

Build Good Habits

Don't develop bad ones! In your twenties and thirties it is tempting to throw caution to the wind because a young body tolerates incredible abuse. Three-pack-a-day smokers pass through this period with an increasingly annoying cough but only an occasional heart attack. Drinkers suffer gastritis and nervous stomachs, but their shrinking liver hasn't yet called attention to itself. Even narcotic addicts don't do badly provided that they escape overdoses and infections. My patients invariably straighten out their lives after their first abnormal electrocardiogram, bleeding ulcer, or positive HIV test, and while it's never too late to begin, a great deal is lost irretrievably by the time your body begins to show wear and tear.

Don't smoke

If you don't, you're ahead of the health and longevity game. If you still smoke, quitting is your most important health goal.

Except for the benefit of school children, I no longer rail against smoking because everyone knows how disastrous it is. Rather, I enjoy boasting that the battle against smoking is one of our triumphs: We're winning. In 1966, 50 percent of men smoked. By 1988 this had dropped below 30 percent, and the decline continues at about 0.5 percent per year. At some time in the twenty-first century, smoking will disappear as a health problem.

Wear a condom

Despite the medical profession's dramatic espousal of safe sex during the past decade, this is not a new obligation on our part but correction of a shameful neglect. Unprotected sex between strangers has been wildly unhealthy since the dawn of humanity; AIDS is only the latest in a series of terrible diseases that result. Until well into the twentieth century, syphilis was far more common than AIDS today and led to more sickness, deformity, and insanity; it even provoked the same discrimination from those who felt that victims were immoral people who deserved what they got.

Syphilis remains a nasty infection and is growing more common among heterosexuals, but the list of sexually transmitted diseases is longer than laypeople realize. It includes the common cold, flu, hepatitis, cancer of the penis and anus (cervical cancer in women), several intestinal and joint inflammations, as well as a dozen traditional VDs, among them gonorrhea, herpes, and warts. Unprotected sex with someone you don't know well is almost as unhealthy as smoking.

Drink lightly

I'm doubtful about even moderate drinking. Thanks partly to our persistent hammering, every heavy smoker knows that he is doomed to sickness and misery. Equally doomed, a heavy drinker doesn't worry as much. Of course, the drinker's family doctor is probably unaware that he has an alcoholic patient because doctors are notoriously bad at ferreting out the information. Another difficulty is that there's no such thing as safe, moderate smoking, but everyone agrees that moderate drinking is fine, so a middle-class alcoholic is certain that he qualifies as a moderate. If you drink every day and would be annoyed if you couldn't, it's not positive that you're an alcoholic, but the chances are good.

Drive carefully; use your seat belt; make sure your next car has air bags

Although my younger patients fear cancer and heart attacks, auto accidents are easily the leading cause of death for white men under forty, and the second leading cause for black men.

Nothing illustrates the inherently unhealthy nature of the male sex better than their propensity for dying in cars. This happens partly because men drink more, but even sober men are touchy, impatient drivers who take foolish risks. Statistics show this clearly. Women and men have the same number of accidents, but in fatal accidents male drivers outnumber females two to one. By middle age, men drive safely; this makes their earlier record even more outrageous. Young men with their good vision and quick reflexes have the same risk of accidents as the very elderly—those seventy-five and older.

Half the time an accident won't be your fault, but whether or not your testosterone is involved, wearing a seat belt reduces your chance of severe injury by half; an airbag reduces it more.

Stay out of the sun

The sun damages your skin, causing premature aging and wrinkles as well as skin cancer. If you obey experts who tell you to sunbathe in moderation, your risk of premature skin aging and cancer will be moderate. The healthiest amount of sun is zero. If you spent your life in a cave, the only result would be a better complexion. If you've read that you need sunlight to produce vitamin D, that's only true if you don't consume enough in your diet. If you eat a balanced diet, sunlight on your skin produces no benefit, only harm.

Brush your teeth after every meal and floss once a day

This sounds like advice one hears on "Sesame Street," but I'm surprised how many men are proceeding blithely on a course that guarantees false teeth in middle age. They nod when I ask if their gums bleed after vigorous brushing as if this were normal, but it's a sign of a chronic gum inflammation. As decades pass, inflammation dissolves the bony sockets holding the teeth. Eventually teeth loosen and fall out.

Flossing is essential. Brushing never reaches debris between the teeth. Brush your tongue along with your teeth. It prevents buildup of harmless but ugly patches and diminishes bad breath.

Don't Ignore Your Diet

Achieving a balanced diet is not difficult; achieving the healthiest possible diet takes more effort, but the benefits of zero heart attacks, less cancer, etc., make it worthwhile. Read Chapter 2.

Besides keeping you healthy, your diet should keep you thin. Most men put on weight after forty. A middle-aged paunch is of some consequence, but obesity in a young man is a serious matter. Like smoking, it causes few inconveniences for decades but big trouble later. Fat young men have a higher risk of heart disease and high blood pressure and a much higher risk of diabetes plus arthritis, back pain, corns, and other tiresome disorders that few young men suffer but that fill the thoughts of my older patients.

Losing weight is simple (although not necessarily easy). You cut your food consumption in half and begin an exercise program, as described in Chapter 2. If you have grown up overweight, obesity is in your genes, so staying thin will always be a struggle. You can make it less of a struggle by persisting in exercise.

Here is why. Losing up to 20 pounds is easy. Almost any diet works; diet pills work long enough to knock off 20 pounds; even a bad case of flu works. After 20 pounds, dieting becomes hard. Alarmed at the loss of fat, your brain assumes that you're starving (during most of human history, that would be the correct impression). In an effort to protect you, it slows your metabolism, so the diet that formerly worked now provides all the calories you need.

You can continue to lose weight by eating less, but this is exactly the wrong time for a dieter to hear such advice. The enthusiasm with which he began has faded, a gnawing feeling of deprivation is becoming hard to bear, and appetite suppressants have lost their effect. Most dieters quit at this point. If diet doctors and diet clinics couldn't charge until clients had lost 20 pounds, they'd be out of business. Exercise is the only solution to this difficulty. I explain why later.

Don't Develop an "Attitude"

Although psychologists warn of the dangers of hiding your feelings, I take the opposite view with young men, encouraging them to hold their tempers. A short fuse contributes to their greater risk (compared to older men and all women) of murder, suicide, auto accidents, and work-related injuries.

Although it seems odd to mention as a health problem, murder is the number twelve cause of death in the United States—and number one for black men in this age group. Eighty percent of murders aren't associated with crime but with quarrels between family members, friends, or acquaintances in bars, the street, etc. Unlike women, men tend to be bad tempered and quick to violence; hormones are definitely a factor. Athletes and body builders who take extra male hormone become more irritable.

Murder is as preventable as heart disease. You prevent it by

- Not owning a gun (probably the major preventive)
- Not carrying a weapon of any kind in public
- Being wary about drinking in male company
- Learning to back down, refuse taunts, and flee challenges.

Exercise Is a Must

Irrespective of the health benefits, it's almost impossible to lose a significant amount of weight without exercise. Apparently the brain decides that an active man can't be starving, so it doesn't slow his metabolism. Active men stay thin; if they become active they grow thin.

If weight isn't a problem, give priority to healthy habits, nutrition, and a calm attitude. Then read the sections on exercise in Chapter 2 and give them some thought. Once you begin exercising, you'll be doing every healthy thing a man can do on his own; plenty of my middle-aged patients have seen the light; a young man who follows all four guidelines is wise beyond his years.

Annual Physicals—Good or Bad Idea?

Medical science offers modest benefits to a young man. Clinics and health maintenance organizations (HMOs) that boast of annual physicals regard them as public relations for younger patients. The battery of tests that accompany the exam serves the same purpose. Everyone enjoys hearing that his blood count, chest X-ray, blood sugar, urinalysis, etc., are normal, but studies show that no lab test or X-ray benefits a young man with the exception of a cholesterol test. A man with a normal level should have the test repeated every five years.

High blood pressure isn't common before middle age, but it's not rare. Despite the almost universal belief, absolutely no symptoms accompany hypertension. Measuring pressure is easy; a doctor's skill isn't required. You should have a reading every few years.

Cancer is the fourth leading cause of death in young men, but this is misleadingly high because accidents are overwhelmingly number one. Cancer deaths are one seventh as common as accidents and half as common as murders.

Only one cancer is worth a special effort. Testicular cancer peaks in this age group and becomes rarer in middle age. Detected early, it's almost always curable, and early detection is easy. A monthly testicle self-examination is as important for a man as the breast exam for a woman. Most lumps are benign, but all are worth a trip to the doctor.

Health Priorities if You're in Your Forties

Despite external signs of aging, this remains a healthy period except for men engaged in wildly risky behavior. Smokers suffer most of the heart attacks and a lion's share of the cancer. Even the dimmest doctor begins to suspect alcoholism in otherwise upstanding patients as liver damage and chronic digestive disorders come to his or her attention. For most men, accidents and murder remain the leading causes of death until they near fifty, when heart attacks and cancer take over.

PRIORITIES

1. Diet   **4.** Attitude
2. Exercise   **5.** Medical care
3. Habits

Focus on Your Diet

As long as you're in good health, good eating benefits you more than anything a doctor can do. Your goals don't change from those of young men: staying thin and keeping your cholesterol down.

You might also think about cutting down on salt. Late in the day, especially if you've been on your feet, you'll notice slight puffiness around your ankles—perhaps only the impression of the elastic in your socks. This occurs in your ankles because veins in the lowest part of your body must endure high pressure when you stand, and as veins age they weaken and leak, so fluid oozes into the tissues. After a night in bed, the puffiness disappears. This is not a sign of ill

CHECKLIST FOR THE MAN
IN HIS FORTIES

_____ Check three times if you've never smoked more than a rare cigarette.

_____ Check if you've smoked more but quit permanently.

_____ Check if you practice safe sex with everyone except long-term relationships. Don't check if you occasionally slip up.

_____ Check if you drink lightly.

_____ Check if you brush and floss daily and have regular dental checkups.

_____ Check if you've lost your temper enough to have a fistfight no more than once as an adult *and* you don't have a handgun in the house.

_____ Check if you exercise as much as I recommend.

_____ Check twice if your weight is near normal.

_____ Check twice if your cholesterol is under 180.

_____ Check once if it's between 180 and 200.

_____ Check once if you're a conservative, safe driver.

_____ Check if you have a regular doctor.

_____ Check once if you're married or have a permanent live-in companion.

_____ Check once if you feel that life has treated you at least satisfactorily: that work is tolerable, money is not a great problem, and you are rarely lonely.

Priorities shift as you pass forty. Avoiding the sun drops out because almost all sun damage occurs during youth, and it's not reversible. Auto accidents become statistically less important, so they're also off the list. If, as an individual, you choose to engage in risky behavior, the danger remains.

Not smoking always brings generous benefits, but with advancing age, health depends to an increasing degree on domestic arrangements, social life, and self-confidence. Lack of a spouse dramatically shortens a man's life; it has little effect on a woman's. Unhappy men get sick and kill themselves at an increasing rate as they get older, but unhappy women soldier on. Medical care begins to influence a man's health.

---

health, and it's also not evidence of high blood pressure (which affects arteries but not veins). You can reduce this puffiness by reducing the volume of fluid inside your vascular system. Consuming less salt (not less water) accomplishes this. This sounds like a paradox, but excess fluid intake doesn't cause edema because the kidneys instantly eliminate it; if you consume excess salt, the kidneys must hold back water to dissolve it.

Blood pressure often creeps up during your adult years, and in this period many readings will rise above normal, so cutting back on salt may kill two birds with one stone.

Developing Good Habits

Unnerved by the first glimpse of a paunch, wrinkle, or bald spot, men who have been sedentary all their lives launch into violent activity and then stumble into my office with their sprained ankles, charley horses, and back injuries. They are on the right track. Healing is usually prompt during this period, and the visit gives me a chance to encourage them. Start slowly with walking or jogging.

The forties mark the last period to obtain maximum benefit from a conditioning program. No amount of exercise will reverse the slow loss of bone and muscle that all men experience beginning in the mid-thirties, but regular activity slows it.

By this period smokers suffer chronic lung disease; breathing tests reveal shrinking lung volume and increasing air flow obstruction in all smokers, including those without symptoms. If you don't smoke at forty, chances are almost nil that you'll begin. If you do, your first priority is clear.

For nonsmokers, safe driving and safe sex are most likely to keep you healthy until middle age. Continue to brush, floss, and stay out of the sun.

During this period you'll wonder if life has been worthwhile. Since it probably wasn't an uninterrupted triumph and since men tend to focus on their defects, you may conclude that you're a failure. When men feel this way, it's a midlife crisis. Women call it depression, a more honest description.

Emotional pain is no less disabling than physical pain, and tolerating it shows as much good sense as walking on a sprained ankle or ignoring chest pain. As with much physical illness, it's all right to try home treatment first, but if confiding in friends or trying to pull yourself together doesn't help, get professional help. Men in a crisis seem to feel that they should rely on their inner strength to pull themselves out of it, but willpower is as overrated here as it is in curing physical disease. Furthermore, medical science does fairly well in treating psychological illness—better than with heart attacks and other serious diseases.

Be straight with the doctor. Don't make an appointment for a head-to-toe physical, because that's what you may receive. If you feel bad, say so. It's true that many doctors aren't comfortable dealing with heavy emotional problems, but they're also not good at plenty of other ailments. If so, they'll know someone who does better.

Getting Good Medical Care in Your Forties

If you don't already have a satisfactory doctor, read the chapter on choosing one (Chapter 12) and proceed. If you find a candidate, make an appointment for whatever introductory exam he or she performs. Don't be examined by a doctor you'll never see again. Overwhelmed by the demand for complete physicals from patients who don't need them, many clinics hire outside doctors or pay their own extra to come in after hours and churn them out. An important goal of your introductory exam is to establish yourself as the doctor's patient. Doctors perform slightly better with their own patients, and you want that edge.

The exam enables the doctor to record your medical history and physical findings. There will be a great deal of tapping, shining of lights, and thoughtful listening with a stethoscope, but the important part of the exam occurs when the doctor inserts a finger into your rectum.

Have a rectal exam yearly for the rest of your life, beginning at forty. At forty your risk of the leading fatal malignancy in non-smokers, colon cancer, begins to rise. Perhaps 10 percent grow within the reach of the finger, but the doctor should also wipe his or her fingertip across a small card and add a drop of fluid that detects tiny amounts of blood in stool. Many colon cancers ooze blood; this test picks them up early. The finger also runs over your prostate to search for lumps that may be cancer, an unlikely finding during this period but more important as the years pass.

Only the most rigorous doctor orders the necessary lab tests (still just one—the cholesterol) and no others, so you'll probably get a battery of blood tests plus a urinalysis and perhaps a chest X-ray and electrocardiogram. Although they turn up little curable disease but a great many alarming abnormalities with no significance, doctors find them irresistible. I discuss the hazards of overtesting later in this chapter.

Confronted with their overtesting, doctors justify many tests on the grounds that they need a baseline, a record to consult when something changes. For example, if a man suffers chest discomfort and his electrocardiogram shows vague abnormalities, it's reassuring that the previous routine tracing looks identical—and ominous when it doesn't. The defect in this argument is that baseline tests help only if you carry copies of them at all times. You can bet that when you have your chest pain, you'll end up at an unfamiliar hospital late at night, and your earlier tracing will be tucked away in a record room across town.

During your forties, make an appointment with an ophthalmologist for a routine exam including a check for glaucoma, and then return at whatever intervals he or she advises. Glaucoma, the result of elevated pressure of fluid inside the eye, causes progressive blindness without other symptoms. Beginning in the 1960s when disease prevention became popular, family doctors tested for glaucoma by touching the eye with a clever instrument called a tonometer. It was easy and painless; when pressure readings rose above a certain level, they referred the patient to an ophthalmologist and felt pleased with themselves. Preventive medicine experts urged doctors to perform tonometry on everyone over forty.

They did so despite increasing complaints from ophthalmologists that almost everyone referred didn't have glaucoma. It turns out that most people with elevated eye pressure don't develop disease, the tonometer missed a good many that do, and diagnosing glaucoma requires a more sophisticated exam than family doctors can perform. The message got across early in the 1980s; today our expensive tonometers gather dust.

Continue to examine your testes. Although it peaks at age thirty-four, testicular cancer remains a threat during this period. You should also buy one of the colon cancer detection kits sold in pharmacies. Simple to use, you drop a pad into the toilet; chemicals in the paper change color in the presence of blood. Test yourself three times a year. Don't panic at the sight of a color change. Anything that bleeds (including hemorrhoids, benign polyps, and ulcers) produces a positive test. Only 5 to 10 percent are cancers; these are mostly small and curable.

HEALTH PRIORITIES IF YOU'RE IN YOUR FIFTIES

A number of my middle-aged male patients decide abruptly to follow my advice, clean up their diet, quit smoking, take up exercise, etc. Most, I regret to say, are practicing secondary prevention: They've had their heart attack. Fear provides a powerful motivation, and these men will benefit, but practicing primary prevention (keeping bad things from happening) is better. Think about it while you're still eligible.

Although your body is showing signs of aging, don't assume that everything is downhill. The common cold and other viral upper respiratory infections grow less common, probably because about a hundred viruses cause these infections, and by middle age you've acquired immunity to most by catching them. Many tiresome ailments burn themselves out in later life; allergies, migraine headaches, acne, and other chronic skin conditions fade in middle age.

Medical care leaps in priority because medical problems become significant (doctors are only modestly useful in disease prevention). If you're already following my advice, this period begins to provide substantial rewards, but never forget that the human body is imperfect, and life is unpredictable. Things go wrong that aren't your fault, so mental attitude plays an increasingly important role.

PRIORITIES

1. Diet   4. Habits
2. Medical care   5. Exercise
3. Attitude

Diet and Medical Care

The diet discussed in Chapter 2 remains the best no matter how old you become. During my training in the 1960s, cardiologists were already lecturing

CHECKLIST FOR THE MAN
IN HIS FIFTIES

_____ Check three times if you've never smoked more than a rare cigarette.

_____ Check if you've smoked more but quit permanently.

_____ Check if you drink lightly.

_____ Check if you brush and floss daily and have regular dental checkups.

_____ Check if you exercise as much as I recommend.

_____ Check twice if your weight is near normal.

_____ Check twice if your cholesterol is under 180.

_____ Check once if it's between 180 and 200.

_____ Check twice if you have a regular doctor and a yearly checkup.

_____ Check twice if you're married or have a permanent live-in companion.

_____ Check twice if you feel that life has treated you at least satisfactorily.

Notice that as your health obligations grow less numerous, some become increasingly important. Accidents, violence, and sexual indiscretions fade, but it's never safe to tempt fate. Medical care contributes more; so does your social and emotional life.

on the benefits of a low cholesterol level, but they warned us not to go overboard with older patients. Middle-aged arteries were already packed with rock-hard cholesterol, they explained. Mere dietary changes wouldn't dissolve it. They added that middle-aged habits were fixed; eliminating favorite foods led to stress and unhappiness, so we should not make your declining years more difficult. I remember encouraging older men with cardiac disease to eat what they pleased.

By the 1970s experts were less certain that lowering cholesterol wouldn't benefit older men, and by the 1980s they suggested that some good might result. Nowadays I encourage men of all ages to lower their cholesterol.

At age fifty, make an appointment for a sigmoidoscopy. If your family doctor doesn't perform this procedure you'll see a gastroenterologist, who will insert a flexible tube the diameter of a forefinger through your anus and 2 feet into your colon to search for tumors and precancerous polyps. This is a good test for early detection; almost every expert recommends at least one. We still debate how often you should have it; most doctors advise every three to five years.

Besides its health benefits, undergoing a flexible sigmoidoscopy teaches you two important principles:

1. New medical technology is fantastically more expensive than the technology it replaces, and

2. Sometimes it's worth it.

An ingenious device developed by the Japanese during the 1960s, the flexible fiber-optic endoscope costs fifty times more than the traditional sigmoidoscope, which is basically a stiff tube with a light at one end. A complete fiber-optic setup costs several thousand dollars, one reason why many doctors don't own one.

In the old days experts complained that we family doctors weren't performing enough rigid sigmoidoscopies and thus missing our patients' early colon cancers. They assured us that, despite its reputation, the procedure wasn't terribly uncomfortable. After statements like that, experts wonder why practicing doctors ignore their advice. The truth is that undergoing rigid sigmoidoscopy was not unlike medieval torture and accompanied by similar groans and screams. I witnessed many and (as a result) performed few.

The new instrument produces much less discomfort. Experts claim that it's a breeze, their usual exaggeration. Having undergone one myself, I found it unpleasant but tolerable.

You must continue your yearly rectal exam as well as regular checks of your blood pressure and cholesterol. No other lab test offers much benefit in detecting early disease, but you'll probably receive plenty.

Prevention for High-Risk Patients—a Gray Area. An aspirin a day lowers the risk of heart attack by almost half in men over fifty, at the price of a slight increase in strokes. An aspirin every other day works as well, although no one recommends this because people tend to forget which day requires a pill. A man over fifty should take aspirin daily unless his risk is low (a cholesterol under 180) or he suffers a medical condition such as ulcers that forbids aspirin.

Twenty years ago we X-rayed smokers to detect lung cancer. Although plenty of early diagnoses turned up, lung cancer spreads so rapidly that smokers who had the test died as quickly as those who didn't, so chest X-rays fell into disfavor.

Although men with a family history of a particular ailment often ask for tests to search for it, the yield is poor. An electrocardiogram is almost worthless in detecting coronary artery disease in someone who feels well. A blood glucose test certainly detects diabetes, but almost all older diabetics are overweight. I tell overweight men to lose weight. Once I detect their diabetes, I prescribe the best treatment: losing weight. Medical students learn and doctors forget a good rule for deciding on a test: If the result won't change the treatment, don't order it.

The exercise ECG illustrates this rule vividly. Many men feel an irresistible urge to clump to exhaustion on a treadmill and then experience deep satisfaction on hearing that their electrocardiogram remains normal. It seems to be a middle-age rite of passage similar to losing one's virginity in high school. Yet a treadmill is a poor screening test. Most men who feel well have a normal treadmill, but there is less here than meets the eye. Fifteen percent of these happy men have severe coronary artery disease, because the test isn't perfect. Many of the rest have the usual coronary disease for their age; the exercise ECG won't detect that unless their arteries are narrow enough to prevent adequate blood flow during exercise.

A positive treadmill requires confirmation with more complex tests, probably including an angiogram. In the end, a minority of these men have endured fear and expense for nothing. Their coronary arteries are normal. The remainder know that they have serious heart disease. They felt fine before the test; they'll never feel healthy again. You might think that they benefit because their disease has been detected, but this is not certain. Doctors can't agree what to do with these men. Naturally, we encourage them to lose weight, follow a low-cholesterol diet, and exercise (carefully), but they should be doing that already. Some will have bypass surgery. Most begin taking aspirin. All worry. Like most laboratory tests, the treadmill gives valuable information when we already suspect that something is wrong, but it's less helpful and often troublesome in subjects who feel well.

The Right Attitude

Too many men believe they have a choice between being either perfect or a terrible person. As a result, they feel good when things go well but crushed when they don't. The fifties are a critical period because life's blows (career disappointments, divorce, financial losses) cause more pain than in earlier years. Less time is available to recover, and if this is the second or third occurrence of the same disaster, you may wonder if you're cursed (in fact you're simply not learning from your mistakes; a sign that you're human). Several blows in a short period convince anyone that he's not perfect.

■ HAZARDS OF OVERTESTING. ■

Even if you could afford it, you shouldn't have every possible test during your annual physical.

A few simple tests (temperature, blood pressure) are almost 100 percent accurate, but complex ones involving chemicals or machines rarely perform as well. We consider 95 percent accuracy acceptable. In other words, the test will occasionally turn out abnormal in subjects who are perfectly healthy or remain normal when it shouldn't. If you think about it, this means that the sicker you are, the better the test works. As you get healthier, the test grows more and more unreliable.

If the only alternative to perfection is being a terrible person, that man is in trouble.

A man who sees himself as a worthless failure suffers a serious medical problem that a doctor can help. Although depression lacks the concrete reality of ulcer or pneumonia, it's a physical disorder: brain disease, just as emphysema is lung disease. It can be fatal; men kill themselves more often as they get older. Yet medical science does well at treatment (better, certainly, than our treatment of emphysema). Drugs cure most depression in a few months (electroshock works more quickly, but it's out of fashion). Counseling diminishes the pain; even the body's healing powers play a role; the brain often recovers.

Good Habits for the Man in His Fifties

Men at this age often become set in their ways, so maintaining earlier good habits becomes easier. You'll notice the benefits both in positive ways (absent paunch, intact teeth, stamina) and negative (big-league diseases—heart attacks, diabetes, high blood pressure—begin appearing among men your age).

Think about the contents of medicine cabinets that you've inspected during parties. When I was young and rummaged through the medicine cabinets of my peers, this rarely turned up anything more interesting than birth control gear plus an occasional diet pill or headache remedy. Today I see an increasing collection of sleeping pills, tranquilizers, laxatives, stool softeners, skin creams, and indigestion remedies. These are not really disease therapy, but they represent a struggle to make the aging body operate as smoothly as it once did. Although fairly effective, in the long run these remedies form habits that are hard to break. Good habits are not only lifesaving, they'll make life run more smoothly. You'll never be constipated, and you'll sleep better.

If you've been slothful all your life, take care of the first four priorities. Think about golf—not a conditioning exercise but strenuous enough to provide evidence that your body is capable of doing better. Then if you want to exercise, buy one of the books on walking or bicycling, and see how you tolerate a regular program. I don't stress more strenuous exercises like tennis or jogging, but if you feel the urge don't proceed without your doctor's approval.

HEALTH PRIORITIES FOR OLDER MEN

You can't prevent everything, so medical care jumps to first priority during this period. You must have a doctor and regular exams. Plenty of things go wrong that we can fix, and finding them as soon as possible usually makes fixing easier.

CHECKLIST FOR
THE OLDER MAN

_____ Check three times if you've never smoked more than a rare cigarette.

_____ Check if you've smoked more but quit permanently.

_____ Check if you drink lightly.

_____ Check twice if your weight is near normal.

_____ Check twice if your cholesterol is under 200.

_____ Check three times if you have a regular doctor and a yearly checkup.

_____ Check three times if you're married or have a permanent live-in companion.

_____ Check twice if you feel that life has treated you at least satisfactorily.

Diet, marriage, and medical care dominate. I felt uneasy dropping dental hygiene, but if you've brushed and flossed throughout your life, you don't need my encouragement to continue. If not, you probably have few teeth to care for. Heart attack incidence peaks in the fifties, so a man who reaches retirement age has passed the time of highest risk, but he should still keep his cholesterol below average. Keeping active remains important but less so than other elements on the list.

PRIORITIES

1. Medical care   4. Habits
2. Attitude   5. Exercise
3. Diet

Medical care

If you reach this period without heart disease, you're not entirely home free, but many doctors stop ordering a blood cholesterol because the elderly don't tolerate cholesterol-lowering drugs and become more reluctant to make radical dietary changes. On the other hand, doctors grow more liberal in ordering other lab tests despite the lack of evidence that they detect enough early disease to help you. Be understanding about this. Remember that your doctor is younger than you; young people believe that old people are sicker than they really are.

The single generally accepted test is a yearly urinalysis. A technician dips a strip containing half a dozen test areas into a urine sample. The areas change color in the presence of blood, sugar, protein, bile, and a few other substances.

Like so many tests, this test is often positive because of minor ailments and negative when serious disease exists, but it picks up enough early kidney disease, urinary tract cancer, and diabetes to compensate. See a more extensive discussion of urinalysis in Chapter 12.

Although the rectal exam remains mandatory, the rest of your yearly checkup is up to the doctor. You must understand why I list medical care first during this period. Prevention is not the reason; we still prevent problems, but fewer as times passes. Early detection is not the major reason; it grows increasingly important, although laypeople exaggerate the number of diseases doctors can detect before symptoms appear.

You need doctors most because during this period *bad things happen*. It's fashionable to denounce doctors for spending too little time on health education and disease prevention. We're undoubtedly guilty. Critics are also fond of telling us that, compared to prevention, treating disease is expensive and inefficient. Although also true, that's what doctors mostly do. Treating sick people has been our role since the dawn of history. That's probably what attracted us to medicine originally. You may have disapproved of this emphasis when you were younger, but now you will reap the benefits.

Since your doctor probably prefers the role of a healer, don't deprive him or her of the opportunity. My older male patients perform badly here. Several times a year one calls to tell me he's suffered a bellyache for about a week. Invariably he wants to keep the conversation centered on constipation, dietary advice, or a medicine to straighten him out. I concentrate on getting him into the office because too often—perhaps a third of the time—this man requires surgery for his gangrenous bowel and may not survive. Had he come in after a day or two, I might have treated him at home. When a 25-year-old tells me he's been coughing for two weeks or tired for two months, I rarely worry. After sixty, this delay may be fatal.

Attitude

A man who reaches sixty-five has an even chance of passing eighty, so old age is often the longest period in life—longer than middle age or young adulthood. Although it can be as satisfying as the others, unique stresses appear.

Some are best ignored. In my experience, few older people worry much about death but rather more about the illness, pain, and inability to care for themselves that precedes it. I can't promise that this won't happen, just as I can't assure a fifty-year-old that he won't have a heart attack, but it's not inevitable. If you follow the advice in this book and make sure you have a good relationship with a doctor (who should be at least twenty years younger than you—to reduce the chance that he or she will retire or die before you), you're doing everything possible. Concentrate on the present.

Concentrate most on not being alone. If you don't have a spouse or companion, find one. Make sure your daily activities or work keep you around people.

Although they don't like it, women tolerate loneliness well, but men deteriorate. Single men and widowers suffer many more heart attacks than married men. Their suicide rate is triple that of married men—and nineteen times more than married women. You might assume this is because a man's health requires a wife to provide decent food, hygiene, and general psychological support, but the presence of any companion will do. Even those whose wives have died (the most stressful event in a man's life) maintain their health if they don't live alone.

Diet

If you're not following a zero atherosclerosis diet, it's still good to begin, but realize that the leading dietary disorder in older men is the one mistakenly believed common in everyone else: poor nutrition. Authorities blame this on lack of money and lack of a wife's cooking, since most men who get into trouble lack both.

Although the belief is correct, these factors merely increase the risk because an excellent diet is cheap and doesn't involve much cooking. Two hours spent cooking quantities of natural, whole foods can provide a week of dinners. Cereal and fruit make up an excellent breakfast. Older men suffer poor nutrition when they become unhappy, set in their ways, and slow to adapt. By reading this far, you've shown that you don't qualify.

Habits

Sensible young men avoid bad habits like smoking and drinking. This allows them to live to an old age, when they must resist the urge to hang onto habits they took for granted, such as going to bed at the same time or having a bowel movement after breakfast.

We don't realize how much our daily lives teem with routine until body functions slow or turn unreliable with age. Sleep becomes shallower, with more interruptions. Digestion and elimination grow more leisurely. Metabolism declines, so we require less food. Erections occur more slowly, but they should never disappear.

Don't try to coerce your body to function as regularly as it once did. Sleep when you're sleepy, eat when you're hungry, and have a bowel movement when the urge appears. Otherwise, wait.

Exercise

Until well after World War II, doctors treated many childhood diseases (such as rheumatic fever and polio) with months of strict bed rest. Nowadays we understand how harmful this was, but fortunately children are tough; they can tolerate long periods of immobility without suffering permanent harm. This is definitely not the case once you pass sixty.

During this period, any incident that leads to prolonged inactivity can herald the beginning of the end. Time and again, one of my older patients suffers a treatable problem such as a broken hip. Broken hips heal; if not, an artificial hip works fine. Yet most of the elderly who break a hip end up permanently enfeebled, not from the injury but from the weeks of enforced bed rest.

Exercise is less a preventive during this period than a necessity to keep muscles and joints in working order. Without it muscles wither, joints stiffen, calcium leaches from bone, and bowels grow somnolent. Stay out of bed. Keep moving. Take up walking.

MANAGING THE MALE TEMPERAMENT

As a man makes his way through life, he is likely to review his progress and ask himself questions such as: What have I done with my life? Where do I stand now? Of what value is my life now to society and to others? He must come to grips with the gap between what he is and what he had always dreamed of becoming.

Men make up only 30 percent of patients seeking psychotherapy. Perhaps the percentage ought to be higher. Many men bury their emotions, never or only rarely able to own up to the pressures and pains of their interior lives. To compensate they take greater advantage of other ways of dealing with life's stresses. Men abuse alcohol and drugs three times as often as women, kill themselves three times as often and commit over 90 percent of violent crimes.

Your Temperament Can Help or Harm You

Defined correctly, temperament refers to an inborn pattern of behavior that often tends to remain constant throughout a man's life. Some men are garrulous and sociable, others withdrawn, still others touchy and critical. Most parents notice these tendencies from an early age and either smile with satisfaction or wrinkle their brows with worry as the tendencies persist.

In the past psychiatrists were confident that severe mental illness such as depression, mania, and schizophrenia represented actual brain disease, with disordered nerve transmission and even visible anatomic abnormalities. When it came to the normal range of human character traits (for example, from pessimism to optimism, shyness to gregariousness, fear of novelty to delight in risks), doctors didn't object strongly when Freudians explained these as the outcome of early childhood experiences. If some aspect of temperament, such as shyness or fear of failure, became too painful, only psychotherapy could help.

Today we are beginning to wonder if a continuum of nerve transmission doesn't give rise to all ranges of temperament, just as blood pressure produces disease at its extremes but normal function in the middle. One might place a person who is profoundly depressed at one extreme. Moving toward the center reveals a chronic pessimist, someone who is often moody, then a normal temperament, a generally cheerful person, moving on to an intensely optimistic enthusiast (hypomania) proceeding into mania: disease at the opposite end of the spectrum. Everyone agrees that temperament between the extremes doesn't represent disease, but it can be an intense source of stress.

Modern society rewards the hypomanic temperament. In business, school, or relations with women, success favors the decisive, positive, sparkling person who exudes confidence and hurries through the day with energy to spare. The talented but colorless individual suffers. A thriving industry of books, seminars, and lectures teach the secrets of success—mostly the elements of hypomanic behavior. These represent the male equivalent of diet books and diet clinics. Much of the advice is reasonable, but following it is harder than enthusiasts claim. Temperament resists change.

Research into both animal and human brain function over the past twenty years has supported this biological approach to personality, but doctors paid little attention until recently, when it became unnervingly clear that drugs could change temperament.

Drugs That Help You Deal with Stress

Safe drugs, that is. Humans have used alcohol, opiates, and cocaine to relieve stress for thousands of years, and they work. Shy people become less shy after a few drinks. Amphetamines make the world appear more hopeful. Unfortunately these drugs damage the brain as they improve temperament, so they are a losing proposition. Modern psychoactive medications such as lithium, older antidepressants, and tranquilizers act to move extreme mood disorders toward the middle without damaging health, but they produce a fair degree of unpleasant side-effects, so few people value them for less disabling emotions.

At the end of the 1980s, psychoactive drugs with fewer side-effects appeared, and psychiatrists did what doctors usually do with improved drugs—prescribe them for less severe illnesses. Newer antidepressants such as Prozac and Zoloft worked no better than older ones for typical depression, but some patients began reporting improvements in qualities besides mood. Uncertain individuals became self-confident. Wallflowers found themselves socializing comfortably. Pessimists realized that the future looked exciting. Not only were they well, doctors heard, they were "better than well." Not every patient underwent such a transformation, but it occurred often enough to startle psychiatrists.

Patients themselves quickly passed the word. The first of these new drugs, Prozac, exploded into popular consciousness in 1989. News magazines featured it on cover articles. Talk shows poured out nonsense along with some intelligent discussion. Following the usual pattern, media enthusiasm ran its course and switched to media denunciation. Stories of Prozac's deranged victims replaced miraculous transformations. The Prozac Survivor's Group was organized. Lawsuits were filed. Moralists warned against chemically tampering with the human spirit. Talk shows poured out nonsense along what some intelligent discussion.

After a year the media lost interest. Stories of catastrophic side-effects didn't pan out, but the good effects remained to disturb thoughtful physicians. Most doctors prescribe Prozac and its relatives for depression and a few other serious psychiatric disorders, but I notice a number of otherwise healthy doctors taking it themselves, a situation that reminds me of their rush to minoxidil when rumors arrived of its ability to grow hair. These doctors would not dream of using tranquilizers (they are not searching for tranquility), but a physician's life is full of stress. Much of this is inherent in the practice of medicine, with its terrible responsibilities and heavy work load. But doctors are no different from other humans, so temperament leads to a good deal of their stress. Experts may denounce cosmetic pharmacology—using drugs to improve minor social disabilities—and most doctors turn down patients who request this. But, in quiet moments, doctors wonder how they'd feel if they were a bit more optimistic, cheerful, and decisive, a bit less compulsive and less upset by failure and frustration.

As I write, your chance of receiving Prozac to relieve stress remains slight, but the subject remains full of debate and controversy. You can read a thoughtful discussion in *Listening to Prozac*, by Peter Kramer (Publisher, Viking, 1993). Fortunately, men can make some changes in the second source of stress.

Mostly from parents but also from friends, the media, and culture, a man learns how a man should behave. Everyone understands the enormous effect of family on a man's coping tactics, but we fail to appreciate how much American society contributes. Confucian society, which still influences China and Japan, teaches that a man owes absolute, unquestioning loyalty to his superiors. To us, this sounds outrageous, but in a rigid social system this philosophy keeps stress at a minimum. Democratic society encourages us to give loyalty where loyalty is deserved but refuse to accept injustice. So an American man feels that he must not tolerate unfair treatment—an agonizing source of stress in many jobs and relationships, where alternatives are limited. In the end, however, learned coping tactics are not immutable.

How Much Stress Can You Avoid? So far, these sections on health priorities have discussed five guidelines in maintaining your health. Not only are they backed by good evidence, but I follow them myself—the diet, exercise, medical care guidelines, etc. That I am in perfect health at my age provides no proof that this advice is correct (individual testimonials are worthless but vivid, so popular health writers and the media depend on them). However, you have the right to expect an advisor to follow his own advice.

My philosophy is that life contains plenty of pain and frustration, but that the good parts outweigh the bad. Since the greatest sources of emotional difficulty in a man's life are (1) dealing with other people and (2) achieving the success in his own goals, I've boiled my advice down to one guideline for each. Plenty of others exist, but these are learnable without doing violence to most men's temperament.

Learn to say no without feeling guilty

Most strong emotions follow interactions with other people, and most of these interactions are verbal. Almost everyone feels inadequate in this area; one consequence is a stream of books and psychotherapeutic schools dedicated to improving coping skills. Best-seller lists for the entire twentieth century have always included catchy titles from *How to Make Friends and Influence People* to *Looking Out for Number One* to *Life's Little Instruction Book*. Although invariably too optimistic about what they can accomplish, they are rarely entirely off base.

Stay away from writers who tell you how to win arguments, negotiations, etc. Not only is this almost impossible to teach, but productive interactions shouldn't involve victory or defeat. It's easier to steer a middle course—to express your wishes honestly while avoiding being manipulated. Almost everyone feels uncomfortable refusing a favor, changing his mind, admitting a mistake, deflecting criticism, or inconveniencing someone who should serve us. Authorities from Ann Landers to Sigmund Freud give advice on overcoming this, but I believe the best techniques come from a school of behavior therapy called assertiveness training. Although not the most fashionable today, plenty of authorities use it. My favorite book on the subject is *When I Say No, I Feel Guilty*, by Manuel J. Smith (Dial, 1975).

Plan to lead a fulfilling life. Be willing to persist in pursuing your goals and to switch gears if your goals change.

Men who want to achieve fulfillment quickly turn to crime or drugs. Those are willing to wait months to a few years turn to books and seminars on achieving fulfillment; as I mentioned earlier, their appeal to men resembles that of diet books for women, and the success rate is similar. Yet it is not pollyannish to state that any man with reasonable life goals can achieve them with planning and persistence, but a great deal of both may be required.

CHAPTER ■ 6

THE MAN GETTING ON IN YEARS

No animal and almost no human dies of old age. We die of disease or trauma, self-inflicted or otherwise. It's true that organ function declines slowly with age, but physiologists estimate that our vital organs would support life adequately until well past 120.

Things happen as you grow older. When those things cause discomfort or a decline in sexual appeal, humans quickly blame aging, a process often regarded as a relentless progression to generalized crumbling and senility. This is an exaggeration. While few bodily processes improve with age, a good part of their decline stems from disease, much of it preventable. You've already learned that heart attacks and strokes increase with age because of the accumulated insults of cholesterol plaques and high blood pressure. Aging itself bears no blame. On the other hand, cancer incidence rises with age partly from accumulated environmental toxins and unhealthy lifestyles, but partly because the aging immune system grows less efficient in destroying malignant cells. Aging bears part of the blame.

This chapter summarizes what to expect as you get older. But first you should know what's irrelevant.

IS THIS A SIGN THAT I'M GETTING OLD?

It's a myth that your body wears out as you age. Only teeth and joints wear out. As it happens, technology performs well in protecting worn teeth with caps, crowns, etc. A good deal more complex, the technology of replacing worn joints will eventually become routine. For now, replacing hips and knees has reached the status of accepted practice, and research is well along with other joints.

Other parts of the body—skin, bone, nerves, eyes, heart, kidney, bowel, etc.—don't deteriorate faster if you use them more. You don't accelerate visual loss by excessive reading, and your heart won't give out sooner if forced to pump more than the average. Using these organs for what they're designed to do won't cause premature aging; only abuse does that.

Following are descriptions of how your body parts age plus advice for slowing this process or, if slowing is impossible, dealing effectively with the consequences.

What Happens to Your Skin

Despite the popular impression, the skin surface (epidermis; see Chapter 9) changes only modestly with age. Cell turnover decreases, so wounds heal more slowly. One positive consequence is that scars that form after an injury appear thinner and less visible. Since they're replaced more slowly, dead surface cells become less efficient at preventing evaporation, making dry skin an increasing problem.

After age thirty caucasians lose about 20 percent of their pigment cells (melanocytes) per decade. Scattered in the basal layer at the bottom of the epidermis in everyone except albinos, melanocytes multiply after sun exposure to produce a protective tan. Depending on their normal distribution, they produce our skin pigmentation and hair color, and their tendency to clump irregularly leads to freckles and moles. You'll learn about these and similar skin conditions in Chapter 9.

Because of the decline in melanocytes, older skin grows more susceptible to sun damage. This same lack of pigment produces gray and white hair, but prematurely gray hair does not indicate premature aging. It occurs in families who otherwise enjoy good health. Balding is a sign of sexual maturity, not advancing age.

Most skin aging changes occur below the epidermis in the living dermis. The dense connective tissue loses elasticity and shrinks, causing wrinkles. Older people bruise more easily, not because of a clotting disorder but because blood vessels in the dermis become delicate, liable to leak after minor injuries. Tissue below the dermis (i.e., subcutaneous tissue) also diminishes. Mostly fat, this serves as insulation, so older people grow more sensitive to cold.

The same decline of the immune system that increases susceptibility to skin cancer diminishes the inflammatory response to solar radiation. Much of the burning and redness after sun exposure results from inflammation, not the burn itself (a large dose of cortisone taken before exposure or even shortly afterward eliminates the discomfort of inflammation). Older people can sit in the sun longer without acquiring a burn, but they shouldn't. More, not less, skin damage is occurring.

To Slow Skin Aging: Stay Out of the Sun. Old Swedes look younger than old Italians. Unlike many health measures, sun avoidance works with high efficiency. A person who complied all his life would probably slow skin aging by 70 to 80 percent, but it's never too late to begin. Authorities advise older patients to keep their skin hydrated by avoiding harsh soaps and by applying emollients after bathing. Although good advice, this has little effect on aging but relieves the consequences (i.e., dry skin, itching).

Cardiovascular System

Until only a few years ago, physiologists agreed that cardiac output, the volume of blood pumped per minute, declines 1 percent per year beginning around age thirty. Then they realized that subtle coronary atherosclerosis is so common that their studies were full of subjects with heart disease. Recent studies of healthy hearts show almost no decline with age. The maximum possible heart rate during exercise drifts down; as I mentioned in Chapter 3, you can calculate the rate as 220 minus your age.

Like the dermis, arteries contain rubbery connective tissue that stiffens with age, increasing their resistance to blood flow. As a result, circulation diminishes slowly. By age eighty, blood flow through the kidneys has dropped by half, through the brain by 20 percent.

To Slow Cardiovascular Aging: Maintain Your Reserve by Exercising. Although this sounds ominous, if your kidney and brain circulation dropped by the amounts mentioned, you wouldn't notice anything because all body functions contain an enormous built-in reserve. The average man going about his business requires one quarter of his possible cardiac output. The unused three quarters allow him to exercise vigorously but also come in handy when a severe illness, accident, or even major surgery puts enormous strain on the heart. Aging hardly affects day-to-day activities but reduces the ability to withstand stresses.

Vigorous exercise reduces your resting cardiac output from 25 to perhaps 16 percent of the maximum. Besides increasing stamina and resistance to trauma, this bigger reserve provides a cushion against the inevitable decline.

What's Inevitable As a Man Ages; What's Avoidable

Inevitable and Unchangeable	Inevitable but can be modified	Not part of aging
Graying hair	Osteoporosis	Atherosclerosis
Farsightedness (need for reading glasses)	Tendency to gain weight	Senility
Replacement of muscle by fibrous tissue	Loss of stamina	Loss of teeth
Slowing of intestinal transport	Baldness*	Constipation
Prostate enlargement	Slowing of erection and ejaculation	Impotence
Wrinkles from shrinkage of connective tissue	Age spots	Wrinkles from sun exposure
Difficulty remembering names	Short-term memory loss	Decline in intelligence
Loss of skin elasticity	Loss of cardiac reserve	High blood pressure
Cataracts	Cancer	Heart attacks
	Declining vision	Blindness
	Declining hearing	Deafness
	Declining immunity	Severe immune deficiency

* Although male pattern baldness grows more extensive with age, it's really a consequence of sexual maturity.

Lungs

As with most essential organs, lung tissue disappears slowly with age. A healthy elderly lung weighs about 20 percent less than it did when young and appears smaller.

Lungs are elastic, and breathing is similar to filling a balloon. You must use muscles to expand the chest, sucking air into the lung, but expiration requires no effort. You simply relax, and the rubbery lung contracts, forcing out the air. Age affects elastic tissue here as it does everywhere else, so older lungs become less compliant. Breathing takes more work, and oxygen diffuses more slowly through the stiffer tissue. Combined with diminishing lung volume, this produces a slowly declining blood oxygen level. The physical work capacity of a seventy-year-old is about half that of a twenty-year-old, but that's still a great deal of work.

You learned in Chapter 3 that feeling out of breath during exercise indicates that the heart can't supply adequate oxygen to the muscles. The lungs themselves continue to provide more than enough. At some point in old age, however, lungs overtake the cardiovascular system as the limiting factor in exercise capacity.

Lungs may represent the limiting factor for life itself. Before the antibiotic era, doctors referred to pneumonia as "the old man's friend," because it quietly carried off so many elderly patients. Even today, if you eliminated preventable cancer and cardiovascular disease, the lungs probably remain the weak point of a healthy older man.

To Slow Lung Aging No specific activity accomplishes this, but pay attention to factors that accelerate the lungs' decline. Don't smoke, and stay away from smokers. If you have asthma or a chronic respiratory allergy, treat it aggressively to obtain the long-term as well as immediate benefits. Keep current on flu and pneumonia immunizations. Mild lung infections and even most pneumonias heal without permanent lung damage, but do your best to avoid them. Don't worry about colds, bronchitis, or minor respiratory infections; they do no harm.

Skeletal muscle

Beginning around age thirty-five, muscle mass declines slowly; muscle fibers shrink and some die. This loss affects larger muscle groups more than smaller ones, so professional athletes fade quickly after forty but concert pianists do well into their seventies and eighties.

To Slow Muscle Aging Keep active. Your body deals ruthlessly with its own structure, quickly discarding what doesn't seem necessary. A young man who wears a cast for a few months knows the impressive atrophy that takes place in muscles underneath. A healthy eighty-year-old forced to stay in bed for a month or two will probably never get out.

Having the largest possible muscle mass gives you the advantage when the decline begins, an argument for exercising when young. Active muscles shrink more slowly, so you should never stop, and it's never too late to begin. This may not prolong your life (women in general exercise less but live longer), but it makes life worth living.

Bone

Muscle cells swell, shrink, age, and die, but they don't multiply. Bone behaves differently. From birth to death, bone resorption and formation (remodeling) occurs constantly, so bone cells have no time to grow old. Until late adolescence formation exceeds resorption, so the skeleton grows. During early adult life skeletal mass remains steady, but after forty resorption slightly exceeds formation, and 0.3 to 0.5 percent of bone disappears every year. An old man has lost 20 to 30 percent of his skeleton. Called osteoporosis, bone loss begins earlier and proceeds faster in women (who may lose half their bone mass), so the subject receives great play in women's magazines. But men also suffer osteoporosis and the increasing fractures that result.

To Slow Bone Aging: Exercise, stand at least three hours per day, and watch your diet.

Bone, like muscle, grows stronger with exercise and atrophies with disuse. Unlike muscle, bone requires weight-bearing exercise (swimming doesn't help). Bed rest is positively catastrophic, especially as you get older. Research subjects who stayed in bed for nine months lost ten years of bone mass. Being relatively young and healthy, they regained it, but that also took nine months.

Despite cheerful advice on exercise programs for the bedridden in some health manuals, this helps muscle and circulation but not bone. When scientists discovered that astronauts lost bone while weightless, they prescribed daily exercise to prevent this, but it didn't work. Like so many other organs, your skeleton functions best when doing its jobs, which is to support your body against gravity. That means standing, and men require a minimum of three hours of standing per day to maintain bone strength. Plenty of young men don't achieve that.

Calcium comes instantly to mind during a discussion of bone and diet. Obviously you're better off with healthy bone, and that requires an adequate calcium intake. However, while calcium influences some bone diseases, osteoporosis is not one of them. Taking extra calcium while you're young doesn't make bone stronger than normal, and more calcium doesn't slow normal bone loss or the excess of inactivity.

As one of its nonstructural functions, bone and its calcium act as an acid buffer, and excess acid intake probably dissolves bone more quickly. Citrus juices have little influence on the body's acid load; the major factors are a high-protein diet and excessive consumption of acid phosphates, a major ingredient in soft drinks.

Your Changing Digestive Tract

Like skeletal muscle that moves your body about, the smooth muscle lining your digestive tract weakens with age, so food travels through more slowly. Swallowed food takes longer to reach the stomach, gastric emptying time may double, and propulsion beyond grows more leisurely. Digestion proceeds normally despite the slowdown, but drug absorption grows less predictable.

Gastric acid production declines with age, probably reaching zero in most men in their seventies. Digestion doesn't require acid, its absence shouldn't cause symptoms, and ulcers almost never develop in the absence of gastric acid.

On the other hand, stomach cancer requires no acid. The leading malignancy in many parts of the world, stomach cancer led in the United States until the 1930s but has declined steadily to about eighth place since then. Dietary changes are probably responsible—most likely our obsession with food preservation and convenience. Americans have large refrigerators and prefer to buy packaged foods containing chemical preservatives. Nations with a high stomach cancer rate are more likely to preserve foods by pickling, smoking, or salting.

To Slow Aging of the Digestive Tract: I have no new advice, but an aging digestive tract shouldn't inconvenience a man who follows the healthy diet discussed in Chapter 2. Although colonic function slows along with everything else, aging does not lead to constipation. Like atherosclerosis, constipation is a purely dietary disorder, and the best diet eliminates the risk of both. The greatest digestive disability of the elderly, lack of teeth, is always the consequence of disease, not aging. Brush, floss, and see a dentist every six months.

Sexual organs

Testes shrink slightly with age and testosterone production declines minimally, but neither change should affect a man's sex life. Sperm production decreases by half from age twenty to eighty but remains well within the normal range. Age should not diminish sexual desire, impotence is never a sign of aging, and a healthy man remains fertile to a very old age.

To Slow Aging of the Sexual Organs: Have sex regularly. The generalized slowing of most functions with age also affects the complicated neural and vascular actions that allow intercourse. Attaining an erection takes longer, and more stimulation must occur before ejaculation—changes that would improve the performance of many impatient young men. A man who maintains a sex life adjusts easily.

However, after a decade or so of inactivity, this slowdown comes as a shock;

many men fail and remain convinced that age has wiped out their sexual ability. Despite the best medical efforts, many never regain it.

Kidneys

After age fifty, kidneys shrink, kidney blood flow diminishes, and filtering ability declines. An eighty-year-old man's kidneys have lost half their filtering units, but the remaining half provides more than enough capacity.

To Slow Aging of the Kidneys: While half your renal function easily maintains normal health, the generous reserve of youth has shrunk, so be conscious of stresses that you once took for granted. Kidneys maintain the balance of salt and fluids within precise limits, partly by making you thirsty when more water is required. With age this sensation grows sluggish, so you may not respond even when dehydration becomes significant. Although some health educators encourage everyone to drink inconvenient quantities of water, little evidence shows a benefit for young people. After sixty, however, make sure you consume two quarts of fluid per day.

Don't drink more. Don't make the fashionable assumption that extra urinating is healthy because it flushes bad things out of your system. Excess urinating is no more useful than excess sweating, defecating, exhaling, or increased production of earwax. Although a harmless tradition, this can cause harm if obeyed vigorously in old age, overwhelming the kidneys' ability to excrete a water load.

Brain

The brain shrinks and has lost 20 percent of its weight by the eighties, but this is mostly from loss of fluid inside the cells rather than the cells themselves. Most body cells seem to dry out with age.

Nerves in the brain don't regenerate or multiply, so the brain cells of a ninety-year-old are those that he had at birth minus those that have died. Fifty thousand to 100,000 nerve cells die daily as soon as we reach adulthood. This sounds gruesome, but experts believe that this represents pruning of excess circuitry rather than essential neurons and isn't responsible for senility or memory loss. In fact, brain function declines only modestly with age. Thinking and reaction times slow slightly, but otherwise, in the absence of disease, the brain has no natural lifetime.

What do you really lose? Global memory loss doesn't happen, but expect to have some trouble remembering names. If this annoys you, that's usually a good sign. When family and friends notice forgetfulness before the patient himself, something serious is happening. Don't expect to lose knowledge, facts, calculating ability, or the specialized intellectual skills of your profession.

Age shouldn't affect intelligence or creativity, but these qualities lose some fluidity—the ability to perform in new situations or to change course and come up with radically new ideas. Geniuses such as Verdi, Goethe, and Titian produced works of genius until their eighties but these were a continuation of past efforts.

To Slow Aging of the Brain: Although people speak of mental exercise as a parallel with physical exercise, the truth is that they're identical. Rats raised in a stimulating environment not only learn mazes faster but have heavier brains and more complex nerve branching. Human volunteers placed on strict bed rest show the same electroencephalographic abnormalities that occur with aging.

Since the brain ages more slowly than most of the body, the benefits of paying it attention may be greater. Every discussion of aging trots out famous elderly geniuses such as those mentioned earlier. Invariably the writer draws the wrong conclusion (i.e., that a creative hobby adds spice to old age). A more substantial conclusion is that men age well who lead stimulating lives when young. Dissatisfied young men not only don't improve with the years, their intellectual skills wither. Titian, Verdi, and Goethe were geniuses in their twenties, and they stayed geniuses.

What Happens to Your Eyes

Well before old age—in the forties—the rubbery lens of the eye grows so stiff that the ciliary muscles can no longer pull it into focus for near objects. Normal or farsighted men find themselves holding reading material further and further away. Reading glasses correct this. Nearsighted men like me have no trouble reading even with a stiff lens, provided that they remove their glasses (which, naturally, make a farsighted correction). When I was young, I could read with my glasses on, but no longer. Although this is no inconvenience at home, I find myself taking my glasses off when browsing in a store or reading anything close, like a map or a menu. When this becomes too annoying, I'll get bifocals.

Receptor cells on the retina diminish with age, so visual acuity declines slowly, but it should never decline quickly and it never declines to zero in the absence of disease. Pupils grow smaller and react more slowly to light. Eye movements are reduced, and for reasons no one understands many old people cannot look upward. Except for declining vision, these should not cause great inconvenience.

Diseases increase with age, but that's true for every part of the body. Cataracts (clouding of the lens) and macular degeneration (atrophy of the central retina) grow more common, and some doctors tell patients that these are a result of aging. Experts are not so certain; some forms of these two disorders are certainly the result of diseases such as diabetes; I suspect that this may turn out to be true for all.

Here are some common, visible eye changes that cause unnecessary worry.

1. Arcus senilis, a gray or whitish ring around the cornea, the clear area in front of the pupil. Made of fatty material, it's evidence for a high cholesterol when present in men under fifty. But almost everyone develops an arcus if he lives long enough, so it has no significance in the elderly and doesn't necessarily indicate a high cholesterol.

2. Bloodshot eyes. With age, the white of the eyes shows more and more visible blood vessels. In the absence of symptoms, this is harmless.

3. Pinguecula are yellow nodules visible on the nasal side of the cornea, less often on the opposite side. Common at any age, they're more common with advancing years and in men who work outdoors. They grow slowly, but doctors don't take action unless they begin to grow over the cornea, at which time the name changes to pterygia.

4. Pterygia. Noticing fleshy tissue encroaching on the cornea, some men mistake this for a cataract. An ophthalmologist can easily scrape it off, but pterygia tend to recur, so treatment isn't essential unless they affect vision.

5. Floaters. These specks that drift across your visual field result from shadows cast on the retina by blood cells or other debris floating in the liquid of the eye. Almost everyone who stares at a uniform surface sees a few. Small, transient floaters have no significance, but see a doctor for one that persists and is easily visible.

To Slow Aging of the Eye: Stay healthy and don't smoke. Smokers have a higher incidence of cataracts and macular degeneration. Radiation probably ages the eye as much as skin, especially by provoking cataracts, so keep the sun out of your eyes. Before and after visual loss becomes apparent, don't worry about wearing out your eyes by too much close work or even working in bad light. This tires your eyes and causes discomfort but no permanent damage. Like fatigue in other areas of the body, rest relieves it. Naturally you should see an ophthalmologist to make sure no correctable problem exists. Glasses don't correct the visual loss of aging; in fact, changes in the prescription in an elderly person are a sign of eye disease.

Your Ears Are Affected, Too

Like vision, hearing diminishes slowly with advancing years but never quickly and never to zero in the absence of disease. Called presbycusis, this decline begins around age forty with gradual loss of the highest frequencies. Except perhaps in musicians, high-frequency hearing loss is almost unnoticeable because the most important sound—human speech—occurs in the middle frequencies. By age sixty-five more than half of men realize that they're not hearing as well as in the past.

To Slow Aging of the Ears: Loud noise ages the ear prematurely, producing an identical progressive, permanent high-frequency loss. Much of what doctors call presbycusis may be the result of chronic noise trauma and thus entirely avoidable. The evidence, as with so much preventive medicine, comes from studies of primitive cultures, which reveal less hearing loss with age.

All uncomfortable noise damages hearing: loud music, firearms, subways, power tools, motors, and factory machinery. To preserve hearing, avoid it all. I've always been puzzled by pedestrians who pretend that the siren of a passing fire engine isn't painfully loud; I always put my fingers in my ears. As a young man I put cotton in my ears when attending rock concerts. The music came through loudly but below the pain threshold. You might think that this diminishes the pleasure, but it turns out that deafening amplified music makes your entire body vibrate; this vibration (not the pain in your ears) gives pleasure.

Once hearing loss becomes apparent, see an otolaryngologist for a hearing test and a diagnosis. If you hear that it's presbycusis, the doctor should provide more or less the following advice.

Eventually you may need a hearing aid, but for a while you can adapt by listening more carefully, watching the other person's lips and face for clues to what they're saying, and positioning yourself against walls to pick up more sounds. You should avoid noisy places because men with presbycusis have trouble discriminating speech from background noise (this isn't so with other forms of hearing loss). People can help by facing you when speaking and enunciating clearly. Be assertive about explaining your problem so speakers take care. Think about buying amplifying devices for the television, radio, and telephone, but while you consider this, think about a hearing aid.

Asked whether he'd prefer blindness to deafness, almost everyone prefers deafness, and so would I because living independently is easier if you're deaf. On the other hand, it's easy to talk to a blind person; someone losing his hearing can grow lonely and isolated. I recall many family occasions when we greeted an elderly deaf relative and then proceeded to ignore him. Including him in the conversation required too much shouting and repeating. This is why I differ from doctors who casually advise you to ask speakers to write down words. If you're so deaf that it requires an effort to communicate with you, some people will find the effort too tiresome. Get a hearing aid. Advances in technology have produced smaller, more accurate devices than existed even ten years ago.

Slowdown in Your Immune System

The elderly seem less able to fight off bacterial and viral infections. Although the decline in organ reserve with age makes the body less capable of withstanding severe stress, the immune system itself loses some vigor. Responding to an infection, it manufactures antibodies more slowly. Lymphocytes, the family of cells that attacks invaders, remain as numerous as ever but react to a challenge less aggressively.

Besides destroying invading organisms, the immune system eliminates native cells that have turned malignant, so the incidence of cancer rises slowly with age.

To Slow Aging of the Immune System: Live an active life. Exercise. It turns out that rest damages the body in more ways than we realize. Healthy subjects kept in bed for months not only weaken (or—a good analogy—prematurely age) heart, muscle, and bone, but their immune system declines.

Travel. Meet a variety of people—and catch as many of their minor infections as possible while you're young! Catching major infections also provides long-term benefits, but that only happens if you're alive to enjoy them, so I don't encourage it.

Urging you to get sick to preserve your health seems paradoxical until you understand that the immune system requires exercise as much as do muscles and bones. You may have heard of the "bubble boy," a child born with essentially no immune system who was raised in a sterile capsule, free of all infectious organisms. He grew into a healthy, normal boy but died of infection when removed after an unsuccessful attempt to reconstitute his immune system. Most readers will be surprised to learn that if a normal newborn were raised in such an environment, free of infections, after about five years he or she would end up as immunologically crippled as the bubble boy. Removed from the bubble, the child would die of infections as rapidly.

Not only does repeated exposure to infections strengthen a young immune system, but an early battle with many organisms ensures that an aging immune system need never encounter them. Measles and influenza make children miserable but hardly ever kill them. One attack of measles provides permanent immunity. Healthy eighty-year-olds regularly die of the flu. They'd probably die of measles, but I've never heard of a case in an old man.

Colds attack children half a dozen times per year. They continue to plague many adults but grow less common as years pass. The reason is that each time you recover, you're immune to that particular cold virus. Although these viruses may seem infinite in number, only about a hundred exist, so you'll eventually run out of colds to catch. Healthy nonsmokers can look forward to an old age with a few minor upper respiratory infections.

One can carry this analogy too far. Some infections (tuberculosis, most sexually transmitted diseases) don't provide permanent immunity, and we still don't understand how to prime the immune system to resist cancer better, but solutions to these will come with time. It remains good advice to catch plenty of routine infections when you're young and healthy.

Despite your best efforts, you might not stay healthy until the day you die. The next section may not apply to you now, but keep it in mind.

HANDLING BAD NEWS FROM YOUR DOCTOR

Chances are that, sooner or later, a doctor will announce that you have a serious disease. Although you can't turn bad news into good news (other writers disagree), and your first thought will be that life must run downhill from now on, it isn't so.

The most feared bad news is a diagnosis of cancer. Most men who hear it are not feeling terribly ill, so distractions like pain and emergency procedures don't cushion the blow. Catastrophes such as an accident or heart attack overwhelm the victim at first, so time must pass before he must deal with its affect on his life. Eventually, however, every man with a serious disease must find a way to continue his life. Although what follows emphasizes cancer, the guidelines apply to any bad medical news.

Unlike accidents or heart attacks, where you may know what's happening immediately, a diagnosis of cancer is usually slow torment. Here is the usual scenario. You or the doctor discover something suspicious. It might be cancer, the doctor admits, but maybe it isn't. The doctor will be reassuring, and you'll want to believe him or her. More tests and perhaps consultation with a specialist will provide more information, the doctor adds. You'll have some days to hope before learning that what you have is indeed very suspicious. Your spirits will be dashed, but perhaps they'll rise again as the doctor assures you that many men with your problem don't have cancer. More tests, most likely a biopsy, will give the answer. This requires another appointment, so you'll have more time to brood.

Although the doctor may have explained otherwise, many patients feel great relief on the day of the biopsy because they believe they will finally know the diagnosis. It comes as another discouragement to hear that several days must pass while the pathologist examines the tissue. Add two days because pathologists don't work weekends, except on urgent cases. Although you disagree, your potentially malignant tissue is not considered urgent.

Another appointment. Time in the waiting room will hang heavy. Your heart will sink with the news that you really have cancer, but you may again find reassurance from the explanation. Doctors try to stress the positive. You hope that the doctor is saying that it's just a small cancer. Perhaps it was caught in time. Has it spread? Finding the answer may require more tests and more delays, or you might not know until after treatment. For some cancers, you won't know until spread actually occurs.

As this demonstrates, learning that you have cancer often comes as a series of blows: bad news followed by the feeling that maybe it isn't so bad, then a second dose of bad news, rising hopes, and another disappointment. Three or four such blows come close to breaking anyone's spirit. Patients sink into despair. Life turns into a depressing series of long waits in waiting rooms for the next bit of bad news. The conviction that meaningful life is over may be reinforced when treatment begins, and you wait to see an oncologist or radiation therapist in the company of other people who look obviously sick. As months pass, most men regain some taste for living, but they rarely escape feeling that something irretrievable has been lost even if things turn out well. I have had this experience myself.

Despite the claims of some writers, a diagnosis of cancer can never be anything but bad news. Yet it's not necessarily the worst disease that can strike. The ten-year survival after a first heart attack is less than that of many cancers, yet heart attack victims pull themselves together and get on with their lives. Victims of cancer must do the same. Here is what everyone with a serious disease must do.

Tell Everyone. They Can Help!

Tell family, relatives, as well as friends and colleagues that you see on a regular basis. They'll find out sooner or later; finding out from you shows your respect for them, but it's also essential for your self-respect.

Cancer patients, men especially, tend to keep quiet, but this is too heavy a burden. For a time it will rarely be out of your thoughts. Having a serious disease makes you feel isolated, especially if those around you don't know. You can become bitter seeing others leading their (apparently) happy lives while you carry this weight—a weight so heavy that you wonder why others don't detect it. But they can't. You must tell them.

Leading Sites of Cancer Incidence—1993 Estimates

Cancer Incidence by Site and Sex*

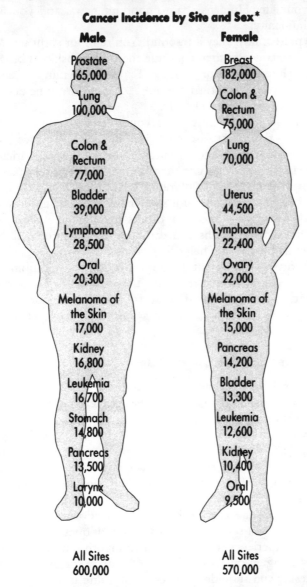

Male	Female
Prostate 165,000	Breast 182,000
Lung 100,000	Colon & Rectum 75,000
Colon & Rectum 77,000	Lung 70,000
Bladder 39,000	Uterus 44,500
Lymphoma 28,500	Lymphoma 22,400
Oral 20,300	Ovary 22,000
Melanoma of the Skin 17,000	Melanoma of the Skin 15,000
Kidney 16,800	Pancreas 14,200
Leukemia 16,700	Bladder 13,300
Stomach 14,800	Leukemia 12,600
Pancreas 13,500	Kidney 10,400
Larynx 10,000	Oral 9,500

| All Sites 600,000 | All Sites 570,000 |

*Excluding basal and squamous cell skin cancer and carcinoma in situ.

Reproduced Courtesy of the American Cancer Society

You're not spreading the news to attract sympathy, although you'll get plenty, some quite annoying. You're telling for the same reason you'd tell any major event in your life. Humans share important news, and you must stay connected with humanity.

Don't try to predict how they'll respond. You're in for surprises. Most will show shock and sympathy and then continue their relationship as before, occasionally showing an interest in your progress. Expect some mindless encouragement ("I'm sure everything will turn out fine . . .") and tiresome tales of other acquaintances with cancer. Listen politely.

Some individuals will disappear from your life! Their first reaction will be no different from those just discussed, but soon you'll notice something disturbing. Perhaps they no longer sit beside you at lunch; if friends, they stop phoning or visiting. If you invite them out, they have other plans. It can be devastating to realize that an old friend is avoiding you, but it happens regularly. This is heartless behavior (if it's any comfort, your friend is certainly racked with guilt), but serious disease in others terrifies some people so much that they flee. After a few months you can approach and reestablish the relationship. Recriminations won't help; forgive them.

A small minority will turn out to be saints, showing genuine concern but without pity or cheery optimism. Later they'll want to know the details of your treatment, and you'll find it easy to talk about your feelings and fears. You'll need a few of these, and it's absolutely unpredictable where they'll turn up.

If You Have Cancer, See an Oncologist

An internist who specializes in cancer, the oncologist will review your records, tests, and biopsies and discuss the next steps. See one even if you have a minor, easily cured malignancy.

The doctor who made the diagnosis—most likely a urologist for the cancers in this book—is primarily a surgeon. If necessary, he or she refers patients for other forms of therapy but is most familiar with what he or she does and tends to prefer surgery when there's any doubt. You want to talk to someone familiar with all possibilities.

Another point is that cancer is probably not your doctor's favorite medical problem, but an oncologist specializes in patients with questions and fears similar to yours. In my experience, oncologists spend more time and have a better bedside manner. Seeing an oncologist is almost routine for most cancers; your doctor may suggest it and shouldn't object if you bring it up.

Ask About Joining a Clinical Trial

Dozens are under way across the country, testing new chemotherapy, new synthetic hormones, and (less often) new surgical or radiological techniques. Your goal in joining is not to benefit humanity but yourself.

Cancer Death Rates by Site, Males, United States, 1930–89

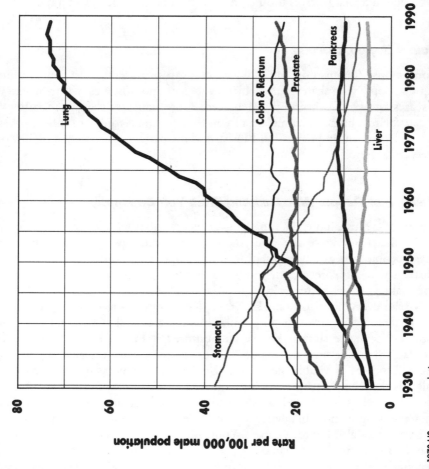

Rates are adjusted to the 1970 US census population.

Source: American Cancer Society, *Cancer Facts & Figures—1993*.

Reproduced Courtesy of the American Cancer Society

Patients almost always recoil when I mention a clinical trial. Why should they take an unproven treatment, they ask. Even if the new treatment is good, they believe, half the subjects must take a placebo for comparison. Why should they risk getting nothing?

This is not how studies operate. A treatment that enters clinical trials has already passed earlier trials. Experts know that it works, that it's relatively safe, and that it may be superior to current treatments. To win FDA approval, researchers must compare their new discovery to *the best* of today's treatments, so everyone in a trial receives top-notch care. As a bonus, therapy in a trial is free.

Join a Support Group

Your spouse/companion and close friends can provide support, but nothing equals people who share your problem. Doctors and hospitals that treat serious diseases know of such groups. Men seem more reluctant than women to talk about their feelings, so let me assure you that no one is forced to speak in these groups. You can sit quietly. But I insist that my patients give them a trial. Most are very grateful.

Beware of People Who Demand That You Be Happy!

Plenty of creative individuals, patients as well as doctors, are eager to communicate their experience and give you advice. I encourage patients to listen to these people just as I want them to join a support group. Any serious illness changes your life forever, but you're not alone. Learning how others handle it will make you feel better.

Read everything you can. However, let me warn you of a persistent, irritating theme that runs though popular literature as well as a number of other disease-experience stories. You've encountered it in old Hollywood movies, where the heroine sinks toward death because, the doctor explains, she has lost the will to live. Inevitably the hero restores it, and she perks up and recovers. I call this the "be cheerful or die" theme.

The enthusiasts would be shocked at my characterization. They believe they're giving wonderful advice. Medical science can fight cancer, they explain, but you must also fight it yourself. Your fight is not only effective, they add, it may be more important than drugs, surgery, or radiation. You fight cancer by keeping a positive attitude, by believing firmly that you will emerge victorious. Having supreme confidence that you will defeat your cancer may shrink it by willpower alone.

Patients are always thrilled to learn that they can cure themselves. Furthermore, it seems to work. A few weeks after the shock of diagnosis, almost everyone feels better emotionally, and whatever treatment the doctor gives improves the disease. But if something goes wrong, patients blame themselves.

"I thought I had this thing licked, but I guess I didn't have the strength" is the sort of comment I hear. Patients are crushed; they're convinced that their own weakness brought this on.

Have you noticed that no one expects a person to cure his own acne, hemorrhoids, or hay fever with willpower? Only serious diseases qualify. Don't take this trendy nonsense seriously. I encourage patients to have a positive attitude because it feels better than being miserable. But you aren't responsible for the success or failure of your treatment.

CHAPTER • 7

WHAT MEN WORRY ABOUT MOST: SYMPTOMS AND THEIR MEANINGS

A person who falls ill wants quickly to give the illness a name—flu, heart attack, hemorrhoids. Although this is human nature and impossible to resist, it's a bad idea. Medical students pride themselves on the speed of their diagnoses, but as they accumulate painful experiences and gain wisdom they learn to relax, gather information, and think carefully before committing themselves.

The first thing you notice when you feel sick is what you feel—pain, fever, upset stomach. Rather than make the obvious connection (vomiting equals food poisoning), consider the symptom and the circumstances surrounding it. You want assurance that it's a self-limited illness that you can treat at home. With the information that follows, you can almost always accomplish that; if any doubts remain, you must put yourself in your doctor's hands.

Don't expect much information on nailing down your diagnosis; self-diagnosis is always dangerous; even doctors have a poor record with their own illnesses.

WHAT DOES CHEST PAIN MEAN?

Sixty percent of all heart attack deaths occur before the victim reaches the hospital, so a quick evaluation of your chest pain can be livesaving. It can also save that piece of heart muscle, because doctors now inject clot-dissolving drugs that can unblock a coronary artery before the muscle dies, but this only works well within the first few hours. Here's exactly the wrong approach, but one I encounter time and again.

After supper one evening a man felt an uncomfortable pressure over his chest. He was middle aged and having trouble cutting down on cholesterol. Naturally he wondered about a heart attack.

"It's probably heartburn," he concluded. The pain felt gassy, and he had belched several times. To check his condition, he climbed up and down his stairs several times. The discomfort did not worsen. "If it were my heart I'm sure I couldn't do that," he told his wife. He belched again. "This is bad indigestion," he concluded, hurrying to the bathroom. Gagging himself with a toothbrush, he vomited. This seemed to improve the pain, but to reassure himself, he began doing calisthenics. By this time his wife had reached his doctor, who phoned the paramedics, who rushed him to the hospital, where he survived his heart attack.

Besides illustrating a typical heart attack, this anecdote helps explain why married men (or men with a live-in companion) live longer than bachelors. Many men waste time investigating chest pain to assure themselves that it's not serious. I encourage some investigation, provided that it follows intelligent guidelines. Unfortunately, most men rely on simpleminded common sense (belching equals a stomach problem) or heroics (if you can exercise, your heart is OK). Use my guidelines instead. Besides saving your life, they'll help detect genuine heart disease before it becomes a real threat.

Another illustration: A man noticed oppressing aching in his midchest while mowing his lawn. Since it disappeared after a few minutes of rest, he didn't worry. When it occurred during a golf game, he mentioned it to a companion.

The partner was aghast. "That sounds like a heart attack!" he exclaimed. "I felt the same way when I had mine!" Since the pain had already gone, the patient shrugged off his friend's diagnosis and insisted on finishing the game. Later he made an appointment with his doctor, who scheduled an exercise electrocardiogram during which the pain recurred.

"You haven't had a heart attack, but your friend was in the right ball park," the doctor explained. "A heart attack happens when an artery supplying part of the heart is blocked, cutting off oxygen to an area of muscle. That area may take several hours to die; during this time it produces the sort of heavy pain your friend suffered.

"None of your coronary arteries seem blocked," he continued. "But the electrocardiogram shows that at least one is very narrow. Enough blood gets through when you're resting, but during exercise the narrow artery can't supply extra blood that the heart needs. Starved for oxygen, the muscle hurts—just as it does during a heart attack. When you rest, the heart slows down. The blood supply becomes adequate again, so the muscle stops hurting and stays alive. This is a common disorder called angina, and you were taking a risk in ignoring it. People with angina have a higher risk of a heart attack."

Most chest pain represents something less ominous than coronary artery disease, but minor problems don't necessarily lead to minor discomfort. Every few months I see a man gasping with pain. Most likely it began a few hours before with a sharp ache that became excruciating whenever he took a breath. After a normal examination of the chest and heart, I can reassure him that the problem is pleuritis, an inflammation of the pleura, the lining of the lungs. Mostly pleuritis accompanies a minor viral infection such as a cold, although it may appear out of the blue. Treatment is aspirin, and the condition disappears in a few days.

Some chest pain is less serious but still deserves a medical evaluation, and most chest pain is trivial, requiring no action at all. Here's what you should know.

Where Does it Hurt?

Remember the textbook description of a heart attack: severe substernal pain lasting twenty minutes, sometimes radiating to the arms, less often to the jaw, neck, back, or upper abdomen. You'll remember better if I explain this word by word.

The pain is *severe*. Vague, niggling chest discomfort is probably not ominous. Many men insist that they are not experiencing pain, but a pressure sensation or even the burning of indigestion. Whatever they feel, it's severe.

Heart pain is *substernal*, meaning located behind the sternum or breastbone in the center of your chest. Although you feel your heart beat on the left side, typical heart pain appears centrally.

Heart attack pain *lasts*. Discomfort may be severe and substernal, but it's more likely angina than a heart attack if it disappears within a few minutes.

Heart pain sometimes *radiates*, but not always. Men with shoulder bursitis of muscle strain often worry needlessly. While pain in the jaw or arm can indicate a heart attack, this is rare in the absence of severe chest pain. I've never seen a case.

Lung Pain. Strictly speaking, this doesn't exist. The lung proper has no pain nerves. Symptoms of pulmonary disease are coughing and difficulty breathing, not pain. The only major pulmonary structure that can hurt is the pleura, and, as the pleuritis example showed, it can hurt badly. The hallmark of pleural disease is increased pain when the pleura stretches. Since it lines the lung, the pleura stretches with every breath, so even minor viral pleuritis can hurt badly—a sharp, stabbing sensation that may disappear when you hold your breath.

Less often, serious lung disease such as pneumonia or a blood clot affects the pleura, but other ominous signs, such as fever, cough, or shortness of breath, should accompany the pain. While breathing aggravates it, pleuritic pain is much less affected by moving the rib cage or chest.

Musculoskeletal Disorders. Anyone with a cracked rib knows what agony breathing becomes, yet pleural disease is clearly not the problem. Even a minor inflammation or injury to the bones, muscles, or ligaments of the chest can cause severe pain on breathing, but it also hurts to bend and twist the body. Making the diagnosis is easy—the affected area hurts when pressed with a finger. Remembering this will keep you from rushing to the doctor for a common trivial cause of chest pain.

Costochondritis. A medical term meaning "inflammation of a rib cartilage," this is simply a form of arthritis—joint inflammation. Although this is not widely known, everyone has fourteen joints in the chest: seven on each side, where the first seven ribs join the sternum. Tracing each rib with a finger, you can feel the joint, a swelling as the rib reaches the sternum. Just as a knee or wrist can hurt after a minor injury or for no reason at all, a costochondral joint can do the same, producing anything from a severe dull ache that resembles a heart attack to sharp pleuritic pain. No matter what the description, if one costochondral joint feels exquisitely painful when you touch, the diagnosis is costochondritis, and treatment is aspirin or other antiinflammatory. Don't press too hard; those joints are normally fairly sensitive, but they shouldn't hurt under modest pressure.

Gas Pains. Your colon extends as high as the rib cage. Traveling across the upper abdomen behind the stomach, it reaches highest behind the left lower chest before making a 90-degree turn to descend to the rectum. This bend occurs behind the spleen, so we call it the splenic flexure. Gas rises, so it collects in this high point. Compressed by the powerful muscles of the colon, trapped gas produces intense pain so often that it has a name: splenic flexure syndrome. I have known men with gas admitted to the hospital for a heart attack or kidney stone—a great relief to the patient later but embarrassing to the doctor. The pain of splenic flexure syndrome occurs just left of the sternum or in the left upper abdomen; an experienced doctor will make the diagnosis. Don't try it yourself if pain is severe.

Other Gastrointestinal Pains. These are tricky. A man may feel the effects of excess acid, ulcers, gallstones, or liver inflammation as chest pain. President Warren G. Harding died of "acute indigestion" in 1923 before doctors understood coronary artery disease, but even today many patients and an occasional doctor think of digestive diseases when the problem lies elsewhere. Nausea, vomiting, and belching often occur during a heart attack. Gastrointestinal pain rarely radiates to the jaw or arms, but this is a feeble clue. Remember the heart attack guidelines: If the pain is severe and lasts, let a doctor know.

Ask Yourself Essential Questions

Location and pattern of symptoms provide clues to the seriousness of the pain, but asking yourself the following questions is equally important.

1. Have I had this before?

You can safely diagnose muscle pain or gas if you've had the same pain before and the doctor has told you that's what it is. Don't do this with a new pain or a familiar one that's much worse.

2. Am I a candidate for something serious?

Heart attacks and angina are so rare in nonsmoking men under thirty-five that they are medical curiosities; smokers should begin worrying after thirty. Once you reach middle age, you can be a thin, active, nonsmoker with a low cholesterol and still run a small risk that only approaches zero as your cholesterol drops below 150.

Where Do You Get Help?

This is not as straightforward as you might think. Follow your doctor's advice if you've managed to make contact. If not, get to the nearest hospital emergency room as soon as possible. Don't assume that every hospital has an emergency room; if you're not certain, phone first. Although you can try, your chance of getting good medical advice is slim. In today's malpractice crisis, an unfamiliar nurse or doctor who talks to you over the phone would be foolish to say anything but "come in."

Do you know the fastest way to get to the hospital? Probably not—the fastest way is to get in your car and go. Have a friend drive. *Don't call an ambulance.* Commercial ambulance services sell routine transportation. They don't handle emergencies. Do call paramedics if your community has them. An emergency number such as 911 will reach someone who knows.

If you arrive alone at an emergency room, go immediately to the check-in desk and tell the clerk that you're having severe chest pain. Don't announce that you're having a heart attack or demand to see the doctor immediately. To an experienced emergency room worker, insistent patients are usually *not* seriously ill, but the words "severe chest pain" produce a quick response.

What Does Stomach Pain Mean?

Entire textbooks teach doctors about the "acute abdomen," a subject far more complex than chest pain. Most urgent chest pain involves a single organ, but a dozen abdominal structures hurt regularly. Although rarely as urgent as a heart attack, it's no less important to make the correct decision because many deadly abdominal pains are cured easily. Once you've had a heart attack, life is never the same. Even if doctors intervene quickly to dissolve the clot before muscle dies, you know that you still have serious coronary disease. But a surgeon who removes your gallbladder or inflamed appendix has removed the disease. You are now as healthy as you were before the pain began. It's no exaggeration to call this a miracle cure—especially if you remember that 100 years ago appendicitis was a death sentence, one that involved several weeks of agonizing dying. Today a bright high school student can remove an appendix.

Men with a bellyache worry too much about ulcers and appendicitis. They should worry more about gallstones and diverticulitis. Although still significant, ulcers and appendicitis have been growing less common since my school days. For unknown reasons, both occur less than half as often as a generation ago, and the decline continues. Gallstones and diverticulitis show no such tendency.

Unlike chest pain, serious abdominal pain almost never demands quick action. A few hours' delay with even a perforated ulcer isn't fatal (in any case, a man with a perforated ulcer finds delay impossible). A few days' delay is a different matter; patients die or sue us if we don't get it right. Fortunately, most abdominal pains represent trivial disease. Use the following guidelines to sort them out.

1. Locate the pain.

A fine landmark, the belly button separates upper and lower digestive tracts (although the colon extends higher, serious colon pain usually localizes below). Coiled centrally and behind the belly button, the small intestine suffers serious disease so rarely that I don't discuss it in this book. Important sources of pain include the following:

- The stomach, located in the upper midline, just below the notch in your ribcage (the medical term for this location is epigastrium). Although school children learn that it churns, mixes, and digests food, the stomach's major function is storage. In its absence, digestion proceeds normally but patients cannot eat a large meal without discomfort.

- The duodenum, the first foot of the small intestine that receives food from the stomach. Most ulcers occur here rather than in the stomach, but no one can separate duodenal from stomach pain.

- The gallbladder, a bag the size of your thumb located below the right rib cage. Oily bile from the liver flows into the gallbladder, which stores and concentrates it, expelling it after meals to help digest fats. Various conditions make the gallbladder hurt, most commonly stones that form in the thickened bile. Harmless while it sits quietly in the gallbladder, trouble arises when a stone flows out with bile and sticks in the duct leading to the small intestine. Pain as the stone squeezes through usually lasts a few hours. Knowing the location, one might guess that gallbladder pain occurs over the gallbladder. This is reassuring when it happens, but pain over the epigastrium occurs as often, so no one should assume that every pain over the middle originates in the stomach.

■ The liver. This is the largest organ in the body and located over the entire right upper abdomen. As a source of acute pain, liver disease is rare in America.

■ The pancreas. It sits deep in the abdomen behind the stomach and duodenum, where it produces digestive juices that flow into the small intestine. Pancreatic inflammation (pancreatitis) usually causes pain in the epigastrium, occasionally to the left.

■ The colon. Colon pain tends to affect the left lower abdomen (diverticulitis as well as garden variety cramps, constipation, and diarrhea) and right lower abdomen (appendicitis). Important large bowel disease rarely hurts above the navel, but remember the left upper abdominal pain of splenic flexure syndrome discussed earlier. The colon also bends 90 degrees behind the liver on the right, but at a more gentle angle, so the gas pain of hepatic flexure syndrome occurs less often.

2. Consider the nature of the pain (burning, aching, gassy) and then don't pay much attention.

Textbooks describe ulcer pain as burning; colic from a stone obstructing a duct rises to a crescendo and then falls momentarily; gassy pain feels like a large ball moving around. The truth is that these are unreliable because nerves supplying your internal organs are primitive compared to those in the skin. Your life depends on a thousand subtle sensations that occur in your fingertips or feet, but feeling from inside your body serves only as a crude warning. As a result, acid burning the stomach may produce aching, gnawing, gassy, dull, or sharp pain and sometimes no pain at all.

3. When does it hurt?

Think about the pain's relation to meals. Food neutralizes acid, so ulcers flare on an empty stomach and subside after eating, but this is not a hard and fast rule.

Gas pains occur during the hour or two after eating, not because food in the stomach produces gas (it doesn't, as you'll learn later) but because the intestines begin to stir and contract in response to eating, squeezing the gas already present.

Folk wisdom and even a few doctors teach that eating provokes gallbladder pain, but this is simply wrong.

Pain that awakens someone from sleep is significant. Nighttime pain typically signals an ulcer because the stomach is empty after midnight, and acid secretion peaks around 2 A.M. Unfortunately, nocturnal pain occurs during almost any stomach disorder, including garden variety indigestion and dyspepsia.

4. What symptoms accompany the pain?

Fever accompanies infection; expect it at some point during appendicitis, diverticulitis, and simple stomach flu but not with an ulcer, gallstones, or gas. The presence or absence or even the height of temperature give no clue to the seriousness of the problem. (You'll learn more about fever later in this section.)

Vomiting occurs when something obstructs the outlet from the stomach. A chronic ulcer can do this; obstruction usually requires surgery. Vomiting also accompanies severe pain such as an acute ulcer or gallstones, but fortunately this is usually less ominous. Most vomiting represents a nonspecific sign that something is not right with the digestive tract. The same is true for diarrhea.

5. Are you at risk?

Diverticulitis occurs in the middle-aged and elderly. A diverticulum is a fancy word for a small hernia—a sac where tissue bulges out. In humans, diverticula occur in the large bowel so often that doctors have given the condition a name: diverticulosis. After a lifetime of eating low-roughage food, the walls of the overworked colon weaken and the weakest areas give way, bulging outward. An older man may have dozens of diverticuli, which cause no problems unless they bleed or perforate through the bowel wall. Perforation produces a painful infection (diverticulitis), which doctors usually treat with antibiotics and a liquid diet but that occasionally requires surgery. If you've eaten a high-roughage diet all your life, your stool remains soft so the colon feels less stress, and you're not at risk.

Although a danger at all ages, appendicitis is mostly a disease of adolescents and young adults. Gallstones occur twice as often in women, but statistics offer cold comfort when the pain is yours.

6. How do you feel generally?

Humans can feel pleasure despite serious disease of lung, bone, eye, and other organs, but a disordered digestive tract takes the joy out of life. Pain in the right lower abdomen accompanied by queasiness, misery, and slight fever points to appendicitis. Severe pain in the same area in someone who feels fine is usually less ominous, perhaps gas or an irritable bowel.

7. How much does it hurt?

Trivial pain generally means trivial disease. Agonizing pain isn't necessarily life threatening because this can accompany ordinary gastroenteritis (stomach flu), but pay attention.

Getting Help

As you've noticed, except for location and severity, these guidelines are remarkably feeble in pointing to a diagnosis. Fortunately, doctors are skilled at making diagnoses. As a patient, naming your illness takes a distant second to deciding whether you must see a doctor or can safely treat yourself and wait.

Treating Upper Abdominal Pain. First, review the chest pain section to make sure you're not overlooking something. Then, if your stomach is empty, fill it. If you don't feel like eating, take antacid, but ignore the absurdly small doses recommended on the label. You need at least two tablespoons of Maalox, Mylanta, or another brand. Don't drink milk; it neutralizes acid no better than water. If pain disappears in five minutes or so, that's fairly good evidence that acid caused it—either a genuine ulcer or the generalized stomach irritation we call gastritis. There's no urgency, but let your doctor know.

Taking antacid makes no sense when the stomach contains food, but it's harmless and hard to resist.

When pain persists, it's all right to take more antacid, but stay away from pain medication that damages the stomach—which includes everything you can buy over the counter except acetaminophen (e.g., Tylenol, Panadol, Anacin-3).

What to do About Lower Abdominal Pain. Over-the-counter drugs are useless. Never take a laxative. Constipation causes bloating and unpleasant fullness but rarely severe pain, and the vigorous contractions induced by a laxative exacerbate any serious colon disease. Don't be fooled by the feeling that a good bowel movement will relieve your pain. An inflamed colon can give this impression, just as stomach or gallbladder pain makes one think that a good belch would help.

Antacids don't help colon disorders. If diarrhea becomes bothersome and persistent, it's all right to take a medication such as Pepto-Bismol or Donnagel. Stay away from narcotic antidiarrheals such as Imodium unless pain isn't a significant problem—but in that case you should be consulting the diarrhea section of this chapter. Don't eat if you have uncomfortable low abdominal pain; if you want to drink, stick to clear fluids such as soft drinks.

Base the next decision on your level of tolerance. If pain grows too unpleasant, regardless of other symptoms such as fever or vomiting, get medical advice. Don't be a hero; I routinely give morphine to patients suffering through a gallstone. Curing appendicitis involves minor surgery before perforation, major surgery afterward. Waiting on diverticulitis can convert a problem requiring antibiotics to one requiring a partial colectomy. Complications rarely occur during the first few hours, but it's a good idea not to let more than a single night or daylight period pass before taking action on significant abdominal pain.

If you've been sensible enough to acquire a family doctor, phone. I often give a patient the option of coming to the more civilized atmosphere of an office if I'm certain it's safe to wait. If you can't talk to a doctor, go to a walk-in clinic or emergency room.

Possible indications of vomiting

As house doctor for most Los Angeles hotels, I deal regularly with severe digestive upsets. A phone call from a guest suffering abdominal pain makes me uneasy because I dislike traveling to a hotel, examining the guest, and then sending him or her off to an emergency room. I'll come, but only after the warning the guest of the possibility. Vomiting reassures me; I know that I can probably treat the patient successfully in the room (vomiting plus diarrhea is even more reassuring).

Nausea

First comes nausea, a sensation of imminent vomiting localized in the throat or chest. Simultaneously the digestive tract grows unnaturally quiet; the stomach relaxes and secretion diminishes. The same autonomic nervous system that controls the digestive tract (*autonomic* means "automatic—beyond your control") affects other organs, so someone about to vomit often grows pale, sweats, and salivates excessively.

Being relaxed, the stomach doesn't expel its own contents. That requires vigorous contraction of the diaphragm and muscles of the abdominal wall. Muscle contraction requires nerve impulses; nerves originate in the central nervous system, so the brain, not the digestive tract, controls the act of vomiting. Irritating drugs as well as toxins from infections and spoiled food stimulate the vomiting center in the brain. Drugs that relieve nausea and vomiting suppress this center. Brain sensitivity varies from individual to individual, so some people vomit more than others.

Causes of Vomiting

Victims tend to blame their last restaurant meal, but this is not likely unless others have become sick. Home cooking causes most food poisoning. An adult overcome with vomiting probably suffers a common viral infection that produces a violent but brief illness, rarely lasting longer than twenty-four hours. I find vomiting satisfying to treat in hotel guests. They feel terrible but recover soon after my visit and give me the credit.

Occasionally someone awakens with dizziness, nausea, and vomiting that disappears if he or she lies perfectly still. In an otherwise healthy adult, the usual diagnosis is acute labyrinthitis—inflammation of the labyrinth, organs deep inside the ear that control balance. When disturbed, they produce intense vertigo with nausea. Most likely another viral infection, the illness rarely lasts more than a day, but let your doctor make the diagnosis. This is an illness where a house call is appropriate.

Naturally, obstruction along the digestive tract leads to vomiting. If the block lies above the stomach, patients regurgitate undigested food. Vomiting partly digested food indicates obstruction just beyond the stomach in the duodenum, the most common site. As obstruction proceeds further down the intestine, pain and abdominal swelling become more prominent than vomiting.

Vomiting can signal local disease of any digestive organ from appendix to gallbladder to liver to stomach; pain often occurs as well. For unclear reasons, vomiting can accompany severe pain in other parts of the body, such as that of a heart attack, kidney stone, or migraine headache. Brain disease, such as tumors or meningitis, produces vomiting, probably by disturbing the vomiting center.

Drugs that directly irritate the stomach (aspirin, erythromycin, ipecac, alcohol) also stimulate the vomiting center; depending on your sensitivity, almost any drug can do the same.

General metabolic disturbances lead to vomiting, so it accompanies gland disease (thyroid or adrenal deficiency, diabetes) as well as derangement in blood volume or mineral level: dehydration, excess water intake, kidney failure, salt or potassium abnormalities.

Treatment

Heroic men vomit, hurry to drink in order to replace the lost fluid, vomit again, then drink again, and finally call me, exhausted, and say, "I can't keep anything down."

Don't do this. Putting anything into an irritable digestive tract makes it more irritable. Leave it alone. Smash a tray of ice cubes with a hammer, then keep a bowl of ice chips on the bedside stand. Rest in bed with a bucket beside you, keeping a piece of ice in your mouth. Once six hours has passed without vomiting, begin sipping a soft drink such as 7-Up, ginger ale, or Coca-Cola.

Sugar water soothes the stomach, and that's mostly what a soft drink contains. Don't drink diet soda. Don't eat anything until you're hungry. Over-the-counter medications (Pepto-Bismol, Emmetrol, Benadryl, Dramamine) suppress nausea modestly but work poorly after vomiting begins, so don't take any until the six hours pass.

Four Common Myths About Vomiting

1. It's important to prevent dehydration and malnutrition.

Although true for infants and the elderly, a healthy man can vomit for a day and fast several days in perfect safety. When doctors hospitalize someone with a gastrointestinal disorder, we write the order "nothing by mouth" and start an intravenous (IV). You'll need an IV if vomiting persists; until that time don't put anything in your mouth except a piece of ice.

2. Vomiting is nature's way of getting rid of poisons.

This is a popular, quasi-religious view of nature. Your body is a wonderful mechanism but full of imperfections; disease regularly produces senseless and positively harmful behavior. After you eat spoiled food, the toxin enters your blood to stimulate the vomiting centers in the brain. By the time you begin vomiting, the toxin has left your digestive tract, but you'll continue until your liver or kidney has eliminated the toxin.

3. Vomiting empties your stomach; vomiting after it empties (retching, dry heaves) is an ominous sign.

To repeat, your brain makes you vomit. You'll continue until it stops sending signals. The presence or absence of food in the stomach makes no difference.

4. Vomiting bile is a bad sign.

Bile normally enters the digestive tract just beyond the stomach, so it often appears in vomiting.

Know When to Get Medical Attention

Ninety percent of vomiting resolves within twelve hours, a reasonable cutoff point, but try to talk to a doctor earlier if you're truly miserable. The presence of fever or diarrhea shouldn't change this, but see a doctor sooner (in fact, immediately) if severe abdominal pain or severe pain anywhere in the body accompanies it. Treat vomiting gross blood as an emergency, but not the appearance of a few small flecks.

While a solid minority of abdominal pains require hospitalization, this is hardly ever so for vomiting. Since we have effective injections that suppress it, the reluctance of doctors to make house calls produces needless suffering because few active vomiters want to leave home. You can find a doctor willing to make a house call in most cities by phoning hotels to find the house doctor who is simply a local doctor willing to come to the hotel. Doctors do it for the money, so they should be willing to see you, but be forewarned that you'll pay well over a hundred dollars.

In the end, you may have to drag yourself to a clinic or emergency room. Fortunately, you'll receive quick attention, not because the problem is urgent but because personnel don't want to keep cleaning up the mess.

WHAT DOES DIARRHEA MEAN?

Like vomiting, diarrhea rarely signals an urgent problem. Unlike vomiting, over-the-counter drugs work fine, making self-treatment more satisfying.

The Nature of Diarrhea

By definition, diarrhea occurs when stool increases in volume or becomes too watery. That this happens only now and then speaks highly of the enormous absorptive capacity of your digestive tract, because a full 9 quarts of fluid enter your small intestine every day: 1 quart of saliva, 1½ quarts of food and drink, 2 quarts of stomach juice, and about 4½ quarts of bile, small intestinal, and pancreatic juice.

After absorbing 8 quarts, the small intestine moves the remaining quart into the colon, which absorbs another 80 to 90 percent. Asked to guess how much he or she excretes, everyone overestimates because a healthy person eliminates only 4 to 8 ounces per day. Even this is mostly water, with the remainder made up of colon bacteria, bile, mucus, cells shed from the intestinal lining, plus a tiny amount of food residue (colon bacteria consume most of the food humans can't digest).

Medical students learn that small intestinal diarrhea differs from large intestinal diarrhea. Because so much overlap occurs in real life, this has mostly academic interest, and doctors pay little attention, but you'll find it helpful in understanding your symptoms.

Since you excrete a cup or less of fluid every day while the small intestine absorbs 32 cups, you'll understand what follows a minor impairment in its function. Small intestinal diarrhea consists of large amounts of watery stool. Many toxins affect the small intestine, the classic being cholera, which produces massive diarrhea. Death occurs from dehydration, but treatment is easy. If a victim takes in fluids fast enough to replace the loss, the disease resolves in a few days. Antibiotics aren't necessary, and antidiarrheal drugs work poorly. Many less severe toxins and intestinal infections attack the small intestine.

With only a quart of residue to work on, an impaired colon can't produce much extra volume. Large intestinal diarrhea shows itself as small amounts of soft stool, the typical pattern of serious disorders such as ulcerative colitis or more garden variety stress-related diarrhea, irritable colon, and some infections.

Keep in mind that the muscular colon controls the actual mechanism of excretion, so a person with colonic disease feels the need to defecate too often. The closer to the anus the disease, the more urgent the feeling, so inflammation of the last part of the colon (the rectum) may lead to loss of control despite only small volumes of stool. With small intestinal disease a person feels an easily controlled urge but excretes a large volume.

Causes of Diarrhea

Unlike vomiting, diarrhea almost never indicates a problem outside the digestive tract. Even the loose stool of anxiety originates in the large intestine, a muscular organ that can become tense and irritable.

Like vomiting, diarrhea usually signals a minor viral infection and disappears in a few days. Travelers worry about dangerous infections, but even the dreaded Montezuma's revenge (from the toxin of a bacterial infection) isn't serious and lasts only a few days even if untreated. Rare in the United States, serious bacterial infections such as cholera and shigellosis produce a violent illness with fever and abdominal pain in addition to diarrhea.

Patients worry about intestinal parasites, and this is not unreasonable; besides those brought back by tourists, American waters harbor native parasites such as giardia that cause a fair amount of disease. However, despite the common belief, profuse diarrhea is not typical. Parasitic protozoa and worms tend to produce vague digestive upsets, weight loss, and soft stool without serious illness.

Fruits and vegetables contain indigestible fiber, which swells and softens stool. Consuming large amounts makes stool even softer but shouldn't cause frank diarrhea. Caffeine stimulates the digestive tract, a quality useful in a morning beverage, but don't blame it unless you've taken more than usual. Among drugs, antacids, antibiotics, digitalis, and thyroid are the leading offenders.

A paradox: Diarrhea can be a sign of constipation, especially in the elderly. Every doctor sees a case now and then. Liquid residue entering the colon encounters a mass of stool or (fortunately less often) an obstructing tumor. After accumulating for a time, some trickles past and exits, so the patient, accustomed to the constipation, complains of diarrhea.

Treatment of Diarrhea

Unlike treatment of vomiting, it's all right to replace lost fluids, although this is not an important early step for a healthy adult (serious diarrhea in infants and the elderly should receive medical attention more quickly). Rehydration solutions such as Gatorade or Pedialyte aren't necessary for ordinary diarrhea. Soda or apple juice work fine.

All narcotics cause constipation, and humans took opium to relieve diarrhea even before discovering the intoxicating properties, and it remains the best treatment. The traditional tincture of opium is so cheap that drug companies don't find it profitable, but they add opium to mixtures like paregoric or brands with similar names (Parapectolin, Parelexir). Loperamide (Imodium) is a good opium derivative available over the counter. The similar and very popular Lomotil remains a prescription drug, but this is the manufacturer's marketing decision, not a mark of superiority.

Bismuth subsalicylate (Pepto-Bismol) works, in general, very well. I recommend the liquid over the tablets. Related to aspirin, bismuth subsalicylate doesn't irritate the stomach, but be aware that it may turn stool black.

The venerable remedy, Kaopectate, mixes kaolin (a powdered clay) and pectin (a sticky carbohydrate extracted from fruit). These are supposed to thicken watery stool, but they probably don't. Another natural remedy, attapulgite (Rheaban, Diasorb, Donnagel, Kaopectate Concentrated) may accomplish this. You'll find activated charcoal advertised for diarrhea, although it works better for gas.

Know When to Get Medical Attention

A typical viral diarrhea lasts three or four days, so there's no reason to go beyond home treatment as long as you're not greatly inconvenienced. Use a week as a cutoff point if you're healthy and feel well, but stick to three or four days if you feel ill. For diarrhea with significant abdominal pain or vomiting, call the doctor after a day.

I don't have to warn about frankly bloody diarrhea; no one ignores it, and this is sensible. Fortunately, it's usually less deadly than frightened patients imagine. Bacterial infections of the colon as well as inflammations like ulcerative colitis produce an impressive blood flow, but these are treatable. Men are less likely to pay attention to soft, black stool, but this indicates heavy bleeding in the upper GI tract, especially the stomach. See a doctor immediately for black (not dark brown) stool.

Intelligent laypeople spend too much time with a fairly useless instrument, the thermometer, while ignoring the most important medical device available for the home—a good scale. Fever, even high fever, is rarely an ominous sign, but this is never true of weight loss. Everyone varies by a few pounds a day, but if you've lost 5 pounds without dieting, see a doctor. A scale helps most when diarrhea drags on without being especially severe. Men with minor ailments or stress-related diarrhea maintain good nutrition. Parasitic infections and serious problems may cause only mild stool changes but a steady weight loss.

WHEN YOU HAVE GAS

No respectable health guide overlooks this subject, a universal complaint rarely mentioned to the doctor and not well handled on those occasions. Because excessive gas is almost never a sign of disease, doctors don't study it during their education, but they should make the effort later because so many patients suffer. Almost every man believes he farts too much, and other forms of gas bother them nearly as often. A doctor who makes the effort can help (and occasionally cure) every patient with reassurance, dietary advice, and drugs.

Researchers on human gas have discovered that the three principal symptoms—belching, bloating, and flatulence—represent separate disorders with different treatments.

Belching

In my experience, belchers blame deranged digestion for their gas. In fact, researchers who analyze belch gas find a composition identical to the atmosphere, so a belch is simply swallowed air. Everyone takes in a small amount of air with each swallow. We consume more in food that contains gas, such as whipped cream, souffles, beer, soda, and meringues. One can easily swallow a pint of air during a normal meal. Anxious individuals swallow air without realizing it.

Gas rises, so most returns from where it came. Very little proceeds through the digestive tract to produce other gas disorders. Researchers proved this by pumping gas into subjects' stomachs and observing that it came back up.

Traditional advice includes chewing with the mouth closed, avoiding foods containing gas, and avoiding talking and drinking large amounts of fluid with meals. No drug eliminates swallowed air.

Men who belch after meals respond well to this treatment. Those who swallow air unconsciously at other times find my explanation hard to believe. I urge them to make an effort to keep their mouth shut for a full four hours and observe how much they belch. No one can swallow much air with the mouth closed.

Bloating Is Different

Normal intestines contain about 6 ounces of air. Intestines of bloaters also contain 6 ounces because excess gas doesn't cause their discomfort. Bloaters' bowels are too sensitive, overreacting to normal amounts of gas and liquid by going into spasm, propelling the contents backward and forward. When researchers pump air into small intestines, normal subjects experience only a vague pressure. Those with chronic bloating feel pain.

Bloating is probably a form of irritable bowel syndrome, the leading gastrointestinal disorder that affects 20 percent of the population. Although never life threatening, it's tiresome enough for those who suffer the various combinations of cramps, gas, constipation, diarrhea, indigestion, and bloating. Suspect irritable bowel syndrome if you're constantly dissatisfied with the state of your digestive tract.

Dietary changes play only a small role in treating bloating because it's a muscular disorder, but patients suspect that certain foods make it worse, so I encourage experimentation. Exercise tones up any muscle, the bowels included, and active people suffer few gastrointestinal complaints. Take a brisk walk after meals.

Drugs have been a mainstay since herbalists discovered the properties of the belladonna plant centuries ago. Extracts contain a powerful anticholinergic, a chemical that blocks transmission of cholinergic nerves, part of the autonomic nervous system that drives your digestive tract as well as other organs. Blocking transmission relaxes the bowel.

That's the theory. Reality is less satisfying. Cholinergic nerves supply many essential organs, so an efficient blocker would not only immobilize the bowel but dry up your salivary and sweat glands, inhibit your bladder from expelling urine, slow your thinking and make you drowsy, and paralyze your pupils. (A side note: *Belladonna* means "beautiful woman" in Italian. During the renaissance, Italian men admired widely dilated pupils, so Italian women used these drops in their eyes to accomplish this. Thus, the name.)

Nervous about making customers ill, drug companies keep the dose of their anticholinergic as low as possible—so low that popular antispasmodics (Donnatol, Librax, Robinul, Bentyl) probably don't work at all, although a few men may be sensitive enough to notice an improvement. More effective are low doses of an antidepressant such as amitriptyline (Elavil) or imipramine (Tofranil). Although the dose is too low to treat depression, unlike anticholinergics low doses of antidepressants often relieve irritable muscles and nerves in conditions such as migraine, chronic low back pain, whiplash, and irritable bowels. Doctors underprescribe antidepressants for these problems, so you may have to suggest them.

Flatulence and Milk

Men expel between a half pint and 2 quarts of gas per day in up to two dozen episodes. Vegetarians expel more. As I've mentioned, swallowed air comes back up, so flatulence originates inside the GI tract from the action of colon bacteria on undigested carbohydrates. Humans digest protein and fats with almost 100 percent efficiency, but the great majority of carbohydrates in our diet pass into the colon unchanged. Bacteria consume it, generating gas: mostly hydrogen, methane, and carbon dioxide (all odorless) plus a small amount of more complex gases that are not.

Foods highest in indigestible carbohydrates include grains (breads and cereals, but not including white and whole wheat bread), legumes (beans, peas, peanuts), dried fruits, bananas, apricots, carrots, and onions.

Although no distinct disease causes excessive gas in a healthy person, many adults have lost the ability to digest lactose, the carbohydrate in milk. If you think about it, milk is baby food. Adult animals don't drink it, and an efficient nature gradually eliminates lactase (the enzyme that breaks down lactose) from a maturing digestive tract. Humans have only consumed milk for a few thousand years, so we haven't had time to adjust. Most of us have some degree of lactase deficiency. Ethnic groups who have drunk milk the longest do the best: those of English and north European ancestry. Ten to 20 percent are severely deficient. Among whites of Mediterranean ancestry plus all other races, this rises to 75 percent. When a lactase deficient person drinks milk, lactose pours into the colon, where bacteria quickly ferment it and produce gas, sometimes accompanied by cramps and diarrhea. Most badly deficient individuals learn what to avoid, but anyone bothered by gas should try a month without dairy products. If necessary, you can buy lactose-free milk. Pharmacies also sell bottled lactase that you can add to regular milk to break down lactose. If milk gives you gas, substituting low-fat or skim milk won't help. These are low in fat, not carbohydrate.

Once you've decided that milk doesn't give you gas, eliminating foods becomes the best treatment. You're lucky if you can identify a few offenders; if not, I encourage a philosophical acceptance of your flatulence. Americans should eat more, not less, complex carbohydrates. Only meat and eggs are gas free.

Despite a generous selection, no drug eliminates gas already present. Advertisements praise simethicone (present in many antacids as well as gas remedies such as Mylicon, Phazyme, Gas-X, Colicon) for its ability to break up gas bubbles, but this is nonsense. Even if it worked, the gas is still there. I suggest activated charcoal, a safe product available without prescription. In good studies, volunteers who took it after a gassy meal produced less gas than those given placebo, and some victims notice an improvement.

How to Deal with Anal Discomfort

The anus is an area men expect to operate flawlessly and about which they complain to doctors with the greatest reluctance after much worrying and worthless self-treatment. Luckily, the most frightening anal symptoms usually signal minor, treatable disorders.

Anal pain means what pain means in any part of the body—injured or otherwise stressed tissue. Pain that's worse on defecating usually indicates an anal fissure, a split in the skin provoked by a particularly hard or wide stool. At least that's the traditional explanation. Many men do notice sudden pain during a difficult bowel movement, but others deny any stool abnormality. The truth is that doctors aren't certain what causes fissures in otherwise healthy men.

A laceration in such an active location seems an ominous problem, but it turns out that anal fissures heal as promptly as cuts anywhere else on the body. Despite the presence of stool, we don't clean the area, yet infections are rare. Doctors treat with stool softeners (Colace, DSS, Surfak), soothing creams (Anusol, Preparation H, Proctocream), and sitz baths (sitting in hot water). These seem sensible, and like so many treatments based on common sense, no evidence shows that they work, but they give patients something to do while nature takes it course. Most stores sell these pills and creams, so you can treat yourself. See a doctor if pain persists a week.

What if You Find a Lump?

An *anal lump accompanied by pain* almost always means a thrombosed hemorrhoid. Men suffering discomfort around the anus blame hemorrhoids, yet when I ask what that is, no patient has yet known. I've concluded that the popular definition of a hemorrhoid is any discomfort around the anus. The medical definition is a varicose vein in the anus. Identical to those in the legs, varicose veins are one of the penalties humans pay for walking on two feet, because standing produces higher pressures in leg and anal veins than walking on all fours. As we age, their thin walls weaken and stretch, leading to swollen and flabby (i.e., varicose) veins. Varicose arteries don't occur because thick muscles make up their walls.

Almost every adult has hemorrhoids without realizing it. Furthermore, when the average hemorrhoid causes symptoms, pain is not among them. The exception occurs when a clot or thrombosis suddenly forms. No one knows why this happens, but every victim knows when. When circulation is blocked in the anus, a high-pressure vessel, blood piles up, stretching the vein painfully and producing a tender lump that the patient can feel and the doctor can see.

Despite this alarming onset, a thrombosed hemorrhoid is entirely benign and doesn't require treatment. The human body does not tolerate a clot for long. Almost immediately, elements in the blood begin dissolving it, and most thrombosed hemorrhoids shrink away in three to four days. Sitting in a tub of hot water for an hour twice a day helps. Unlike fissures, which are probably too far up to benefit, the hot water reaches the swollen vein. Creams and suppositories don't help.

For instant relief, a doctor can slice open the vein and extract the clot. Hearing this suggestion, most men quickly decide to wait. They should realize that surgery is easy, almost painless, and the results are dramatic. I encourage everyone with severe pain to allow the doctor to get rid of the clot on the spot.

An *anal lump without pain* often represents a wart no different from a wart elsewhere. These spread, so you should have treatment. The doctor may paint the wart with a corrosive substance or kill it by freezing with liquid nitrogen.

A large hemorrhoid may dangle and protrude, but it shouldn't hurt unless thrombosed. You will eventually want protruding hemorrhoids eliminated; except for the largest, this is easily done in the office by half a dozen simple techniques. Finally, although anal cancer is rare, it rarely hurts, so see a doctor for any painless anal lump.

Is Anal Itching Bad?

Don't blame *anal itching* on poor hygiene. Like the opening at the opposite end of the digestive tract, the anus maintains a surprising resistance to local germs and dirt. Vigorous attempts to clean cause far more irritation than neglect (similarly, mouthwashes are also useless).

Make sure diet isn't responsible. Coffee, with or without caffeine, produces the most itching of any food. Try two weeks' abstinence if you can stand it. If this doesn't help, try two weeks without dairy products. The remaining possibilities include beer and large amounts of vitamin C—more than a gram a day. If itching remains, feel free to experiment by stopping any new food. Try cutting out spices, which have taken the blame for digestive irritation since the dawn of history. Traditional health beliefs are usually wrong, but not always.

If a companion notices or a mirror reveals pink spots inside the buttock, you may have a common fungal infection similar to that which attacks the groin. Apply an antifungal cream (Micatin, Lotrimin) twice a day for two weeks. If itching disappears, continue for a total of two months. If not, a fungus is not responsible.

A common and maddening affliction, stress-related anal itching is a difficult diagnosis. Don't make it until you've ruled out the other causes and seen a doctor at least once and perhaps several times, because a sensible doctor also hesitates to blame stress. Cortisone creams relieve itching, but don't use them without a firm diagnosis because they relieve itching no matter what the cause. Cortisone suppresses itching from a fungal infection, but the fungus continues to grow; it suppresses itching from harsh soaps and chemicals, but the skin damage will continue.

Always frightening, *anal bleeding* only occasionally represents serious disease. A fissure can bleed slightly, and a leaky hemorrhoid vein can turn the toilet bowl red. Although both are benign, let your doctor know. Colon cancers often ooze blood, but rarely enough to detect with the naked eye. Heavy bleeding in a younger man probably stems from infection (dysentery) or inflammation, such as ulcerative colitis. In an older man, the usual source is a bleeding artery in the bowel wall or diffuse bleeding from ischemic colitis—blockage of circulation to the colon. See a doctor quickly.

Although I mentioned loose, black stool (the medical term is melena) in the diarrhea section, it's worth repeating. Blood remaining in the digestive tract darkens to maroon to black over a period of hours and acts as a laxative. Typically, a bleeding ulcer produces melena, and it's always an urgent problem.

DEALING WITH A FEVER

Awakening one morning feverish and achy, a man suspects that he has the flu. Unwilling to surrender to a minor illness, he prepares for work but out of curiosity puts a thermometer in his mouth. It registers 103°. Hurrying to the doctor, he discovers that his diagnosis was correct. Treatment is plenty of fluids, acetaminophen, and (as long as he feels ill) rest.

Several times a day during the flu season, I explain that a fever of 103° or 104° won't harm a healthy adult and often accompanies an acute illness like influenza. Healthy adults exaggerate the danger of fever (except now and then when they underestimate it). They work hard to lower it and worry if they fail, despite my assurance that treatment is rarely essential.

The Body's Thermostat

Deep in the brain, an area called the hypothalamus regulates basic behavior such as appetite, thirst, emotions, and the sleep–wake cycle as well as body temperature. Sensing the temperature of blood flowing nearby, special neurons send out signals to conserve heat (by constricting blood vessels in the skin), generate heat (by increasing muscle activity—shivering), or dissipate heat (by sweating and dilating blood vessels). These actions occur continually throughout the day to maintain our temperature within narrow limits.

All mammals and birds possess a similar hypothalamic thermostat. Normal temperature for mammals varies between 96° and 103°; much hotter creatures, birds average between 105° and 110°. Maintaining a warm temperature allows for tremendous activity compared to lower animals, especially in cool weather. Anyone visiting the reptile house in a zoo knows how boring it can be, with the inhabitants content to remain motionless for hours. The price of our high temperature is a ferocious appetite. A 150-pound human must eat *twenty times* as much as a 150-pound crocodile.

The Mythical "Normal" Temperature

When reliable thermometers appeared in the mid-nineteenth century, researchers tested normal adults and agreed that 98.6° Fahrenheit orally marked the average. Everyone knows this; every thermometer contains a distinct mark at this point on the scale; almost everyone, doctors included, are surprised to learn that it's wrong. Average is 98.0° or even less. All recent studies confirm this. Everyone varies by several degrees per day, with 96° to 99° the normal range.

Following a daily rhythm, our lowest point occurs in the morning around 6 A.M., with the peak in the evening. Like many biorhythms, temperature follows the rising and setting of the sun, not our level of activity. Men who work at night and sleep during the day keep the same cycle.

"I always run a low temperature," a few patients insist despite this explanation, but a level under 95° always indicates serious disease (usually exposure). Hypothermia victims grow stuporous at a body temperature as high as 90°; most lose consciousness at 85°; most die below 80°. The record for survival in accidental hypothermia is 61°, and subjects in experimental studies have survived 48°.

Age and sex affect your temperature. In one study the average rectal temperature at eighteen months was 99.8°, and half the subjects measured 100° and higher. Slowly cooling with age, girls stabilize at age twelve to thirteen, and boys continue cooling until around eighteen. As a result, a man's temperature averages 0.7 degrees less than a woman's.

Causes of Fever

Fever occurs when the hypothalamus resets the thermostat. For example, it might set "normal" temperature at 102°. With blood flowing through at 98°, neurons react as if the body were too cold, sending out signals to step up muscle activity. Shivering occurs until the blood reaches 102°.

Some variation occurs without disease. Digesting a meal raises it 1 to 2 degrees. A woman's temperature goes up 0.5 to 1 degree after ovulation and remains up until menstruation, the result of increasing progesterone. A marathon runner may finish at 105°, but this is not really "fever" because the hypothalamus hasn't reset; the runner is generating heat faster than he or she can cool.

Genuine fever follows bacterial and viral infections, immune reactions (allergies, after a vaccination), tissue inflammation (colitis, arthritis), tissue death (heart attacks, hemorrhage, after surgery), and even the action of natural hormones (thyroid, progesterone).

Except for hormones whose action we don't understand, these natural hormones stimulate immune cells to secrete substances (interleukins, prostaglandins, interferons) with many actions, one of which resets the hypothalamus. Drugs that reduce fever, such as aspirin and acetaminophen, block the action of these substances.

Is Fever Good For You?

Almost all authorities say yes, reasoning that any action of the immune system must serve a useful purpose. During experiments immune cells kill bacteria faster at higher temperatures. One important cell, the T-lymphocyte, works best at 103°. Cancer researchers shrink tumors with heat. Early in this century, doctors used fever to treat syphilis and some forms of chronic arthritis. Patients sat in a heated box; occasionally doctors infected them with malaria.

Experiments on lizards (useful because researchers can change their temperature at will) provide more evidence. The warmer the lizard, the better it fights off an infection. Giving aspirin to an infected lizard increases mortality.

When a Fever is Ominous

In an intact immune system, fever is a sign of relatively good health. The very old and feeble have difficulty generating heat, so any temperature becomes a matter for concern. The same is true for anyone with weak immunity. Patients with AIDS or leukemia and those undergoing cancer chemotherapy or radiotherapy should report any fever. The newborn's immature immune system reacts unpredictably; fever during the first month of life is always a serious sign.

Should You Treat Your Fever?

Yes, if it will make you feel better.

This sounds like I'm contradicting the authorities, but those same experts aren't certain how important fever is as an immunological weapon. No longer in vogue, fever therapy was dangerous and never worked very well. Medical journals have reported good results from hyperthermia treatment of cancer for twenty years, but no one advises practicing doctors to use it. One must take the lizard experiments seriously, but doctors don't notice human infections getting worse when patients take medicine to reduce fever.

The most important treatment is not drugs but keeping cool. Wrapping in blankets is a bad idea, although it's hard to resist when you're shaking with chills (at which time, remember, your temperature is rising).

Drink plenty of fluids to replace the extra water evaporating from your hot skin. Dehydration not only makes you feel worse, it maintains your fever by cutting off the water the body needs to cool itself. Drink enough juice or soda to produce slightly more than normal urination.

No prescription drug works better than aspirin or acetaminophen (Tylenol, Datril, Panadol) for the average fever. Newer antiinflammatories such as Advil, Nuprin, or Motrin do the same but provide no advantage to compensate for their higher cost.

Within an hour of taking the drug, you may break out in a sweat. Despite the popular belief that this is beneficial, sweating simply means that the body is cooling. Fevers always rise and fall, so a falling temperature is not good, and a rising temperature is not bad; they are simply what happens. When the drugs wears off, shivering may return—also not a harmful or beneficial symptom but the body's way of generating heat. To avoid unpleasant swings of sweats and chills, try keeping the fever suppressed by taking the drug regularly every four hours.

Know When to See Your Doctor

Although a sign of illness, fever alone is rarely a reason to see a doctor. Hearing this, many patients appear uncomfortable, and I often experience the following exchange:

> *Patient:* "But what if I go up to 104°?"
> *Doctor:* "Does a high fever worry you?"
> *Patient:* "Of course."
> *Doctor:* "Then don't take your temperature."

I urge healthy men to follow a simple rule: Sickness makes you sick. See a doctor if you feel bad. If you don't feel very sick, you're probably not sick regardless of your temperature.

When asked for guidelines, I suggest that a patient phone if fever reaches 103° and come in if it passes 104°. At 104° he'll feel sick. Asked for a danger point, I place it at 106°, a level that begins to impair brain function; most often a seizure marks the first sign. Permanent brain damage occurs quickly after 108°. Although this is a frightening fact, adults rarely suffer a fever above 106°, and this usually requires a disorder that damages the hypothalamus, such as heat stroke, encephalitis, or cerebral hemorrhage. Victims of flu and other common infections shouldn't worry. Remember that these guidelines are aimed at healthy men; they are also not written in stone. I encourage patients to call whenever they're worried; all good doctors do the same.

How to Handle Back Pain

Medical writers love primitive cultures as examples of healthy behavior, and I do it myself. Primitive cultures don't suffer high blood pressure because they eat so little salt; they have almost no constipation, appendicitis, and bowel problems because they consume so much roughage; obesity is rare because they must struggle to find enough to feed themselves as well as their parasites.

It turns out that primitive cultures don't have back trouble, either. The reasons are worth considering because they summarize good back care. Primitive people

- Sleep on the ground,
- Squat instead of sit, and
- Lead active lives.

Since these are preventive measures, I'll elaborate after a discussion of why backs hurt and how to treat the pain.

Why Your Back Hurts

While a leg muscle is the size of your forearm, a back muscle resembles your little finger. Obviously not designed for heavy work, human back muscles are too weak to hold us erect. Four-legged animals don't require strong back muscles, and humans stood up only a few million years ago, so evolution hasn't had time to adapt those muscles to a much greater work load.

We stand because the spine sits directly on the pelvis. With our upper body balancing heavily on an area the size of a silver dollar, back muscles serve to make minor adjustments in posture, allowing us to twist and turn, the same function they perform in four-legged animals. But this is risky because now and then humans lift improperly, bend too much, or otherwise move the upper body off center, forcing back muscles to support a heavy weight. Mostly they succeed but they are at the limit of their strength, so strains and injuries occur regularly. Simple muscle injury causes most back pain in otherwise healthy men.

Easily strong enough to bear weight, vertebral bones need a cushion at intervals to absorb shocks. To accomplish this requires the famous disks, a source of so much blame. A superb hydraulic system (its nucleus contains 80 percent water), a young intervertebral disk can flatten, bulge, and otherwise distort in response to stress and then quickly snap back to shape.

Like many tissues, disks grow stiff with age. Although this deprives the back of flexibility, a worn, rigid disk can't hurt because it contains no pain nerves. Problems occur when a brittle disk breaks or ruptures (it can't really "slip"). A broken piece hurts if it presses a pain-sensitive structure such as a ligament. If it presses a nearby nerve, one may feel pain shooting down one leg. This is sciatica, because the sciatic nerve originates in the low spinal cord and supplies the leg.

Finally, like all bones, each vertebra joins its neighbor through joints lined with cartilage and filled with lubricating fluid that permits movement. Because of their angle, the joints at the five lowest vertebra (called lumbar) permit only bending forward and backward. Just above, the twelve thoracic vertebra have joints that make bending forward and back impossible but permit them to twist and to bend side to side. Old joints become worn and rough, so arthritis receives plenty of blame for back pain in the elderly, but muscle injury remains important.

Bones themselves slowly lose mineral after about age thirty-five. Called osteoporosis, this is one disorder in which male enjoy a great advantage. Past age sixty, the vertebrae of many women become so fragile that occasionally one collapses under normal stresses. Called a compression fracture, this sounds catastrophic, but pain is the usual consequence. Men also suffer osteoporosis, but less dramatically and at a later age. Doctors theorize that the drop in estrogens at menopause accelerates bone loss in women, but it's also possible that men suffer less because they are more active (exercise strengthens bone as well as muscle) and because male bones are bigger than female bones when mineral loss begins.

Getting Treatment

Even without treatment, 90 percent of backaches disappear in a week or two. Injuries must heal; nothing accelerates healing; proper treatment prevents you from interfering with healing as well as relieving pain.

If your back hurts, take it easy. Do this even if pain is agonizing, although it's useful to talk to your doctor. Men routinely call friends or an ambulance to carry them off to an emergency room, where they receive useless X-rays, drugs they could buy at the local supermarket, and instructions to rest. Even with an acute slipped disk, you won't be hospitalized without signs of nerve damage, such as a weak leg or difficulty urinating. A few days' rest takes the edge off most low back pain, whether it's an injury, slipped disk, or joint inflammation.

Pain medicine relieves pain; it doesn't affect healing (I'm sorry if this seems to insult your intelligence, but I must make statements like this because a large fraction of my patients confuse cures such as antibiotics with symptomatic remedies. They believe, for example, that aspirin cures a headache, cough medicine shortens a cold, hemorrhoid creams eliminate hemorrhoids, etc.). If you want less pain, take ibuprofen (Advil, Nuprin, Medipren, Motrin IB). Although instructions limit you to one or two 200-milligram tablets, I suggest three.

If you see a doctor for your backache, he or she will probably prescribe a similar drug such as Naprosyn, Anaprox, Feldene, Ansaid, Clinoril, or Orudis. You may even receive ibuprofen itself—sold as a prescription under the name Motrin. *None are superior to over-the-counter ibuprofen.* You can buy ibuprofen without a prescription because the FDA has judged it safe enough. Similar drugs will make the switch when their makers decide that over-the-counter sale will be profitable and win FDA approval.

Heat relaxes muscles and relieves spasm. Cold deadens pain. Cold helps the acute pain of an injury for up to a day; use heat thereafter. A hot-water bottle works as well as a heating pad, and hot baths are fine. More popular in Europe, "plasters" and other wrappings impregnated with drugs generate heat but otherwise offer no advantage. Similarly, local therapy such as Ben-Gay or Therapeutic Mineral Ice produce either heat or cold. These contain drugs such as aspirin, but applied to the skin they probably don't work. Massage without an ointment also generates heat and feels just as good.

Ideas for Preventing Back Pain

We go back to the three healthful activities of primitive cultures.

1. They sleep on the ground.

Victims of chronic back pain prefer to sleep on the floor, and experts approve. The average man doesn't have to go this far, but good sleeping habits prevent trouble.

Sleep on a firm mattress that doesn't sag. Any mattress can be stiffened by putting a board underneath. The best sleeping position is on your side with legs bent and head supported on a pillow. Sleeping on the back is all right provided that your knees are bent. Bending the knees relaxes back muscles; you can do this by putting a cushion under your knees. Sleeping on the stomach forces the back into an unnatural curve, stressing joints and ligaments. Orthopedic beds or special mattresses aren't necessary unless a specialist recommends one.

2. They squat instead of sit.

Squatting is a natural position in which the spine remains balanced over the pelvis. An unnatural position, sitting throws the upper body out of balance. Advanced cultures will not discard their chairs, but they should use them carefully.

- Stay away from stools or benches without back support.
- Seat backs must be firm and extend down to touch the upper part of the low back to prevent the buttocks from slipping under the backrest.
- Use the backrest. Slouching forward stresses the back. It's hard to resist overstuffed furniture or a favorite chair that's developed a hollow into which your buttocks fit, but these are like junk food—agreeable at the time but with unpleasant long-term consequences.
- Make sure your knees rise slightly higher than your hips with feet flat on the floor. When they remain lower, the low back pulls away from the backrest, increasing muscle tension. If you're short, put books under your feet.
- When driving, adjust the seat so you reach the pedals while you knees remain bent. Sit back while driving. If you drive a great deal, buy a firm, flat backrest that doesn't project into the lumbar curve.

These principles also apply to standing. Military posture with shoulders thrown back is as unnatural as sitting. To stand in the healthiest manner, tuck in your chin and tuck in your buttocks. This encourages the spine (which is never straight) to assume its most natural curve. Primitive African cattle herders remain erect the entire day, but they stand on one foot at a time. If you stand for long periods, put one foot on a stool and alternate every five or ten minutes. As you hip muscles tire, the pelvis tilts forward, increasing the lumbar curve and straining low back muscles. Bending the leg relaxes muscles on that side.

3. They lead an active life.

If you already suffer, it's fine to follow a specific back exercise program pre-scribed by a doctor or physical therapist. If not, you should have other health priorities. Stick to the advice about exercise in Chapter 2. Any man who follows professional sports knows that the best athletes suffer crippling back injuries, so experts traditionally warn against contact sports, weight lifting, volleyball, down-hill skiing, squash, and any overenthusiastic exertion. They are risky, but life is short, so I don't discourage any exercise in an otherwise healthy person.

DEALING WITH HEADACHES

Although considered a woman's complaint, the most common pain that afflicts humans brings about 1 out of 8 men to the doctor every year, (the figure for women: 1 out of 5). Despite the popular impression, medical science doesn't do badly here, provided the patient remains persistent. Since headaches occur ep-isodically, sufferers tend to put off doctor visits when they feel well. Don't do that if attacks have become tiresome despite over the counter remedies. During the initial visit, the doctor will examine you; no abnormalities should turn up. He might or might not order a few tests, but he will almost certainly write out a prescription. Give it a chance, but don't assume that this represents all that medical science can offer. In my experience, doctors relieve a minority of head-aches on the first try. Although this is a large minority, too many sufferers continue to suffer unnecessarily. At least a dozen entirely unrelated headache treatments exist: If one doesn't help, let the doctor know and try another. Eventually one should work.

What is a Tension Headache?

A nervous animal's first action is to raise its head to look for danger. Human's can't do this because our heads are already as high as they can go, but this maneuver remains embedded in our genes, so neck and scalp muscles contract when we become uneasy. The head remains in place, and the persistent muscle strain produces pain over the back of the head, temple, and perhaps forehead. This is the familiar tension headache. Without treatment it lasts hours to days and rarely includes other symptoms.

Most headaches, including most seen by a doctor, belong to this category. When severe, patients prefer to call them "migraines," a diagnosis with dignity. "Tension headache," to the laymen, implies neurosis, weakness, difficulty in han-dling stress. In fact, many well adjusted men suffer muscle tension headaches. Not a personal failing, they are evidence that no one is perfect. If over-the-counter therapy provides relief, doctors have little to offer. It not, we can help, first with stronger pain remedies, then with prophylaxis mentioned further on.

If You Have a Migraine Headache

For unknown reasons migraines tend to affect women, but men make up 25 percent of victims, not a trivial number. Also called vascular headaches because scalp arteries seem responsible, patients typically describe pain as pounding or throbbing in contrast to the steady pain of muscle tension. According to the traditional explanation, migraine occurs when these arteries relax and become tender, stretching and pulsating painfully with each heartbeat. Anything that relaxes blood vessels (cigarette smoke, alcohol, hunger, fever, certain foods) provokes vascular headaches, but they often appear out of the blue.

The leading source of pain, the temporal artery, travels vertically up the side of your head. You can feel its pulse in front of your ear. Since 80 percent of attacks affect a single artery, a migraine is usually a one sided headache (migraine is from the Greek for "half skull"), accompanied by nausea, vomiting, and intolerance to light. It lasts a few hours to a day or two and rarely strikes more than once a week. Someone who suffers daily headaches probably doesn't have migraine. Most people know that flashing lights or other visual phenomena can herald a migraine, but this only occurs in 10 to 15 percent of victims.

Although pain remedies work for a migraine, drugs that stiffen the pulsating artery work better. Doctors have prescribed ergotamine for this purpose during most of this century, and it remains the best drug to abort an attack. A patient should take it as soon as he feels the migraine getting started; taken during a full-blown attack it doesn't work as well. Ergotamine acts quickest as a sublingual tablet or inhaler, but many patients prefer the tablet or suppository. These forms usually include caffeine, also a blood vessel stiffener.

If migraines remain disabling despite treatment, you need prophylaxis: a drug taken daily to reduce the frequency of attacks. Literally a dozen good ones exist, so you should be able to find one that works for you. They include several classes of blood pressure medication (which have little affect on normal blood pressures), low dose antidepressants, nonsteroidal anti-inflammatories (such as Motrin, Naprosyn, Anaprox), low dose ergotamines taken daily, and certain antihistamines. If a few months on one doesn't satisfy you, move on to the next. Don't give up, and don't let your doctor give up. In the past, experts carefully explained that migraines and tensions headaches were separate disorders with specific treatments, but we are no longer so certain, and it turns out that many of the same prophylactic drugs help chronic tension headaches, too.

If all fails, it's appropriate to try complex but sometimes effective remedies such as biofeedback, acupuncture, or chiropractic. Although touted as simple, natural, and less expensive than drugs, the opposite is the case. Treatment requires repeated visits and (in the case of biofeedback) intensive practice and concentration. However, they sometimes make both tension and vascular headaches tolerable.

A Man's Migraine: Cluster Headaches

Affecting men in about 90 percent of cases, the typical victim of this migraine variant awakens from sleep with an intense, steady pain localized around the eye and temple on one side. Pain lasts five minutes to several hours, often accompanied by a stuffy or runny nose and eye tearing on the same side. Attacks recur almost nightly for weeks then stop for months or years—hence the name *cluster*. By no means rare, cluster headaches are not as common as ordinary migraines, so some doctors don't think of them. One of my first triumphs as an intern was informing a local doctor of the diagnosis on a man he admitted for a possible cerebral hemorrhage.

Onset occurs so abruptly that "early" treatment isn't a possibility, but inhaled ergotamine sometimes stops an attack. If not, inhaling pure oxygen helps, and some victims keep a tank at their bedside.

Lithium and several antiseizure drugs work for prophylaxis as well as several drugs used for common migraine. Because a man may remain free from attacks for years, daily medication becomes tiresome. If this is so, a doctor can usually cut short a cluster by prescribing a large daily dose of cortisone, then tapering gradually to zero over two weeks.

Other Headaches: Caffeine Withdrawal

A mildly effective remedy for vascular headaches, caffeine stiffens arterial smooth muscle, an action that increases its addictive potential. Adults who skip their regular morning coffee not only miss its stimulation but soon notice an annoying throbbing headache. People who drink a great deal of coffee at work may suffer headaches over the weekend when they drink less. Caffeine works miracles with these headaches. I suspect that so many pain remedies (Excedrin, Fiorinal, Norgesic) contain caffeine because withdrawal makes up an element of many headaches.

What Are Food Headaches?

Some men get a headache from chocolate, others after eating cheese, Chinese food, or a hot dog. These foods can trigger migraine because they contain chemicals that relax blood vessels, but they are also the source of garden variety headaches. Major offenders include the additive nitrite in hot dogs and lunch meat as well as monosodium glutamate in Chinese food. Avoiding additives and processed food may not solve the problem because several natural substances have the same action: tyramine in cheese, nuts, and red wine and phenylethylamine in chocolate.

Lack of oxygen

Relaxes blood vessels to enable them to carry more oxygen to tissues. Traveling to a high altitude or in an unpressurized plane often causes a headache for this reason. Those who work in poorly ventilated garages or areas with a faulty heating system suffer headaches as the only sign of chronic carbon monoxide poisoning. Carbon monoxide binds to red blood cells, preventing them from carrying oxygen. Heavy cigarette smoking may cause carbon monoxide headaches in the smoker and sometimes in those nearby.

Heat and fever headaches

The body cools itself by increasing blood flow to the skin and scalp, so anything that generates body heat can produce a headache in a sensitive person: fever, exercise, even a hot day. Relief occurs by lowering skin temperature with aspirin, acetaminophen, a cool bath, or a cold compress.

Other Types of Headaches

Several conditions are universally but incorrectly blamed for headaches. They include:

High blood pressure

Men and women with ordinary high blood pressure suffer no more headaches than the general population. The only way to determine blood pressure is to measure it with a blood pressure cuff. Good studies confirm this, but laypeople and a surprising number of doctors believe otherwise.

Sinus problems

An acute sinus infection produces severe pain over the infected sinus, and victims quickly seek out a doctor. Chronic infections cause a nasal discharge or post-nasal drip but little pain. Sinus congestion leads to a congested feeling over the nose and face but no severe pain.

Allergies

Hay fever can lead to sinus congestion and a stuffy head, but a bad headache is something else. Foods, aromas, smoke, etc., trigger headaches by a direct chemical insult. Avoidance is the only tactic; these aren't allergies, so allergy treatment doesn't help.

A brain tumor or stroke

In the absence of other symptoms (local weakness, personality change, seizures) the chance is remote that a brain tumor is causing your headache. A cerebral hemorrhage usually produces severe pain, so victims rarely hesitate to see a doctor. Headaches from catastrophic disease rarely present in a subtle manner, but it's a good rule to let a doctor evaluate any new or different headache as well as one that's worse than any you've experienced.

Eyestrain

Eyestrain causes discomfort while eyes are under strain and disappears when they rest. If you need glasses or your present glasses have the wrong correction, you won't see as clearly as you should, but this is unlikely to cause recurrent headaches. See your doctor before your optometrist.

CHAPTER ■ 8

STRICTLY
MALE MEDICAL
PROBLEMS

Many a man, but no sensible woman, reaches middle age without seeing a doctor, and this difference stems almost entirely from their respective genitals. Hers require regular attention. A woman in perfect health should see the doctor yearly for a pap smear and breast exam. Sexually transmitted diseases harm women more than men, but even women practicing safe sex suffer a host of noncontagious urinary and a vaginal disorders provoked either by intercourse or the vulnerabilities of their genitourinary tract. (You can read about some in Chapter 10.) Finally, healthy women see doctors to either prevent, cut short, or nurture pregnancy.

Witnessing their female friends' seemingly endless need for medical care, young men congratulate themselves for possessing genitourinary organs requiring so little attention. In general, young men are right to feel good, although their time will come later (see the sections in this chapter on prostate disorders).

Yet they pay a price for this good fortune. After decades of no care or of visits for a respectable inconvenience such as a respiratory infection or injury, the first yearly rectal exam beginning at age forty seems a depressing milestone marking the end of youth. It's also undignified. As a result, many men decide to wait. Undignified exams are no news to women, so doctors detect their colon and genital cancers at an earlier stage.

We also detect testicular cancer at an alarmingly late stage in men who should be examining themselves. You'll learn about that further on. Three of the following sections may teach you more about the prostate than you want to know, but the prostate is second only to the heart in amount of medical attention it requires throughout a man's life. Two sections contain better news: The penis and male breast cause relatively little trouble, but you know less about them than you should.

WHAT TO DO ABOUT TESTICULAR LUMPS AND TUMORS

An innocent penile wart quickly brings the average man to the doctor's office. Provided that it's painless, a lump on the testes can grow to impressive size before provoking the same concern. Almost all of these lumps are harmless, but 6,000 American men per year develop testicular cancer, the most common malignancy in the fifteen to thirty-four age group. If you have to have cancer, this is a good choice because we cure close to 100 percent of early testicular cancers, and early detection is easy. Later we don't succeed as well.

Testicular Cancer

Risk Factors and Prevention. Sex and sexually transmitted disease have no influence. Men born with undescended testes run at least ten times the risk— even in the normal testes if the other was undescended. Undoubtedly some congenital abnormality is present because surgical correction doesn't change this risk, although it makes a tumor easier to detect. Since only 10 percent of men with testicular cancer have had undescended testes, those without this history should not feel protected.

Being black or oriental is good news here because the risk is only one quarter that of whites. This racial difference persists in other nations, evidence that genetics play a larger role than the environment.

Now and then a man insists that he suffered an injury to the testes and then noticed the tumor. This association of injury with cancer has existed for a century (some women with breast cancer make the same connection). Most doctors remain skeptical, although a few researchers have produced tumors in rats and fowl by injuring various organs. One theory (also present for a century) explains that after an injury the patient pays more attention to that area, so he is more likely to detect something. This is not terribly convincing, but I see no reason why an injury should lead to cancer. On the other hand, scarring and atrophy that occur long afterward may produce changes that encourage malignancy. Men with atrophic testes and those who have suffered mumps orchitis seem to have more risk.

No way exists to prevent testicular cancer; early detection is your only protection.

Diagnosis. Blood tests and X-rays play no role in screening. Currently, doctors detect half of testicular cancers during a routine exam or after a man develops symptoms of spread. This should never happen, because men should detect their own. Every man should examine himself monthly.

Examining Yourself Pays Off

The usual questions men ask about their testes have nothing to do with cancer, but I'll answer them here.

1. The testes should be approximately the same size; an abnormally small one has probably atrophied as the result of an old infection (see the discussion of orchitis page 158).
2. One testis always hangs lower. If it didn't, you couldn't bring your legs together.

Examine yourself monthly and in a warm place; the scrotum contracts tightly when it's chilly. During a bath or shower is ideal. Roll each testis between your thumb and fingers. It should feel like a hard-boiled egg about one and a half inches in diameter; the pair shouldn't vary in size by more than one quarter inch. Running up the back, you should detect the epididymus, a thin cord the diameter of a piece of spaghetti. You're better off if you can identify this cord because any mass attached to the epididymus (or lying free) is almost certainly benign. This is less certain for a mass on the testis itself. The epididymus joins the thicker spermatic cord at the top of each testis.

If you find a new lump or any new irregularity, you can perform a simple diagnostic test with a flashlight in a dark room. Shine it through the scrotum from behind. If light easily passes through, the mass is probably filled with fluid—typical of a harmless hydrocele or spermatocele, which I'll discuss further on. Exceptions occur, so do this to reassure yourself, not as an excuse to stay away from the doctor. Provided that you're gentle, testis shouldn't hurt, so frank tenderness isn't normal, but it's also not typical of a malignancy.

Only a few percent of testicular masses turn out malignant, but doctors treat them all as cancer until proven otherwise. Fortunately, a skilled urologist can confidently diagnose most benign masses in the office. When suspicions remain, he or she explores the scrotum in the operating room to closely examine and feel the testes. If any doubt persists, he removes that testis and spermatic cord. Doctors don't biopsy a testis because the chance of spreading malignant cells is too great.

Symptoms. Although an occasional patient complains of pain or heaviness, almost all testicular cancer begins as a painless mass. A man performing self-exam is unlikely to develop other symptoms (back pain, cough, weight loss) because these indicate metastases.

Staging. To determine the extent, every man receives a CAT scan and chest X-ray as well as blood tests that check most organs, but specifically the liver. As with prostate cancer, tumor markers secreted by malignant cells give useful hints, so doctors check for substances with names like alpha-fetoprotein and beta-hCG.

The stages:

Stage I: Tumor confined to the testes
Stage II: Tumor spread to the nearby lymph nodes
Stage III: Distant spread

Treatment. Unlike our maddeningly slow improvement in curing many cancers, progress with testicular cancer has proceeded so rapidly that this section may be obsolete by the time you read it, but the general principles will remain.

Unlike prostate cancer, several different cells in the testes can become malignant, and treatment varies depending on the cell type. In all cases, of course, the affected testis has already been removed.

Radiotherapy to the abdomen and groin cures almost everyone with the most common tumor type, called seminoma, provided that it's in stage I or early stage II. Radiotherapy works less well for advanced seminomas, but this is an area of dramatic advance since the 1980s, when experts switched to chemotherapy. As I write, the cure rate for advanced seminoma has passed 80 percent.

For other cell types grouped as nonseminomatous tumors, the usual treatment for stage I disease is surgery to remove nearby lymph nodes, and the cure rate approaches that of a seminoma. With so much progress in chemotherapy, some doctors skip this surgery entirely. Most men suffer a recurrence, but for the minority who do the cure rate with chemotherapy is excellent. Chemotherapy with or without surgery cures most advanced nonseminomas.

Benign Testicular Masses

1. Varicocele. You're unlikely to mistake this clump of varicose veins above a testis (usually on the left) for a solid mass, but it's happened. Since the clump results from veins that swell under high pressure, it should disappear when you lie down. I discuss varicoceles in the section on infertility in Chapter 10.

2. Hydrocele. Fluid often accumulates in one scrotum, forming a cystic mass separate from and in front of one testis. A large hydrocele may seem to surround the entire testis, and a tense cyst feels like a solid mass. Hydroceles are harmless, but a doctor should confirm the diagnosis because the cyst rarely conceals a tumor. Treatment isn't necessary, but for diagnostic purposes the doctor may extract the fluid (which should be clear and yellow) with a syringe or order ultrasound, a test which accurately separates solid tissue from liquid.

3. Spermatocele. Smaller than a hydrocele, this is a cyst attached to the epididymus just above a testis. Most are freely movable and measure less than half an inch in diameter. Treatment isn't necessary, but a doctor can shrink the cyst by aspiration, which should produce milky fluid containing dead sperm.

Hernias. *Hernia* is a medical term meaning "protrusion of tissue through an abnormal opening," so hernias can exist throughout the body. It may sound odd to discuss the subject in a section on testicular masses, but that is where almost all of a man's hernias make their appearance.

If you remember Chapter 1, testes first appear in the fetal abdomen at eight weeks, gradually descending to reach the scrotum during the eighth month. Once testes leave the abdominal cavity, it's important that they don't return, so the passage into the scrotum closes. Unfortunately, this is another defective design, so the passage remains open in 20 percent of men. Almost all go through life without a problem, but occasionally a piece of bowel slips into the opening. Since it's an "abnormal opening," this fits the definition of a hernia—in this case an inguinal hernia, *inguinal* being a medical term for groin.

Traditionally men notice an inguinal hernia after heavy lifting, a reasonable connection because any action that increases abdominal pressure (exercise, vomiting, persistent constipation) can push an organ through any available opening. Hernias also increase with age as the general slackening of tissues enlarges the passage.

Because their abdominal organs rest in close proximity to two potential openings, males suffer 90 percent of inguinal hernias.

Painless hernias are generally harmless. A man may notice only a lump in the groin or a soft mass in one scrotum which disappears on pressure, especially if he lies down. Occasionally an amazing amount of bowel descends into the hernia; textbook photos show men with a scrotum the size of a football. Provided that one can easily reduce the hernia (i.e., push it back), there is no urgency about repairing it, but all hernias must be repaired. If a piece of bowel becomes jammed tightly into the opening (strangulated) so that blood supply is cut off, this is an emergency because the bowel quickly becomes gangrenous.

See a doctor if you think you have a hernia; do the same for any groin pain during exertion that quickly resolves, even if no lump is present.

How to Handle Painful Testicles

Epididymitis

In the leading cause of a painful testicle in adult men, the testicle itself is normal. Pain arises in the epididymus, the beginning of the spermatic cord, which originates at the bottom of the testis and coils behind it. Sperm rest in the epididymus until ejaculation, when they travel up the cord and empty into the urethra inside the prostate. Because of this proximity, men with epididymitis always complain of pain in a testicle.

Cause. Bacterial infection is the culprit, usually by the same gonococcus or chlamydia responsible for urethritis. Experts theorize that high pressure in the urethra forces infected urine backward up the spermatic cord to the epididymus. Sexual arousal remains the leading source of pressure, but older men occasionally suffer when bacteria spread from an infected prostate.

The Usual Course. Epididymitis almost always attacks on one side. Pain begins gradually, rising to an unpleasant crescendo over one to three days. Although pain may appear abruptly, this is more likely to indicate torsion (discussed later). A man may experience other symptoms of an infected urinary tract such as fever, discharge from the urethra, or urinary burning, but mostly he notices pain.

Diagnosis. A doctor's examination reveals a normal testicle, but the cord-like epididymus behind it feels swollen and tender. If a stoic patient delays coming in, the entire scrotum may be swollen and painful. We order a urinalysis and perhaps a culture to search for signs of infection; results are usually negative, but we make the diagnosis despite this.

Treatment. On the rare occasions when gonorrhea turns up, we treat that. Otherwise, doctors give an antibiotic that covers both gonorrhea and chlamydia such as doxycycline, tetracycline, or erythromycin. We treat an older man with trimethoprim-sulfamethoxazole (Bactrim, Septra, Cotrim) when we suspect an infected prostate as the source of his epididymitis.

What Does Torsion of the Testicle Signify?

Mostly a disorder of boys and teenagers, torsion occurs less often than epididymitis in adults, but a man must consider both possibilities when he feels pain. Delaying with an infected epididymus is merely unwise; after a few days of torsion, the testicle is dead.

Causes. If you remember the embryology of sex glands discussed in Chapter 1, testes and ovaries begin from the same primitive tissue deep in the abdomen of the tiny fetus. In a developing girl, ovaries remain where they began, but in a boy the testes descend gradually into the scrotum (this is essential to keep them cool; sperm die at body temperature, so a man with undescended testes is sterile).

As a result of its long descent, each testicle hangs suspended from a spermatic cord that supplies arteries, veins, and nerves as well as a tube for carrying off sperm. This design allows the testicle to twist back and forth, and occasionally one twists too far and becomes stuck. No one knows why this happens; activity isn't responsible because torsion often occurs during sleep. Cold weather increases the risk, so local muscle contraction may play a part. The incidence drops rapidly after age thirty, one benefit of the general loss of flexibility that comes with age.

The Usual Course. A typical torsion begins abruptly with excruciating pain, often accompanied by vomiting. No one with this onset delays seeing a doctor; unfortunately one third of cases begin gradually. Torsion cuts off the blood supply, so it's an emergency. See a doctor immediately for any severe testicular pain. Restoring the blood supply within six hours saves 80 to 100 percent of glands. After two days this drops to 20 percent.

Diagnosis. We suspect torsion if the history is typical. Examination is difficult because the affected side is swollen and tender. It's reassuring to feel an enlarged, painful epididymus and ominous to see one testis tilted out of position, but the only reliable tests are either an ultrasound or a radioactive tracer scan, both of which measure blood flow. In torsion, these show no flow in the affected testis; flow is normal or increased in an inflammation such as epididymitis.

Treatment. In torsion, the left testis always rotates counterclockwise, the right clockwise, so a skilled doctor can unscrew a twisted gland, but even if successful, surgery is essential. The surgeon restores the testis to its normal position and then fixes both glands to the scrotum to prevent futures twisting.

Orchitis—Inflamed Testes

Orchitis is an inflammation of the testes, and it's rare except for the orchitis that complicates mumps. A diagnosis of mumps terrifies many of my adult patients, who assume that they have a good chance of becoming sterile. This is possible, I assure them, but less likely than they believe.

Cause. The mumps virus usually affects the parotid (a salivary gland) in children, producing gross swelling behind the jaw with fever and generalized illness that lasts about a week. Now and then the virus infects other organs, most commonly (for unknown reasons) the testes. This almost never happens before puberty.

The Usual Course. Mumps is not more severe in adults, and despite their fears orchitis affects only 20 to 30 percent of patients. Only 10 percent of infections involve both testes. Symptoms begin suddenly three to four days after the parotids swell, with high fever and a tender, swollen testicle. The illness resolves in a week or less, and about half the affected testes shrink over the next two months. An atrophied testicle usually produces less sperm, but a man with one normal testicle loses no fertility. Even bilateral orchitis doesn't guarantee sterility, although the prognosis is not good if both glands atrophy a great deal. There is no treatment.

Prevention. Mumps immunization works well. An adolescent who can't remember having mumps should make sure he's had the vaccine.

THE MALE ORGAN

Although this seems like an essential male organ, may animals do without it. Male and female birds, for example, share an identical opening, called a cloaca, that serves all excretory and sexual functions. Semen, eggs, and body waste pass through the cloaca, and it works fine.

Unlike other male organs such as the prostate, the penis remains surprisingly trouble free throughout life. Infections enter through the urethral opening, but most spread through sex and are easy to prevent. This is not the case for other bodily orifices, such as the nose and mouth, which pass a host of tiresome, unavoidable, and occasionally serious infections. As a conduit for urine, the penis provides a more convenient exit than the female equivalent as well as almost 100 percent protection against bladder infections—a persistent problem that women suffer as a result of their shorter urethra. As an organ of impregnation, it almost always works perfectly; impotence rarely results from disease in the penis itself. Finally, penile cancer is not only rare, it's mostly preventable.

You can read about infections in Chapter 10, on sexually transmitted diseases. Impotence is discussed in Chapter 11, including most of what you should know about penile anatomy and function.

The Foreskin and its Controversy

If you are among the 80 percent or more of American men circumcised as an infant, this is not a pressing part of your health education, although you'll encounter the subject if you have children. For the remainder and for most foreign readers, your foreskin is the source of a fair number of penile problems and the center of a small but surprisingly emotional controversy.

An ancient ritual among Jews and Moslems, newborn circumcision isn't performed routinely for nonreligious purposes in most countries, but the United States is an exception. For most of this century, doctors justified it as a health measure to improve hygiene as well as prevent infections and penile cancer. Like many beliefs held by both doctors and laypeople, this belief was based on common sense—meaning that everyone assumed it worked so no one bothered to prove it. Similar vague reasoning justified tonsillectomies, once performed on so many children.

Inevitably, some doctors noticed the lack of scientific proof, and by the 1970s many began to oppose routine circumcision. Medical organizations that took circumcision for granted grew uneasy. In 1971 the American Academy of Pediatrics announced that there were no valid medical indications for newborn circumcisions. Doctors took notice, and the rate of circumcision began to drift downward—from almost 90 percent to under 60 percent by 1990.

Ironically, during this period genuine evidence appeared for circumcision's benefits. Studies showed that uncircumcised boys suffer ten to thirty-nine times more urinary tract infections in infancy and 2½ times more from boyhood to adolescence. Although treatable, a small percentage of infections end in permanent kidney damage. Minor infections, as well as most sexually transmitted diseases, occur more frequently in uncircumcised men. As a result, some experts began publicly to favor the operation; in 1989 the Academy of Pediatrics changed its mind and announced that circumcision provided potential benefits.

To my amusement, the parties in this debate have switched the basis of their arguments. Those in favor now cite scientific evidence. Opponents appeal to common sense, insisting that vigorous penile hygiene prevents all the aforementioned complications. The pages of solemn medical journals occasionally resound with sarcastic exchanges as doctors accuse each other of greed, quackery, and unscientific thinking.

I am mildly in favor of routine circumcision, performed shortly after birth under local anesthesia by a skilled doctor. Afterward, I don't recommend it unless the boy or man suffers frequent annoying infections under the foreskin. But he must wash the area daily.

Cancer of the Penis

Accounting for 1 in 250 male malignancies in the United States, cancer of the penis is a greater health problem over much of the world, making up over 10 percent of male cancers in China and other Asiatic nations. Israel enjoys the lowest rate—one in a thousand.

Risk Factors and Prevention Does Circumcision Help? Jews have almost no penile cancer. Circumcision provides almost 100 percent protection, a statement supported by the fact that almost all penile cancer occurs on the glans or inner surface of the foreskin. Experts theorize that chronic inflammation aggravated by poor hygiene plays a role, perhaps encouraged by a virus (penile cancer, like cervical cancer in women, may be a sexually transmitted disease). This suggests that men who wash under the foreskin regularly can eliminate their risk, but studies to confirm this would be difficult to perform, so none exist.

Symptoms and Treatment. Any red spot, pimple, crust, or bump that remains after a few weeks is worth bringing to a doctor's attention, especially on the glans or foreskin. Almost all will turn out to be minor disorders and infections, but those are early signs of cancer.

I have seen only one man with this cancer, but his penis was half eaten away by a large ulceration, an unpleasant experience for me and a bad decision by the victim, although I sympathize with the fear that made him procrastinate. Despite affecting an organ with a rich blood supply, penile cancer tends to remain localized for a long time, so doctors cure most early tumors and preserve the penis with radiotherapy or surgery.

What do Abnormal Erections Mean?

Although uncommon, disorders producing a prolonged erection exert a gruesome fascination, so I'll mention two.

In *priapism*, a man's erection remains, usually growing increasingly painful. In 40 percent of cases the patient suffers a distinct disease that affects penile blood flow (such as sickle cell anemia), local infections or injuries, leukemia, a spinal injury, or cocaine use. The remaining 60 percent occur in healthy men, often after prolonged sexual stimulation but not always. Most experts believe that the erection persists because venous drainage becomes obstructed, causing a buildup of increasingly viscous blood within the corpora cavernosa (Chapter 11 describes the structure and blood supply of the penis).

Priapism is an emergency; if allowed to continue for several days, scarring and fibrosis inside the penis leads to impotence. Heavy sedation followed by ice-cold enemas may relieve the erection. If not, doctors evacuate the sludged blood into a needle inserted through the glans.

Peyronie's disease affects middle-aged and older men and begins more slowly. Erections become painful and the erect penis appears bent, often so bent that intercourse is impossible. The man may feel a firm, lumpy area along the shaft: fibrous plaques that contain calcification. No one knows why these form, but they resemble those that appear elsewhere. A plaque in the palm that produces a bent finger is called Dupuytren's contracture.

Half of Peyronie's cases eventually disappear, so doctors who prescribe vitamins, hormones, drugs, or cortisone injections report cures, but these may work no better than a placebo. Surgically removing the plaque may produce impotence, but stubborn cases may require this.

DEALING WITH PROSTATE PROBLEMS

Although men worry about them, serious diseases of their genitals are uncommon, with the exception of VD. A penis and testes may work more slowly as you get old, but they're unlikely to malfunction or seriously inconvenience you.

This is not true of the prostate, an organ the size of a small walnut resting just under the bladder. Although a sex gland, the prostate produces no hormone and isn't essential for intercourse; it manufactures half your ejaculatory fluid, which it secretes into the urethra running conveniently down the middle.

Throughout adulthood, the prostate is prey to obvious bacterial infections, subtle infections, and frustrating inflammatory ailments that were once considered bacterial but probably aren't. After middle age, benign and malignant growths become more prominent.

The Many Faces of Prostatitis

1. Acute bacterial prostatitis: the worst but the easiest to treat.

A man who experiences acute prostatitis never forgets it. Mostly attacking younger adults, it begins suddenly with fever, chills, body aches, and sometimes pain in the prostate—felt in the low back or around the anus. Bacteria usually spread to the nearby bladder, causing the same symptoms that women suffer during a bladder infection (a trio every medical student memorize): frequency, urgency, and dysuria (i.e., frequent urination, an uncontrollable urge to urinate, and burning on urination).

Diagnosis and Treatment. Once we suspect an infection, we confirm it with a rectal exam that reveals a painful, swollen prostate. Unlike our exam for chronic prostatitis (discussed later), we don't massage the prostate to squeeze out pus. It's too painful, and we can find the germs by culturing a urine sample. The usual culprits are bacteria that live around your genitals and rectum, so infections probably occur when germs travel up the urethra into the prostate. No one knows how to prevent acute prostatitis, and it's not sexually transmitted.

Some patients are sick enough to need hospitalization and intravenous antibiotics. If not, acute prostatitis responds quickly to oral antibiotics, usually trimethoprim-sulfamethoxazole (Septra, Bactrim, Cotrim). When urine culture results return in two days, we switch antibiotics if the bacteria turn out to be resistant, but this is rare.

Prostate infections are more stubborn than those in other organs, so treatment must continue for at least a month. Some patients complain of mild urinary irritation for months after a cure, but this disappears eventually.

2. Chronic bacterial prostatitis: stubborn and not so easy.

Although caused by the same bacteria as acute prostatitis, symptoms are less unpleasant. The downside is that symptoms occur again and again. More common than acute prostatitis, it affects adults of all ages.

When their infection remains in the prostate, patients feel fine or notice only a tiresome ache in the low back, anus, or testes; when it spreads to the bladder they suffer frequency, urgency, and dysuria. Fever or severe illness are rare. Sexual function isn't diminished. The drugs that work in acute prostatitis also work here, but not for long.

To say that chronic bacterial prostatitis occurs when bacteria persist despite treatment doesn't give you more information (that's what *chronic* means: persistent). No one knows why this happens.

Diagnosis and Treatment. A simple urinalysis is often normal. Fortunately, a chronically infected prostate is not as tender as an acutely infected one, so we get better information by massaging it with a finger to force some fluid into the urethra. A urinalysis after a massage is more revealing.

This works fine for the first infection or two, but after a few recurrences, we want to make sure you don't have a deceptive problem somewhere else in the urinary tract. To localize the infection, we perform the traditional "three-glass urinalysis," which medical students learn but may forget unless they become urologists.

The Three-Glass Urinalysis: What it Means. You shouldn't have this test during an infection (some doctors forget this) because the germs are everywhere, so the test doesn't localize. Once you've had a course of antibiotics and feel fine, a doctor can determine if bacteria persist somewhere. To prepare, avoid sex for five days to ensure a prostate full of secretions. You should also have a full bladder, but if you arrive on time for the appointment and wait until the doctor is caught up, that should be no problem.

The first glass: Urinate directly into the container. That washes out any infection inside the penis to check for a subtle urethritis, such as NGU (see Chapter 10).

The second glass: Urinate into the toilet until your bladder is half empty; then collect another ounce in the glass. This midstream specimen represents urine from the bladder and kidney.

Following this the doctor massages your prostate. Any secretion that oozes from your penis is a bonus that is collected in a separate container.

The third glass: Finish urinating and collect the last ounce, which concentrates prostate secretions. We sometimes skip this step if we obtain plenty of fluid directly from the massage.

Other tests are less revealing, but after a few infections, you'll get an X-ray called an IVP (intravenous pyelogram), where dye injected into a vein is excreted quickly by the kidneys, outlining the urinary tract. Sooner or later a urologist will look inside with his or her instruments to search for obstructions such as a narrow urethra or enlarged prostate; obstructions encourage infections. Sometimes they turn up, but usually not.

Treatment. The primary treatment is long-term antibiotics. Therapy can be frustrating because a chronically infected prostate is not fiercely inflamed. The severely inflamed acute prostate makes a patient miserable, but inflamed tissue is leaky, so antibiotics from the blood pour into the prostate and quickly kill germs. Although victims of chronic infections suffer less, antibiotics penetrate their prostates very slowly. A large dose for three months is typical, and some doctors treat for longer.

The best drugs are trimethoprim-sulfamethoxazole and doxycycline (Vibramycin, Doryx, Vibra-tabs). Used for many years with relatively few side-effects, these antibiotics have another advantage that some doctors rarely consider: They're cheap. I stress this because a new class of antibiotic, called the fluoroquinolones (Cipro, Floxin), appeared in the late 1980s. Wildly expensive but excellent for many obscure infections that I never encounter, fluoroquinolones also work for common ones including prostatitis, and it's reasonable to try one if several attempts and older antibiotics fail.

Despite vast advertising and great popularity, no evidence exists that Cipro or Floxin are superior to doxycycline, but doctors are no different from the average American in their eagerness to try new developments. You may want to quote me to your doctor if he or she decides to start you on one of these first. Three months of Cipro will set you back well over $1,000.

One course of doxycycline (Septra, etc.) provides permanent cure perhaps 30 percent of the time. Several courses after several recurrences raise this to 50 percent. Frustrated patients ask about surgery. This works in some limited cases—for example, if a prostatic stone provides a site of infection. Otherwise the chance of success is one in three.

When it's clear that nothing will eradicate the infection, we can reliably suppress recurrences by prescribing a smaller dose of antibiotic daily for the rest of your life. Although this is safe, you shouldn't begin without absolute proof that you have a chronic bacterial infection, so you'll have many prostate massages with cultures and a thorough urological exam. This is necessary because antibiotics are useless in an even more common but similar disorder, nonbacterial prostatitis.

3. Nonbacterial prostatitis: the most common kind.

Unfortunately, this is the largest category. Victims suffer pain in the usual areas of the anus, low back, and testes as well as frequency, urgency, and dysuria, but we never find an infection.

Many theories try to explain this—a sure sign of our ignorance. Some experts blame microorganisms that are difficult to detect, such as chlamydia (see Chapter 10), but attempts to prove this have failed. On the other hand, nonbacterial prostatitis tends to attack younger, sexually active men, so this theory remains popular. Another school teaches that these prostates are abnormally congested, perhaps because their outlets are obstructed. Finally, there is speculation that nonbacterial prostatitis is an autoimmune disease in which the body attacks itself, similar to some forms of arthritis.

Diagnosis and Treatment. This is a "diagnosis of exclusion." We search for something easier to treat; if nothing turns up, we call it nonbacterial prostatitis.

X-rays and a urological exam are normal. Examination of prostatic fluid reveals white blood cells, a sign of inflammation. But inflammation is simply a reaction of the body to a host of disturbances. White cells occur during infection but also during allergic and autoimmune reactions, generalized irritation, and simple injuries.

On the chance that chlamydia or another obscure infection is responsible, you'll probably get a month of antibiotic, most likely doxycycline or tetracycline. Erythromycin attacks the same organisms, but in the proper dose (500 milligrams four times a day) it's hard on the stomach. Trimethoprim-sulfamethoxazole doesn't kill chlamydia.

Urologists traditionally recommend regular sex to keep the prostate drained (the excess congestion theory is particularly popular with urologists). As a supplement, they perform regular prostate massages. Studies to prove that massage helps aren't impressive, but a handful of my patients are convinced. Finally, we prescribe hot baths, antispasmodics, tranquilizers, and the same antiinflammatories that women take for menstrual cramps: ibuprofen (Motrin, Advil, Nuprin, Medipren) and their relatives.

All this is less futile than it sounds. Provided that both doctor and patient are persistent in running through these remedies, most victims feel some relief.

4. Prostatodynia.

A medical term for painful prostate, this is the diagnosis when we encounter the aforementioned symptoms but no abnormalities after prostate massage or urinalysis. Urologists theorize (and their tests occasionally hint) that muscle spasm is responsible, so they prescribe hot baths as well as prazosin (Minipress), baclofen (Lioresal), and other muscle relaxants with fair results.

Nowadays no doctor in his or her right mind suggests that menstrual cramps are psychosomatic, but we have no inhibitions toward male genital pain, so experts freely recommend tranquilizers and psychotherapy. Since a skilled psychotherapist makes any medical problem more bearable, go along if the therapist is good and you can afford it. But try simpler treatments first.

PROSTATIC ENLARGEMENT

Strictly speaking, prostatic enlargement is not a disease but an inevitable part of aging. Tiny in boys, the prostate grows to adult size during puberty under the influence of male hormone. Between ages twenty and forty-five it remains stable and then undergoes a second growth spurt. By age eighty, almost every man has benign prostatic hypertrophy (BPH).

Testicles are required for BPH because castration prevents it. Also essential, testosterone has little affect on the prostate until converted into dihydrotestosterone, a more powerful male hormone that's responsible for most androgenic action throughout the body. With advancing age, the prostate seems to convert more testosterone into dihydrotestosterone, but other hormonal changes also play a role, so experts don't understand completely why hypertrophy occurs.

No matter how swollen, an aging prostate would cause no difficulty if it weren't for a clumsy flaw in the design of the urinary tract: The urethra runs through the prostate, which surrounds it on all sides, a path that guarantees trouble.

Symptoms

Trouble comes suddenly when the enlarged prostate completely obstructs the urethra. Although a frightening experience, acute urinary retention is easy to relieve by inserting a catheter, and after a few days the prostate usually shrinks enough to allow urination. An occasional complication of prostatitis, acute urinary retention marks the first symptom of BPH in about 10 percent of men. The rest become gradually aware that something is not right as their growing prostate slowly constricts the urethra.

Most often in his sixties (65 on the average for whites, 60 for blacks, later for orientals, who suffer less BPH), a man notices a weaker urinary stream. It doesn't carry as far and may look thinner. Perhaps he must strain several seconds before the bladder generates enough pressure to overcome resistance and begin emptying. If it can't maintain pressure, the stream stops, often with dribbling or squirting, so the man must resume straining. Once aware of these symptoms, most men realize that they had been coming on slowly for some time.

Although annoying, a weak stream is not necessarily an ominous sign, and BPH doesn't always progress further. Many men are never inconvenienced enough to consult a doctor, but you should go because other conditions (cancer, infections) produce the same symptom.

As the urethra continues to narrow, men prefer to sit on the toilet, partly to pass time until the bladder builds up pressure, partly because sitting relaxes pelvic muscles around the urethra. Eventually the bladder reaches its limit; despite a maximum effort, it can't empty completely.

When a man with BPH has residual urine, his problems increase. Retained urine invites infection, but even without infection life begins to revolve around the bathroom. A full bladder normally triggers the urge to urinate, so a man with a bladder always partly full feels the urge more often. Matters are made worse because an overstrained bladder may become irritable, contracting when it isn't full, so a victim may hurry to the bathroom, urinate only a little, and assume that his obstruction is worse than it is. Since frequency is worse at night, he may find himself getting up every hour or two (nocturia).

At this point, few men have the stamina to stay away from the doctor. This is fortunate because pressure from a swollen bladder eventually overcomes the one-way valves in ureters, tubes that carry urine from the kidney. Backup (reflux) of urine obstructs outflow from the kidneys, making them swell and eventually causing permanent damage. Men with BPH once died of kidney failure; this shouldn't happen today.

Diagnosis

A urinalysis detects infection but is otherwise unhelpful. Blood tests show kidney damage in the most severe cases.

A rectal exam gives better evidence. To the doctor's finger, a normal prostate feels like a rubbery lump with a groove down the middle—similar to the tip of your nose. Enlarged, it can grow as large as a baseball, and the groove disappears. You should realize that the doctor is feeling the rear of the prostate, which pushes into the rectum. No matter how massive, this does no harm because only the forward lobes of the prostate surround the urethra. Determining the degree of obstruction requires more sophisticated tests.

A residual urine over 150 cubic centimeters (about 5 ounces) is abnormal. Traditionally doctors measure by inserting a catheter after urination; today a bladder ultrasound can accomplish this more comfortably but at greater cost.

An experienced doctor can estimate obstruction by watching a patient urinate into a graduated flask and timing the rise with the minute hand of a watch. Nowadays, of course, electronic instruments can measure flow rate and bladder pressure.

An intravenous pyelogram (IVP) outlines the entire urinary tract, so it detects swollen kidneys, obstructed ureters, and stones. Experts debate whether an IVP is useful in uncomplicated BPH, but urologists routinely order one.

Occasionally blood appears in the urine of a man with BPH. This triggers a cystoscopy, an office procedure performed under local anesthesia in which the urologist inserts a flexible tube through the penis and inspects the urethra, prostate, and bladder. Bloody urine from BPH is not an ominous sign, but the urologist must make sure that the sources isn't another disorder such as a bladder tumor. Although not essential for the average enlarged prostate, cystoscopies are often done because urologists want to look directly at whatever they're dealing with.

Treatment

Don't assume that surgery is inevitable. Only 10 percent of men who reach forty require surgery for BPH by age eighty, so the odds are heavy that you can get by on less.

Once you notice a weaker urinary stream, see your family doctor. A urologist isn't necessary for early BPH, but your doctor must make sure that BPH is what it is. Although the leading cause of a weak stream, prostatic hypertrophy is the first on a long, long list.

Then expect the traditional advice about avoiding spices, excessive alcohol, and irritative foods. Like most traditional advice, no evidence exists that it works, but it's harmless and gives patients a sense of self-control. The truth is that anyone having trouble urinating quickly discovers what makes it worse, so my patients come to their own conclusions. Experiment with food and make your own rules.

Don't experiment with fluids. Drinking less in an effort to avoid trips to the bathroom encourages infections; drinking more to flush out the tract makes the overworked bladder work still more. Drink about two quarts of fluid a day as recommended earlier.

Drugs Can Improve Urine Flow

Prostatic hypertrophy is an aging process, and like all aging processes (hearing loss, cataracts, osteoporosis, muscle atrophy) we'll find ways to slow them or ease the consequences, but stopping the cold is unlikely. Until recently drugs to shrink the prostate either worked feebly or worked well but caused intolerable side-effects. Modest progress has occurred during the past few years, so I believe the future holds promise.

Alpha-blockers. These drugs don't shrink the prostate at all but relax smooth muscle in the urethra and bladder outlet. Unlike muscles that moves your limbs and body (striated muscle), smooth muscle works without conscious control in tissue such as the bowel, stomach, urinary tract, genitals, and arteries. Relaxing arterial smooth muscle became a big priority in the 1940s, when we realized that high blood pressure was a deadly disease and not merely another vital sign like fever and pulse rate.

Early drugs lowered blood pressure dramatically by relaxing arterial smooth muscle, but they relaxed smooth muscle everywhere. In fact, they relaxed everything. Patients became drowsy, dizzy, constipated, impotent, and they stopped sweating and salivating. It took a lot of encouragement to keep patients with high blood pressure on these pills. Older hypertensives couldn't tolerate them, so they were impractical for BPH.

As time passed, newer drugs lowered blood pressure with fewer and fewer side-effects. With one exception, they don't work by relaxing smooth muscle, so they don't help BPH. The exception is a class called alpha-blockers, developed in the early 1980s. Members of this class, such as prazosin (Minipress), terazosin (Hytrin), or doxazosin (Cardura) modestly improve urine flow and diminish frequency and nocturia. Side-effects, mostly dizziness, aren't common. Costing several dollars a day, these are not cheap, but many men find that they make life more pleasant. I prescribe these first because, unlike hormones (discussed next), alpha-blockers work quickly. Any improvement will be apparent in a few days.

Hormonal Therapy Can Help. As I mentioned, castration prevents BPH. Nowadays no one is exploring possibilities of this treatment, but nineteenth-century doctors were more adventurous. An 1896 study of sixty-one men found that fifty improved dramatically after their testes were removed. Despite these encouraging results, no one recommends castration today. Less heroic ways to block testicular hormones have become a real possibility.

Several FDA-approved drugs do this. Leuprolide (Lupron) reduces pituitary hormones that stimulate the testes. Flutamide (Eulexin) blocks the action of male hormones throughout the body. Although both shrink the prostate, they are breathtakingly expensive, and they produce impotence and a reduced libido. Helpful in prostate cancer, they are rarely used for BPH.

As the history of antihypertensives shows, drugs work better with fewer side-effects as their site of action becomes narrower, and this is happening with BPH therapy. In 1992 the FDA approved finasteride (Proscar), the first drug that has no effect on testosterone but blocks its conversion to dihydrotestosterone. Unless an unexpected problem turns up, finasteride should replace all other drug treatments. Although the best drug, it works slowly, requiring three months to produce the maximum shrinkage (about 28 percent). Ninety percent of men enjoy a significant improvement in urine flow as long as they take the drug, and they must take it indefinitely. Side-effects, including impotence and decreased libido, are surprisingly rare. The major inconvenience is cost—several dollars per day.

Blocking conversion of testosterone to dihydrotestosterone holds promise for treating disorders such as male baldness and acne and perhaps excessive hairiness in women. It may also have a role in treating prostate cancer. Studies of all these possibilities are in progress.

Overcoming Obstruction: Balloon Dilatation. Since the early 1980s, cardiologists have been threading a long tube into their patients' coronary arteries and then blowing up a balloon to unblock them. Despite the skill required, angioplasty is now routine, and patients prefer it to coronary bypass surgery.

Threading a tube into the bladder requires much less skill, so unblocking a urethra doesn't seem difficult. Yet despite widespread publicity in the media, it doesn't work terribly well. Arteries respond better because they are lined with rock-hard cholesterol; once stretched, they tend to stay stretched. The rubbery prostate isn't so cooperative.

Researchers who measure urine flow after dilatation usually find a small improvement that fades within a year. Despite this, a minority of urologists remain enthusiastic, and patients almost always feel better. I can understand why. Given a choice between surgery and dilatation, I wouldn't think twice, and neither would most men. I encourage patients to try it.

Overcoming Obstruction: Hyperthermia. Heat shrinks the prostate, but the amount required damages other tissue. With the development of a surface-cooling device to protect the urethra, urologists have begun heating enlarged prostates with a transurethral microwave probe. Treatment takes an hour and requires only local anesthesia.

With some effort, you can find a urologist who uses hyperthermia, but most don't because it's still an experimental procedure (so medical insurance won't pay). As I write, clinical trials are underway at medical centers around the country. The results seem promising, and when researchers announce the outcome in a few years, hyperthermia may become routine.

Overcoming Obstruction: Tubes and Stents. In previous centuries the elderly carried a straw or metal tube to use whenever urination became impossible. Such "in and out" catheterization encourages injury and infections, so doctors frown on it today. With all our mechanical ingenuity, you'd think we could design a permanently implanted hollow rod (stent), perhaps with a one-way valve, to keep the urethra open no matter how much the prostate swells. It seems simple, but apparently it isn't. Even when they don't provoke infections, foreign bodies in the urinary tract lead to stones, inflammation, and a rapid buildup of calcium deposits. Research continues.

When Surgery is Recommended

In our lifetime, surgery will be the best treatment BPH. We try not to wait for kidney damage or complete blockage before recommending it, but this is rarely necessary. Men themselves make the decision when their symptoms become too tiresome. See your doctor regularly to check the status of your urinary tract, and decide for yourself.

Prostate Surgery: The TURP. Ninety-five percent of BPH operations are a transurethral resection of the prostate (TURP). Popular since the 1940s and performed on 400,000 men per year, it's the most common surgery on people over sixty-five. Unlike earlier prostate operations, the surgeon doesn't open the abdomen to reach the prostate, so both operation and recovery time are shorter.

Transurethral means just that. The urologist inserts an instrument called a resectoscope through the urethra into the bladder. Under direct vision, he or she manipulates a wire loop to slice off pieces of prostate. An electric current in the loop cuts the tissue and cauterizes blood vessels to reduce bleeding, but plenty of bleeding occurs. To keep the field of vision clear, a stream of fluid washes blood and pieces of prostate into the bladder. At the end, the surgeon evacuates the tissue and fluid and inserts a catheter for two or three days. The operation should take less than half an hour and can often be performed under local or spinal anesthesia (ask for these if the doctor doesn't mention them; you may prefer to sleep, but local anesthesia is safer).

The urologist sends the prostate pieces to a pathologist for a microscopic examination; cancer turns up in 10 percent. If this sounds high, remember that most TURPs are performed on the elderly, so it's probably the expected risk.

Complications—Immediate. The TURP is not a major operation, so serious complications aren't common. In the hands of a good urologist, the death rate is about 1 in 250—high for routine surgery, but remember that many patients are in their seventies and eighties, with other medical problems. As in other surgery on the elderly, the operation itself causes fewer deaths than the heart attacks or strokes that it provokes. If you're in good health, this risk approaches zero.

During surgery, every patient absorbs about a quart of irrigating fluid, the equivalent of drinking a quart of water. Most men tolerate this, but absorbing too much leads to the leading complication: the TURP syndrome. A mild case produces mental confusion with nausea and vomiting, but it can lead to high blood pressure, heart failure, and seizures. Keeping operating time short minimizes the risk. Most urologists stop and change to another procedure if they can't finish in an hour.

Bloody urine diminishes after several days but occasionally persists off and on for a month. Sometimes I see a frightened patient discharged a few weeks before with normal urine who suddenly sees a gush of blood. Unless he is passing clots or has a clot obstructing the urethra, no treatment is necessary, and bleeding usually stops in a few days. Phone the doctor if this happens.

What You Can Expect Afterwards. A good operation, the TURP satisfies over 90 percent of patients. Their urine flows as freely as it did twenty years earlier. Men occasionally suffer urgency and loss of control for several weeks, but permanent incontinence occurs only rarely—in less than 1 percent.

Working inside the prostrate instead of outside, the urologist is less likely to injure nerves to the genitals, so the risk of impotence is small—perhaps one or two in a hundred. However, surgery distorts the walls of the urethra, making the path of the ejaculate unpredictable. Half or more of patients ejaculate backward: into the bladder instead of out the penis. Although this sounds distressing, retrograde ejaculation doesn't interfere with erection or the sense of orgasm. Men are usually sterile, but a doctor can recover sperm from the urine for artificial insemination.

As years or decades pass, about 20 percent of men require a second operation either to correct narrowing of the urethra from scar tissue or to remove more prostate as it continues to grow.

Alternatives to the TURP: Open Prostatectomy. Because of the dangers of fluid absorption, a TURP shouldn't take more than an hour, so a urologist whose patient has a very large prostate performs an open prostatectomy through an incision in the low abdomen or between the legs. The urologist does the same if he or she wants to correct a bladder abnormality at the same time or if the urethra has a stricture too narrow for the resectoscope.

Open prostatectomy takes longer; more bleeding occurs, and a catheter remains for seven to ten days instead of two or three. Otherwise, it works as well as a TURP with similar long-term results.

Alternatives to the TURP: Transurethral Incision. In this simpler operation, the urologist makes two incisions along the prostate near the bladder neck. Cutting prostate muscle in this area relieves obstruction as well as the TURP, with fewer complications and a shorter hospital stay. Although less effective for the biggest prostates or those with an enlarged median lobe, transurethral incision works well for selected patients. Since it's underused, ask the urologist if you're a candidate.

Removing the entire prostate during BPH surgery would be a nice bonus, eliminating the risk of prostate cancer. Unfortunately, a complete prostatectomy is too complex, so it's never done for benign hypertrophy. Having BPH doesn't increase your risk of cancer, but it also doesn't decrease it, so pay special attention to the next section.

WHAT YOU SHOULD KNOW ABOUT PROSTATE CANCER

The most common malignancy in nonsmoking men, prostate cancer ties for second in deaths with colon cancer. Like most malignancies, cancer of the prostate is a disease of aging, rare under age fifty but increasing steadily thereafter. Examining prostates of men over fifty who have died from other causes, pathologists find cancer in 30 percent. This rises to 40 percent at ages seventy to seventy-nine and two thirds for those aged eighty to eighty-nine. This is less alarming than it sounds because many prostate cancers grow very slowly.

Risk Factors and Prevention

Some cancers (lung, skin) are easy to prevent, but prostate cancer is not among them because it's not clear what causes it. Studies to find who is at highest risk have turned up little to help me in advising patients; being male and growing old are definite factors, but there's nothing you can do about that.

Diet. Despite this, some tantalizing facts emerge. American blacks have a death rate almost double that of whites, yet the incidence in Nigerian blacks is only one sixth that of U.S. blacks. More significant, prostate cancer mortality in Japan is one seventh of ours, but when Japanese move to the United States their rate quickly rises. Everyone theorizes (meaning that no firm proof exists) that dietary differences are responsible. Japanese and Nigerians eat little animal fat but a large amount of green and yellow vegetables. Americans do the opposite, blacks to a greater degree.

I agree with experts on cancer prevention, who urge you to eat less fat and more vegetables. If you're truly serious, eliminate meat entirely. Vegetarians have the lowest risk of most cancers.

Chemicals. Prostate cancer is among the few malignancies *not* associated with smoking. Among industrial chemicals, cadmium is the leading prostate carcinogen; men exposed while working on batteries have a much higher rate. Working the rubber, textile, and fertilizer industry increases the risk, but not dramatically.

Hormones. Alcoholics with cirrhosis have less prostate cancer, perhaps because their damaged liver results in a lower level of testosterone. Although this helps our understanding, it doesn't suggest a practical way to prevent prostate cancer; liver damage, not alcohol, is required.

Men with prostate cancer appear more sexually active and more fertile than average. This could mean that they have increased hormonal activity, but this is equally consistent with an infectious cause (discussed later).

Infections. Cervical cancer in women behaves exactly like a sexually transmitted disease and a virus is the most likely culprit. The more sexual partners a woman has, the greater her risk. Data on prostate cancer are much vaguer. Viral particles turn up when researchers examine malignant prostate tissue under the electron microscope, but this is true for many cancers.

Experts are certain that viruses are involved in many malignancies. They've proved this for a few very rare tumors plus one that is universal, warts, but they're getting close with more common ones (not, unfortunately, prostate cancer, although viruses may play a role).

The Future: We'll Do Better When We Know More. Writers like to discuss basic research and future developments when they don't have good news about the present, and that's the case with preventing prostate cancer.

The last twenty years have produced a flood of knowledge on the biochemistry and genetics of cancer. This frustrates laypeople, who are more interested in practical advice and treatment, but the best scientific progress occurs when we understand exactly what's going on. During the nineteenth century, infectious diseases and mental illness were the worst public health problems. Toward the end of the century, scientists discovered that germs cause infectious diseases. By the middle of the twentieth century, infections had become a minor medical concern. We don't understand mental illness nearly as well, and progress has been more modest.

Once we know what causes cancer (and not just factors that encourage it, like fatty foods or hormones) breakthroughs will follow.

Let's Hope for Some Screening Tests

Everyone would love a test for early prostate cancer as superb as the pap is for cervical cancer or even as good as the mammogram for breast cancer. None exists as I write, but several seem on the horizon, and I predict that one will be added to the annual rectal exam before the turn of the century.

During the late 1980s, urologists held strong opinions on transrectal ultrasound and a blood test called prostatic-specific antigen (PSA). Although excellent for evaluating the progress of prostate cancer and the response to treatment, they explained, they should absolutely never be used in a man without symptoms. They weren't sensitive enough (i.e., they missed too many small tumors—false negatives) or specific enough (i.e., they gave too many abnormal results in normal prostates—false positives).

Research continued; by the early 1990s experts still warned us not to rely on these tests, but they were wavering.

Transrectal ultrasound is an attractive candidate: harmless, more objective than a rectal exam, and (as high-tech exams go) cheap. A probe in the rectum beams sound waves through the prostate. The waves pass through a normal prostate, but any change in density should produce an echo that bounces back to a detector. Reading the pattern of echoes, the doctor can decide if something ominous is present.

Unlike CAT scans or magnetic resonance, ultrasound is old technology, dating from the sonar of World War II. It is superior to X-rays for detecting gallstones and safer for checking a growing fetus. Cardiologists routinely order ultrasound (the echocardiogram) to detect abnormalities in the heart.

Urologists have long used transrectal ultrasound to reveal how far an existing prostate cancer has spread and to measure its change in size after treatment. As the instrument grows more sensitive, we'll use it to detect early cancer, and plenty of studies are in progress.

Prostate-specific antigen (*PSA*) is a protein secreted exclusively by prostate cells and usually elevated in prostate cancer. The more extensive the cancer, the higher the PSA—again usually. After treatment the level falls, so doctors check it regularly during follow-up.

Since its discovery in the early 1980s, researchers have studied PSA for early detection. Results so far are intriguing and perhaps useful. When healthy men were found to have a moderately elevated PSA level (up to 2½ times normal), a biopsy revealed cancer in 22 percent. When PSA was over 2½ times normal, two thirds had cancer. A rectal exam alone would have missed 32 percent of these. The downside is that 20 percent of men with prostate cancer have a normal PSA, and we find an elevated level in 30 to 50 percent of ordinary BPH.

Using PSA for screening today would subject those men to an unnecessary prostate biopsy, but many doctors have begun to use it as a supplement to the rectal exam. No organization included it as part of a routine exam until the American Urological Association did so in 1992, urging men to have a PSA yearly after age fifty. This provoked an outcry from many nonurologists, but the American Cancer Society came around a few months later, so the tide is turning. I have the test myself and give patients the choice, but evidence that the benefits outweigh the risks remains borderline.

Recognizing the Symptoms of Prostate Cancer

There are no symptoms in early stages. Unlike prostatic hypertrophy, which affects the area around the urethra, cancer arises on the periphery, so a tumor can grow large before it interferes with urination. Symptoms, when they occur, include a weak stream, frequency, nocturia, and occasionally bloody urine. These are no different from those of BPH, but they tend to come on more quickly—a few months instead of a few years. About a third of victims come to the office because of progressive fatigue, weight loss, or bone pain—symptoms of widespread disease. To make sure you're not among them, pay attention to the next section.

Diagnosis

Malignant tissue is dense, so a doctor running a finger over the rubbery prostate feels a rock-hard lump or an irregularity in texture (only about half of lumps are malignant; the rest are stones, infections, and local areas of benign hyperplasia). After finding an abnormality, the doctor takes a biopsy by inserting a needle into the suspicious area, either through the rectum or the low abdomen.

Hearing the diagnosis after a routine exam will be shocking, but your chance of cure is better than if you'd waited for symptoms. Get a yearly rectal exam beginning at age forty.

Staging

Obviously treatment of a small cancer differs from one that has spread, so every patient undergoes a battery of tests to evaluate the size and extension of the original tumor and check for spread outside the prostate, which we call metastases.

The simplest blood tests detect anemia as well as abnormalities in the kidney, liver, and bone. The doctor will also order one of the prostate tumor markers, most likely the PSA. Like most simple tests, these work better at providing hints than definite answers. Normal results on the entire battery are a hopeful sign, but a minority of cancers have spread despite this.

Everyone receives a chest X-ray and transrectal ultrasound, as well as an IVP to outline the urinary tract. Equally routine is a bone scan, in which injected radioactive tracer concentrates in areas of increased bone activity. Although more sensitive than an X-ray, a positive scan doesn't prove the presence of bone metastases because other abnormalities (injuries, infections, arthritis) also con-centrate tracer, but a negative scan is evidence against spread. This is good news because when prostate cancer spreads, it spreads to bone over three quarters of the time.

Despite their impressive size and great expense, CT and magnetic resonance scanners have no distinct role in evaluating the prostate; some doctors use them to define the size of a tumor, although transrectal ultrasound seems better.

Doctors are anxious to determine if nearby lymph nodes contain cancer, so some patients undergo lymphangiography, in which dye is injected into lymph vessels in the feet, and X-rays outline the vessels and lymph glands as dye passes through the pelvis. A simpler technique is to aspirate tissue from lymph nodes through a long needle; a complicated one is to open the abdomen surgically and sample nodes directly. Surgery is more accurate and more risky, but no tech-nique identifies all affected nodes. Some experts skip this step except for patients being considered for a radical prostatectomy (discussed later).

The stages:

Stage A: These are cancers that turn up on prostatectomy but can't be felt on a rectal exam. In the past, doctors prescribed no treat-ment if only a few tiny areas of cancer appeared, but studies showed that 16 percent of these spread after eight years, so we are now more aggressive with younger patients.

Stage B: Cancer detected on rectal exam but confined inside the prostate, with no evidence of metastases. Despite the best stag-ing tests, some have spread to nearby lymph nodes, but most may be curable.

Stage C: These extend outside the prostate capsule without evi-dence of metastases. Lymph nodes are affected half the time.

Stage D: Distant metastases, usually to bone. Lymph nodes are always involved.

The Best Treatment: Surgery

A treatment for stages A and B, surgery produces a fifteen-year survival equal to men with no prostate cancer. Although this sounds excellent, there's less here than meets the eye. Prostate cancer grows slowly, and most patients are old, so many die of other causes while their cancer remains. As I write, evidence that treating prostate cancer with either surgery or radiation prolongs life long enough to make it worth the risk and side-effects is surprisingly thin. Your doctor (probably a urologist) should discuss the pros and cons of every treatment, but you must also consult an oncologist (a doctor who specializes in cancer but performs neither surgery nor radiotherapy) to hear the most unbiased opinion.

During the operation called a radical prostatectomy, the surgeon removes the entire prostate and seminal vesicles as well as part of the spermatic cord. Dating from the early 1900s, the original operation is safe with a mortality of about 1 percent, but impotence afterward is almost certain. Nearly everyone suffers urinary incontinence during healing, but control returns after six months in nearly everyone.

In the 1980s, surgeons modified the radical prostatectomy in an effort to avoid damaging nerves to the penis. This reduces postoperative impotence to 20 percent with no obvious increase in recurrences. However, since we wait fifteen years before considering prostate cancer cured, we can't yet be certain of this. Your surgeon will have the latest evidence.

Another Form of Treatment: Radiation Therapy

Radiation works by damaging tissue, and it's most harmful to active tissue. Cells are most active when they divide, so rapidly dividing cells such as cancers are more sensitive than those that reproduce slowly. In the end, radiation damages all tissues to some extent, so radiation therapists must be as careful with their beams as surgeons with their knives.

Although other techniques of delivering radiation exist, external-beam irradiation is what most people visualize. A machine similar to an X-ray camera generates the beam, which is focused carefully on a target. A radiation oncologist calculates the proper dose for an individual tumor, and then technicians deliver it in a series of treatments. A typical course might be three times a week for six weeks. You'll see an accurate depiction of preparation for radiation therapy in the movie *The Doctor*, although I hope you'll be treated with more consideration than its hero.

Radiotheraphy works for stages A and B. Surgery works better for A and smaller tumors in stage B, so we recommend radiation only if a patient is very old or can't tolerate an operation. Radiation becomes the choice in stage C and for larger tumors in B because the chance of lymph node spread is high. A therapist can radiate a wider area of nodes than a surgeon can remove.

In selected patients with localized stage B or C, a surgeon removes nearby lymph nodes and then implants seeds of iodine 125 throughout the prostate. This iodine's radioactivity has a long halflife of sixty days—meaning that it isn't terribly intense but the radioactivity lasts a long time: over a year. Called interstitial irradiation, it avoids major surgery and produces few side-effects, especially impotence, than the external beam.

Finally, we can combine interstitial and external-beam therapy. Instead of iodine, the surgeon implants gold 198 into the prostate. Much more energetic with a halflife of only three days, the gold delivers is radioactivity in a few weeks. Using gold alone would produce too much tissue damage, so gold delivers only part of the dose. Later an external beam provides the rest.

The Side-Effects: Radiation Therapy. During the first weeks, patients should notice nothing. Then skin in the path of an external beam begins to itch and burn. This disappears after treatment; the doctor will prescribe a cortisone cream. With either external or internal radiation, structures near the prostate receive less radiation but enough to cause side-effects in some patients. Bladder irritation produces frequency and urgency. One third of patients notice rectal pain or diarrhea.

Acute side-effects are temporary, but permanent damage occurs just as it does after surgery. Twelve percent of patients suffer chronic rectal inflammation, and about 10 percent have bladder damage that produces obstruction as well as the symptoms listed earlier. Incontinence is rare, and the rate of impotence is 30 to 40 percent—less than with traditional radical prostatectomy.

Hormone Treatment

Deprived of male hormone, the prostate shrinks. Although removing the testes (orchiectomy) is unacceptable therapy for benign hypertrophy, matters are different when cancer is involved. Adopted in the 1940s, it remains the best treatment for stage D. Eighty percent of patients feel better; if they suffer anemia, bone pain, or urinary obstruction, this diminishes. Compared to years of hormone treatment, orchiectomy probably costs less, and it eliminates drug side-effects. The operation itself is simple, requiring only a few days in the hospital.

Although I'd choose it myself, I understand why many men refuse orchiectomy. As an alternative, we deprive the prostate of male hormone with drugs. Estrogens accomplish this—not directly but by suppressing pituitary hormones that stimulate the testes. In the past we used high doses, which led to the same complications women suffered on old, high-dose birth control pills: fluid retention, heart attacks, and blood clots. Lower doses seem to work as well with fewer (but still some) side-effects.

Estrogen side-effects are reduced to zero with newer synthetic hormones, which are unrelated to estrogens but also block the pituitary. Leuprolide (Lupron) and goseralin (Zoladex) are currently in use, and others are being tested. Given a choice, patients prefer these despite a side-effect not apparent with estrogens, hot flashes. Impotence occurs, but this is also true for estrogens. These new drugs are expensive; a month costs around $1,000, and they must be given by injection.

Antiandrogens are another alternative. Rather than suppress testosterone, they block its action on the prostate. Theoretically antiandrogens produce fewer unpleasant side-effects as well as less impotence, and this may turn out to be true once researchers refine their knowledge. Today we combine flutamide (Eulexin), the first approved antiandrogen, with one of the pituitary blockers to produce a more complete suppression. Antiandrogens as well as other hormonal agents are rarely used alone except in clinical trials. Ask about trials in your area.

Chemotherapy

Unlike hormones, chemotherapeutic drugs kill cells. Like radiation, they produce their greatest damage on rapidly dividing cells; unlike radiation, they can't be focused, so they act throughout the body.

Despite a fearful reputation, chemotherapy cures most victims of a few malignancies such as childhood leukemia. It's helpful in others but doesn't play a significant role in prostate cancer, except in an occasional advanced case after hormones lose their effect. Discuss the pros and cons with your oncologist and ask about clinical trials. As I mentioned in Chapter 4, participating in a clinical trial usually assures you of the best treatment.

Don't Forget Follow-Up Care

Although many malignancies are considered cured after five years, some prostate cancers grow so slowly that no one can agree on a cutoff date; fifteen years is the most popular. After treatment the doctor will see you periodically for the rest of your life. A typical schedule includes a visit every three months for a year, every six months for five years, and then yearly. The doctor always performs a rectal exam and checks the blood level of a tumor marker (which, if high, drops after successful treatment and usually rises with a recurrence). Some visits include a bone scan as well as chest and abdominal X-rays. Transrectal ultrasound's role is still uncertain, but it's so popular that you'll probably have it.

WHAT TO WATCH FOR IN THE MALE BREAST

At some point in their lives, half of all men notice more breast than seems manly, so it's an organ worth knowing about. Rudimentary compared to a woman's, these are not simply the symmetrical nipples that men hardly notice—in contrast to their intense concern for other reproductive organs. Under each nipple lies a trace of genuine breast tissue, including milk ducts, as responsive to hormones as a woman's, capable of swelling and becoming malignant. Occasionally an overstimulated male breast secretes fluid (called witch's milk in a baby), but despite legends, significant milk production doesn't occur.

Breasts of both sexes share a similar nerve supply, so stimulating the male nipple produces sexual arousal second only to stimulating the penis.

Abnormal Breast Swelling

The medical term for this is gynecomastia. In the early stages the man notices a rubbery, movable button just behind the nipple. Later a firm swelling becomes visible; often one breast is larger. A painful breast usually means an infection, although mild tenderness occasionally occurs with gynecomastia. Don't confuse gynecomastia with the enlarged breasts of obesity. Those contain fat and feel softer than real breast tissue (but obesity encourages gynecomastia).

Why Breasts Swell. They do so from estrogen stimulation, so a man who takes extra estrogen (once prescribed to suppress prostate cancer; still used by transsexuals) grows breasts. A surprising paradox: The body synthesizes female hormones from male hormones, so athletes who consume extra male hormones develop gynecomastia. Because fat normally converts male hormones to estrogen, obese men sometimes suffer gynecomastia. Serious liver disease such as alcoholic cirrhosis leads to gynecomastia, probably because liver cells normally inactivate estrogens.

If a man's estrogen level remains normal but male hormone falls, the relative estrogen level increases. This occurs after infections and other diseases of the testes as well as castration. Drugs cause most breast swelling in otherwise healthy men, sometimes by altering hormone levels but often for unknown reasons.

Physiological gynecomastia. During three periods in a man's life, his breasts swell as a result of normal (i.e., physiological) hormonal changes. Although we don't call this a disease, many men are not pleased.

1. Newborn boys show breasts for the first few weeks of life as a result of their mother's estrogen.
2. Both male and female hormones rise during puberty, but male hormone may lag behind. As a result, most adolescent boys show some gynecomastia, often enough to alarm him or his parents and lead to a good number of doctor visits. Treatment is an explanation plus reassurance that it rarely lasts more than a few years.
3. After age sixty-five, 40 percent of men notice gynecomastia, probably because their testosterone level declines faster than their estrogens. Increasing obesity also plays a role.

Diseases That Make the Breasts Grow. Although this include dozens of genetic, malignant, and hormonal disorders, all occur too rarely to discuss in this book. The only common disorder is alcoholism. Liver damage isn't required; alcohol itself suppresses testosterone production, so anyone who drinks regularly can develop gynecomastia. Once cirrhosis appears, breasts are usually obvious.

Estrogen in the Environment. Chickens fed estrogen to encourage growth produced an epidemic of gynecomastia in Puerto Rican boys, and similar incidents have occurred. Estrogens are not routinely used in American meat production, but they're cheap. Anecdotes in the medical literature tell of gynecomastia in a man who used an estrogen-continuing hair cream and after sex with a woman treated with a vaginal estrogen.

Drugs and Gynecomastia. Like impotence, this is a highly unpopular side-effect, so doctors rarely mention it when prescribing a drug. Although not common, drug-induced gynecomastia is not terribly rare, and a surprisingly number of drugs are responsible. This effect is not serious and easily reversible, so don't avoid a good treatment until a better one appears.

Digitalis, commonly prescribed for heart disease, bears a distant chemical resemblance to estrogen and occasionally produces this side-effect. Tetrahydrocannibinol, the active ingredient in marijuana, also vaguely resembles estrogen, although its structure doesn't resemble digitalis. Chronic marijuana and hashish users develop gynecomastia.

One of the oldest and cheapest antiseizure drugs, phenytoin (Dilantin) remains popular because it doesn't make patients drowsy and its many side-effects, although annoying, are not fatal. Besides suppressing seizures, Dilantin stimulates the conversion of testosterone to estrogen.

Cimetidine (Tagamet), the first effective suppressor of stomach acid released in the United States, quickly became a best-seller, but not because it dramatically relieves ulcer symptoms. All major medical drug advances (penicillin, vitamin B_{12}, thyroid, cortisone) are wildly overprescribed for ailments they don't affect; most Tagamet is given for garden variety digestive upsets unrelated to excessive acid. Newer acid suppressors outsell Tagamet today, but it remains an excellent drug. Furthermore, its patent expired in 1994, so the price has plummeted compared to its rivals. Tagamet also suppresses testosterone to a slight extent, an action that rivals may not share but not a reason to avoid it.

Two fairly important drugs interfere with testosterone action. One is a new and effective antifungal antibiotic, ketoconazole (Nizoral); the other is spironolactone (Aldactone), often used in blood pressure remedies and diuretics to reduce potassium loss in the urine. Other everyday drugs that cause gynecomastia include Valium, metronidazole (Flagyl), ranitidine (Zantac), and theophylline (Theo-Dur, Theo-Bid). No one is certain why, and it happens only rarely.

Treatment. Active treatment is rarely necessary because most gynecomastia disappears in time or after discontinuing whatever caused it. Occasionally some swelling remains; a man who feels that this is cosmetically unacceptable can have plastic surgery.

Drugs exist that block the action of estrogen. Doctors prescribe tamoxifen and danazol to treat breast pain and breast cancer in women. Men with stubborn gynecomastia from an obscure hormonal abnormality may benefit, but these drugs are too expensive and risky for most cases.

Men Can Get Breast Cancer Too

One percent of all breast cancer occurs in men. Since this is the leading malignancy in women, with over 150,000 new cases per year, 1 percent is not a trivial number. Male breast cancer is about one fourth as common as penile cancer. The mortality rate is greater in men because they lack the frightening awareness that's almost universal among women. A soft lump behind your nipple is probably gynecomastia; a hard lump points to cancer. Either is worth a trip to the doctor.

CHAPTER ▪ 9

A MAN'S SKIN

Disadvantaged compared to women in other medical areas, men benefit when it comes to skin. Smooth, soft skin plays only a minor role in male sexual attractiveness, so we are spared the intense and often futile energy that women devote to preserving a youthful complexion.

While a little roughness is acceptable, men dislike wrinkles, blemishes, flaking, itching, pimples, and lumps as much as women. All are preventable to a surprising extent; skin maintenance requires less effort than muscle, bone, or the cardiovascular system.

A MAN'S NORMAL SKIN

Skin to the layperson means epidermis, the surface. The topmost of two layers, it marks the boundary between you and the rest of the universe over most of your body. With protection as its major function, the epidermis measures a full 1.5 millimeters thick over the palms and soles, shrinking to a few tenths of a millimeter on the face to only one tenth on the eyelids.

Epidermis originates in a single layer of living cells at its base. Cells move upward, fill with a tough protein called keratin (which also forms nails and hair), die, flatten out, and reach the surface. Contact with the environment rubs off many, but even protected areas shed continually. A normal epidermal cell lasts four to six weeks. The epidermis contains no nerves or blood vessels. Except for the basal layer, all the tissue is dead. Hair, skin oil, and sweat pass through the epidermis to exit, but they originate from glands or follicles below.

With this knowledge, you'll realize that everything that happens within the epidermis is temporary. Injuries and burns heal without scarring. Diseases leave no trace, and any blemish or lump that a doctor scrapes off will not return.

Beneath the epidermis, and twenty to forty times thicker, lies the dermis. Glands and hair originate here, nourished by a rich blood supply. Collagen is the principal tissue, a fibrous protein that also makes up ligaments and tendons. We also called this connective tissue because it anchors most body structures and fills in the gaps between them. Healthy connective tissue is loose and flexible; aging, injury, and sunlight make it stiffen and shrink. Keep this in mind when I discuss wrinkles. Damage to the dermis is permanent; healing produces scarring. Ointments, superficial scraping, and other surface treatments have no effect on the dermis.

Cleanliness and a Man's Skin

For obscure evolutionary reasons, orientals have little body odor, and they have always believed that white people smell bad. White people did not concern themselves with body odor until well into the nineteenth century, when piped water became available. Until then, polite people kept their hands and faces clean, but rarely washed their bodies.

Health beliefs and practicality go hand in hand. Until a century ago, bathing required hours of labor, heating water over an open fire and filling a portable iron tub. Repeating this work was too tedious unless one had plenty of servants, so everyone in the family took turns in the same water.

Pre-twentieth-century Western physicians considered bathing harmful. Only the rich could afford this regularly (although few took advantage), and doctors have traditionally believed that whatever the rich do is excessive and unhealthy. Today Americans bathe daily; not all Europeans follow this custom, a shock to the noses of many North American tourists.

That Americans bathe so often without harm speaks highly for the toughness of their skin. Cleanliness (except beneath the foreskin) contributes little to personal health. Except for eliminating visible dirt, bathing is not essential for personal attractiveness—specifically, a good complexion. Soap and water harm skin far more than dirt.

Guidelines for Bathing

Although a daily bath or shower with vigorous scrubbing is overkill, most men never suffer the consequences. However, to take the best care of your skin, follow these guidelines.

To avoid socially unacceptable smells, use soap on your armpits and feet and between your legs, but not elsewhere. Keep the bath or shower short. Dry by patting lightly with a towel. Woman routinely apply a moisturizing cream to compensate for the drying action of bathing. Although this seems unmasculine, men should do the same. Consider this preventive care because as you grow older your skin becomes drier and tends to itch and flake more readily. By age sixty, a man who wants to take the best care of his skin bathes once or twice a week, washing daily only the three areas mentioned.

Although hard to believe, we bathe our children too often. Their skin is the most delicate of all; it's never oily because humans don't produce skin oils until after age eight. Bathe a child under six months with soap once a week, with a quick sponge bath at other times.

How to Deal With Body Odor

Sweat contains water, salts, glucose, and a few other simple chemicals—all odorless. The action of skin bacteria on your oils and dead surface cells plus the passage of time leads to your characteristic smell. Bacteria work fastest in the warmest areas: armpits, groin, and feet.

Body odor isn't inevitable even among Caucasians. Many men who wash these areas daily and change their underwear have no problem and need not use a deodorant. To determine if you are among them *ask someone else*, someone you trust. No one can detect his body odor (or breath odor). Every doctor sees hundreds of patients with foul body odor or breath. They are invariably unaware. We also see dozens who complain that they smell or have terrible halitosis. They are invariably wrong (smelly feet are the exception). A conviction that you smell is a serious delusion unless others agree.

Using Deodorants and Antiperspirants. A deodorant is simply a perfume, a substance used for thousands of years to give the body a pleasant fragrance. An antiperspirant contains a metallic salt, usually aluminum chloride, that shrinks the skin and blocks sweat secretion. When buying, read the label. A container that says only "deodorant" contains no antiperspirant, so it doesn't prevent wetness.

If you prefer a deodorant, apply it in the morning. A man who uses an antiperspirant should wash at night and apply before going to bed. The armpit produces almost no sweat at night, so the chemical has time to penetrate the skin and act. Applied in the morning when sweat is flowing, much of the antiperspirant washes away.

An ideal underarm product would eliminate perspiration for long periods without the irritation produced by metallic salts, which have been used for decades. No such product exists, and few chemists are searching for one because of a peculiarity in our laws. Current law classifies a deodorant as a cosmetic, a substance easy to test and market, but an antiperspirant comes under the heading of a drug. To introduce a new drug requires approval of the Food and Drug Administration after extensive animal and human testing. Cosmetic companies shy away from the expense, preferring to invent new odors for their deodorants while sticking to the established antiperspirants.

Heavy Sweating and Heavy Smells. For a man who pours sweat from his armpits, palms, or feet, a doctor can prescribe concentrated aluminum chloride solutions with names like Drysol and Xerac-AC. Similar prescription products work for sweaty, smelly feet, but I suggest soaking for fifteen minutes a day in a pan of formaldehyde—one teaspoon of a commercial solution in a pint of cool water.

The Man With Dry Skin

Dry skin lacks water, not oil. Your dead epidermis contains water, which is kept from evaporating by a layer of natural oils. Most dry skin affects the hands, arms, and lower legs. The epidermis of the face is so thin that water from the dermis can keep it hydrated. A man who believes his face is dry probably suffers a skin condition such as seborrhea or sun damage.

Three conditions cause most dryness:

- Age: Older skin produces less oil, so moisture evaporates more quickly.
- Washing: Soaps and detergents efficiently remove protective oil.
- Low humidity: Conveniences like air conditioning and central heating lower humidity, so much that skin dries out despite natural oils.

Putting moisturizing cream on dry skin is a poor method. You must first replace the missing water, and *then* apply a protective coat. The best time is right after a bath while skin is damp. Even bath oils work best when applied directly to the skin. Poured into the bath water, most remains there.

The best coating is heavy enough to prevent evaporation of all water underneath. Lard and other animal fats served well for centuries. Equally fine but odor-free is petroleum jelly (e.g., Vaseline), but most people don't like the oily feeling. Unfortunately, pure fats or oils protect skin the best, but all feel greasy.

Fortunately, chemists working with emulsifying agents discovered ways to mix oil and water together to produce a creamy liquid that's much more pleasant. A suspension of water in oil is called a lotion and forms the basis of modern skin conditioners. Good examples are Lubriderm, Keri, Moisturel, and Neutrogena, but I suggest trying the largest generic skin cream sold in your local supermarket. Some lack the pleasant feel and quick disappearance of the brands, but they work as well at much less cost. Apply it daily.

If you have extremely dry skin, never wash with water. Buy a waterless cleanser such as Cetaphil or Aquanil. Apply it, rub to make a lather, and then wipe off with a soft cloth.

The Man With Oily Skin

Skin normally exists under a layer of oil, and excessively oily skin causes no disease (it doesn't cause acne, for example). However, if your only problem is a complexion that seems too oily, wash more often. Soap removes skin oils. Avoid moisturizers. You can buy astringents, usually continuing alcohol. Applied after washing, they remove oil and dehydrate the skin, tightening it temporarily. This feels pleasantly tingly but has no permanent effect.

How You Should Care for Your Scalp and Hair

Unlike skin cleansing, vigorous washing is appropriate for the scalp because it attracts dirt. Twice a week is adequate, but daily shampooing won't harm the normal scalp. You've probably heard reassurance that hair pulled out during scrubbing would have been lost anyway and grows back. It's true; you'll learn why hair falls out permanently later in this chapter.

It's fine to wash your hair with the same bar that cleans the rest of you. If your hair looks fine afterward, don't bother with a shampoo. Advertisements warm solemnly against dull soap films that render hair repulsive to the opposite sex, and it's true that soap reacts with the minerals in hard water to produce a film. If you notice one, you can wash it off with an acid rinse such as vinegar or lemon juice. If this seems too much trouble, try a detergent. All shampoos are detergents, but so is ordinary dishwashing liquid. Buy a product that appeals to you, but realize that almost all features are worthless hype. Even shampoos formulated for dry, average, or oily hair have little practical importance. In studies, patients asked to choose which shampoo worked best for their type couldn't tell the difference.

Caring for Your Beard

Shaving removes a thin slice of epidermis as well as beard hair, but this is harmless and quickly replaced. A man can shave his entire life with little harm to his complexion. On the other hand, several minutes per day of shaving over a lifetime adds up to considerable time one could spend in productive activities. A beard is one facial feature that's almost never unattractive in a young man and grows more attractive with age and grayness. Maintenance requires less than a minute to snip dangling hairs with a scissors and shave quickly around the edge to keep it neat.

Men who shave should soften the hair as much as possible beforehand. Wet the beard and apply a shaving soap (almost everyone uses an aerosol, but shaving cream works better). Do this during your daily wash, and save shaving until last. Shave in the direction that hairs grow, and don't stretch the skin with the other hand. With a skillful technique, a man can shave without going over the same area twice. Never forget the age of your blade. For the first few shaves with a new blade, barely touching the skin shears off the hairs. Thereafter you can gradually increase pressure. Use the blade until a single pass doesn't remove all hairs.

Aftershave lotions provide a pleasant smell but serve no essential purpose. The alcohol they contain doesn't disinfect the skin or prevent infection, and any burning they produce means that you're removing too much epidermis.

An electric shaver works fine for a light or light-colored beard and for those men with curly hairs that grow back into the skin after shaving, producing unsightly pimples. Black men often have this problem. One can often free hairs by brushing the face with a toothbrush after shaving; if this doesn't work, one can free them individually with a small hook. Growing a beard offers a permanent solution.

Ear and Nose Hair

Like body odor and bad breath, these are features that almost every American considers unattractive. You can buy small shavers designed for ears and special scissors for nose hairs.

MEN WORRY ABOUT BALDNESS

My grandfather kept a magnificent head of white hair until his death at age eighty-six. Unfortunately, he was my father's father, and baldness passes through your mother's genes. Although my father also died with this hair, my mother's father was balding at forty, and so was I. If you don't know the status of your maternal grandfather, the scalps of your mother's male relatives will predict your future.

Cause

Eunuchs never lose their hair. Although it's never caught on, castrating a man before he loses his hair is a guaranteed preventive because male pattern baldness requires functioning testes. Men grow bald because testosterone shrinks their hair follicles. For unclear reasons, this only happens to follicles on top of the head, not to the beard or to the fringe around the side.

Despite the popular belief, men don't grow bald because hair falls out. Everyone loses 100 hairs a day because a normal hair falls out every few years, and a new one grows to replace it. As a balding man's follicles shrink, each new hair is smaller and thinner than the one that preceded it, but even a naked scalp grows a thin fuzz.

Diagnosis

During several years at a university student health service, I regularly saw students convinced that an ominous disease was taking away their hair. Usually my examination was normal, but I sometimes noticed thinning at the crown or a receding hairline—the beginning of male pattern baldness. Following good medical practice, I asked about their health, the drugs they were taking, and their hairdressing habits (excessive heat or styling methods that apply traction injure or pull out hair, but this is usually obvious).

Answers were invariably negative. Everyone admitted that they were under stress and "didn't eat right," but this never makes hair fall out. Too little or too much shampooing, tight football helmets, and excessive combing are also innocent. Stroke victims don't lose their hair, so poor circulation isn't responsible. Bacterial and fungal infections as well as a host of skin disorders destroy hair, but the affected scalp looks abnormal.

Medical books are full of subtle diseases that make hair fall out, but they are so rare that I haven't seen one in twenty years of practice; in any case, they produce other signs of illness which a doctor can detect by questioning. If you feel well and your scalp looks normal (dandruff doesn't count), thinning hair equals male pattern baldness.

Home Diagnosis

Count hairs for twenty-four hours. Don't shampoo during this time, but collect every hair from the pillow in the morning plus whatever remains after gentle combing several times a day. Save them in an envelope. More than 200 indicates a genuine disorder that increases hair shedding. Sometimes the cause is obvious—a recent severe illness or high fever increases hair loss temporarily—but it's worth showing your doctor.

No male patient of mine has brought in that many, but proof of male pattern baldness is not pleasant news. No sooner had they reached adulthood, patients complained, than the first sign of old age was appearing. I reassured them that baldness is not a sign of aging but of sexual maturity. It begins when puberty ends. Men in their twenties may not notice because a thinning hairline isn't obvious for years, and almost no one looks at the top of his head.

If they were not reassured, my final weapon was the result of an informal poll, which I am convinced is accurate. Men should realize that—women don't object to baldness in a man. Only men are upset by it.Women take as much interest in a man's appearance as vice versa, and among sights that turn many off (exceptions always exist) are flabbiness, shapeless buttocks, poor posture, an obnoxious manner, nose hair, and ugly clothes. I haven't found a woman who thinks baldness is unsexy.

A parallel exists. Women spend a great deal of energy choosing their shoes, many of which are amazingly uncomfortable. Yet, as we know, men never notice, and we certainly don't judge a woman's appeal by her footwear.

In the end, most of my health-service patients accepted my explanation, but a solid minority demanded to see the dermatologist. That was awkward. Our dermatologists came in only two afternoons per week and the appointment book was filled a month in advance. As a result, our medical director warned us not to bore them with routine acne, warts, and other problems that any doctor can handle. In fact, a dermatologist has no special expertise for a man losing his hair, and I never referred anyone because I needed help. I referred men who insisted that my diagnosis was wrong and that only an emergency visit to the dermatologist would prevent them from going entirely bald.

Such patients are one of the prices dermatologists pay for their large income. Ours listed sympathetically, then prescribed vitamins, a medicated shampoo, and plenty of rest. Forced to refuse a referral, I was faced by angry male patients who were convinced I was condemning them to a future of wigs and hair transplants. Many rushed off to a private dermatologist, where they received sympathy, vitamins, and other shampoos.

Treating Baldness

By the mid-1980s I stopped dreading these encounters because I could offer minoxidil—not yet FDA approved for baldness but a nice source of income for pharmacists who ground up the tablets and dissolved them in whatever they had on hand.

Doctors knew that minoxidil grew hair back in the 1970s. That's why they didn't use it! A powerful blood pressure remedy, it produced plenty of side-effects besides unwanted hair, and other drugs worked as well without so much unpleasantness. Although family doctors like me hardly ever prescribed it, this wasn't so for cardiologists.

Around 1980, a number of formerly balding cardiologists became remarkably hairy. They weren't talking, but we suspected them of consuming large doses of minoxidil on the side. Although it obviously worked, this luxurious growth brought disadvantages. According to gossip, the morning shave of a newly hairy cardiologist included not only the beard but also the nose, forehead, ears, cheeks, and probably the palms and soles.

All this hair caught the attention of the Upjohn Company, the maker of minoxidil, which sensed a bonanza. Its researchers knew that the FDA would never approve swallowing such a powerful drug to treat ordinary baldness, but they might look kindly on rubbing it into the scalp. This proved to be the case, and the lotion passed approval in 1989.

Preventing Baldness

Rubbed into the scalp twice a day, minoxidil lotion (Rogaine until the patent expires early in the twenty-first century) blocks the action of testosterone on hair follicles.

Enthusiastic health writers downplay one feature of prevention that I deal with all the time: It's often boring. Once a man has his heart attack, I can persuade him to change his diet radically or take up regular exercise, but young, healthy men show less enthusiasm. Preventing baldness takes no less fortitude; begin using minoxidil at age eighteen and continue for the rest of your life. Waiting for baldness may motivate you, but you might be too late. Minoxidil reverses the shrinkage of hair follicles provided that they haven't shrunk much, but it's better at preventing shrinkage in the first place.

Treating Baldness

Minoxidil works best as a treatment when the first sign of baldness appears at the top of the head. Faithful twice-a-day application fills in the gap about half the time. You should notice a change in six months. The thinner the hair, the less well minoxidil works. It's worthless on bare scalp, but since it's a much better preventive, regular use should stop further hair loss. It resumes if you stop, so treatment is a lifetime commitment.

Can You Do Better?

I was surprised that minoxidil appeared in a 2 percent solution because I and other doctors routinely asked pharmacists for 5 percent. I suspect that Upjohn was so anxious to win approval (and avoid lawsuits—an obsession with drug companies no less than doctors) that it started with the weakest possible concentration.

Give two percent a year's trial. If you're not satisfied, ask your doctor to write a special prescription for a 5 percent solution. Then find a pharmacist (most likely an older one) who "compounds" (i.e., mixes up prescriptions from raw ingredients). With two and a half times as much drug plus the pharmacist's fee for compounding, you will pay several thousand dollars for a year's supply. But you'll see more hair.

A MAN'S ACNE

Along with freedom from baldness and prostate enlargement, eunuchs have no acne, a disorder that cannot exist in the absence of male hormone.

Almost all teenagers suffer to some degree, and heredity plays a modest role.

A child of parents with acne runs ten times the risk of severe acne compared to one whose parents had none. Both sexes are affected, but men experience the worst cases. Although most acne recedes after age twenty, some continues well into adulthood. A number of men first notice pimples during their twenties and must deal with them throughout life.

This is a disease of advanced Western society and its diet. Poor countries suffer much less, but not because their food lacks additives, sugar, fat, and other unhealthy elements. As far as acne is concerned, the most important missing dietary element is nutrition. Starvation suppresses sex hormones and acne. That's why women with anorexia nervosa have smooth complexions and no periods.

Cause

Acne is a disorder of the pilosebaceous follicle—a hair follicle that also contains glands that secrete sebum, your natural skin oil. As you'd predict, these occur over the face, neck, back, chest, and shoulders.

Male hormones control the pilosebaceous follicle. As mentioned in Chapter 1, boys produce little sebum. With the rise in male hormones around age eight, the follicle grows and sebum production rises. Unfortunately, this follicle is among the many imperfectly designed parts of the human body. A crucial weak point is the canal that carries both hair and sebum to the surface. It's lined with the same epidermis that covers your skin, so dead cells slough continually. Normally this debris flows out with sebum, but beginning in early adolescence the lining swells, and dead cells stick together after shedding. As a result, many pores become plugged. Acne begins with a plugged pore.

The Three Forms of Acne

1. Comedos. An obstructed pore looks like a small bump. Doctors call it a comedo (or comedone); everyone else calls it a whitehead or blackhead, depending on the color. Follicles often unplug spontaneously. In the past, a brisk market existed for a little instrument called a comedone extractor, which sucked out the plug. Today some physicians open their patients' comedones with the tip of a scalpel, but most prescribe creams; they work well. Squeezing your comedones is a bad idea. Sometimes it succeeds; sometimes it ruptures the follicle, leading to the next and more advanced form of acne.

2. Papules and Pustules. Sebum piles up inside the obstructed follicle. Germs that normally live there multiply in the abundance of fatty sebum. These cause no harm unless an overburdened or squeezed follicle ruptures, releasing material into the surrounding epidermis to induce a small infection. The smallest leads to a raised, red bump, a papule, but the traditional curse of acne is the red bump with a white dot of pus in the center: the pustule (pimple). Ordinary papules and pustules remain in the epidermis and heal without scarring in a week or two. Squeezing pimples is another bad idea that risks spreading the infection more widely, leading to nodules and cysts.

3. Nodules and Cysts. A few unfortunate victims (mostly men) suffer fiercely overactive glands whose rupture produces large pimples that coalesce into boils and extend to the dermis. These leave scars.

Important Myths About Acne

Having learned the facts, you'll realize that poor hygiene doesn't cause acne. Pores plug from below, not as the result of dirt on the skin. The black of a blackhead isn't dirt but a chemical change in the sebum plug. Keeping clean is fine, but aggressive scrubbing accomplishes nothing except to encourage follicles to rupture.

Although regularly blamed, oily skin isn't responsible. As long as sebum flows freely, acne won't appear. Once on the surface, sebum does no harm, so washing it off doesn't help. Superficial drying agents like alcohol don't affect sebum flow. Dermatologists warn patients to keep creams and moisturizers off their face, but this is merely common sense; little evidence exists that bland creams aggravate acne. It's true that men who work with grease and oil suffer more acne, but this results from irritants in the oil, not the oil itself.

Treatment

Medical science does very well with acne, and any man making a modest effort should have almost none. Except for severe cases, begin with—

Benzoyl peroxide 5 percent, a powerful antibacterial that kills germs within the follicle. Available for several decades, you can buy it without a prescription as Oxy-5 or OxyClear.

Wash with ordinary soap, then dry and apply the benzoyl peroxide cream to the entire face or other affected area twice a day. Apply once a day if it's too irritating; if irritation persists, apply without washing first or try 2.5 percent cream. Remember that benzoyl peroxide works by suppressing germs; it doesn't eliminate pimples already present, so don't expect dramatic improvement. Look hard at your acne before beginning treatment, try not to think about it for six weeks, and then look hard again. If you're not satisfied, see a doctor for prescription remedies. You'll receive one or more of the following.

Tretinoin (retinoic acid, Retin-A) is the best agent for preventing follicle obstruction. A relative of vitamin A, it thins the epidermis, speeds shedding, and reduces stickiness of dead surface cells. As a result, pores drain freely, and existing plugs of blackheads and whiteheads are pushed out.

Applied nightly as a cream or gel, Retin-A inflames normal skin. Some men can only tolerate it every other day, a few not at all. I tell patients to expect their acne to flare after a few weeks but that improvement should be obvious after two months. Skin treated with Retin-A becomes more sensitive to the sun, so patients should apply sunscreen and wear a hat with a broad brim.

Antibiotics Can Help. Excellent at suppressing follicular bacteria, oral antibiotics are probably the first choice for severe papulopustular acne. Doctors overprescribe them for milder forms because almost everyone, patients as well as doctors, believes that pills work more powerfully than creams; also some men lack the will to rub cream over their face twice a day.

Treatment begins with a large dose, usually of tetracycline, the most popular antiacne antibiotic. This doesn't affect existing pimples, so improvement takes several weeks, after which the dose is lowered gradually. Therapy even at a low dose must continue indefinitely, but side-effects are rare.

Topical antibiotics (usually erythromycin or clindamycin) don't penetrate as well, but the combination of Retin-A at night to keep follicles open with a topical antibiotic in the morning works well enough for most acne to make pills unnecessary.

Isotretinoin (Accutane). Until the 1980s, all acne remedies worked temporarily, suppressing pimples only while treatment continued. None cured them until Accutane appeared, one of the few new drugs that deserved its media enthusiasm. Another derivative of vitamin A (which doctors once prescribed for severe acne in large, toxic doses), Accutane poisons the sebaceous glands. They shrink, and sebum output drops; some of this shrinkage is permanent.

Taken for the worst cystic acne, Accutane usually works wonders. A four-month course slowly eliminates ugly cysts and nodules, and improvement often continues after treatment stops. About 30 percent of men require a second course. As doctors gain experience, many prescribe it for stubborn garden variety papulopustular acne. Accutane is only approved for cystic acne, but after the FDA approves a drug for one disorder, doctors are free to use it for whatever they want.

Although magnificently effective, Accutane may be the most disagreeable drug given for a nonfatal disorder. Besides drying and shrinking sebaceous glands, it dries the entire surface of the body. Almost every patient suffers cracked lips, itchy, flaking skin, watery eyes, and sometimes nosebleeds and hair loss. These should resolve after treatment, and most patients endure the discomfort because the end result is so good. They are also willing to put up with the expense—about $1,000 for a four-month course.

Other Treatments That Can Help. Dietary restrictions helped in the past by giving the man a sense of control and the physician something to blame when treatment didn't work. No evidence exists that food exacerbates acne, and today's treatments should please almost everyone who complies.

Plenty of over-the-counter and fold remedies rely on drying, peeling, scrubbing, scraping, and otherwise attacking the skin. Ingredients include alcohol, sulfur, resorcin, and salicylic acid as well as various harsh cleansers. According to the theory, this aggression unblocks obstructed pores, but any comedo plugs removed would probably have popped on their own.

Artificial ultraviolet lamps as well as ordinary sun exposure improve acne but cause skin cancer, so we use them much less than in the past.

Understanding Wrinkles and Sun Damage

Old-fashioned women and more than a few feminists detest wrinkles—and with good reason, because they are often perceived as the mark of a woman past her prime. As men know, this does not hold for men. Just as most women don't object to gray hair or a receding hairline in the opposite sex, a weathered face marks us as men of the world. Elderly male celebrities from Cary Grant to Sean Connery entered their seventies with undiminished sex appeal.

Obligatory in a book aimed at women, guidelines on preventing wrinkles may seem superfluous in this book until you realize that wrinkles appear as the result of two unrelated processes: (1) normal aging and (2) skin disease.

Why Wrinkles Appear

Some people view aging as a process of dehydration—that you dry out, shrink, and wrinkle like a plum becoming a prune—but this is a poor analogy. Although aged skin loses water more readily, dry skin flakes and peels but doesn't wrinkle. Keeping skin hydrated is worthwhile, but it won't prevent wrinkles, so I discussed hydration in the section on skin care.

Remembering my description of normal skin, you'll realize that wrinkling can't be a phenomenon of the epidermis because epidermal cells shed continually. Any localized blemish disappears in a month or so. Permanent changes must originate in the dermis underneath. Bathed in body fluids and laced with blood vessels, the dermis never dries out. Wrinkles occur when dermal connective tissue shrinks, crinkling the epidermis.

Avoidable Wrinkles

Victorian finishing schools taught ladies to avoid laughing, frowning, squinting, smiling, etc. on the grounds that facial movements encourage wrinkles, and there is truth in this. Chronic schizophrenics and the severely retarded, both of whom rarely change expression, maintain smooth complexions into old age. A person who sleeps with his or her face against the pillow develops a permanent sleep line down the center of the cheek.

Smokers develop crow's feet ten years earlier than nonsmokers, probably because they squint so much when smoke drifts into their eyes. Chronic disease accelerates aging with its accompanying wrinkles, and smoking is a chronic disease no less harmful than uncontrolled diabetes or high blood pressure.

For most men, sun exposure represents the leading source of premature skin aging. Ultraviolet radiation penetrates past the epidermis, damaging the living dermis, making it stiffen and shrink. When I report that sun exposure causes premature skin aging, this is not colorful writing meant to attract your attention but the literal truth. Examined under the microscope, the skin of an old man looks identical to that of a young man suffering chronic sun damage.

Preventing Wrinkles

Looking at an old photograph of a crowd, you can easily determine whether it's pre- or post-1960 by one feature: hats. Before 1960 men wore them; afterward they didn't. President Kennedy single-handedly crippled the hat industry by going bareheaded. Since that time, the incidence of skin cancer has climbed. While no one has studied the subject, wrinkling has probably increased, too.

Of all antiaging and disease preventive practices, wearing a broad-brimmed hat is easily the cheapest and one of the most effective. I wish hats would return to fashion. Keep one by the door and wear it when you leave anytime during the day. Ultraviolet rays penetrate clouds, so wear it in any weather.

Some rays bounce off water, snow, and buildings, so a hat's protection isn't 100 percent. Every man should apply a sunscreen daily. Read the label and buy one with an SPF (sun protection factor) of 15 or more. Men apply too little because their face shines when they apply enough. The shininess fades in an hour or two, so putting on the cream before breakfast enables you to arrive at work with dignity.

Traditional sunscreens contain para-aminobenzoic acid to block UVB, those ultraviolet rays which experts have blamed for sun damage. Over the past decade, experts have begun to suspect that UVA, formerly ignored, plays a significant role. As a result, newer sunscreens contain oxybenzone and Parsol 1789, which block both UVA and UVB. Like most new products, these cost more, but I advise using them until experts make up their minds.

Wrinkles, Sun Damage, and Retin-A

Although most men are unaware, Retin-A made a tremendous splash during the late 1980s, when researchers reported that it improved skin texture and eliminated fine facial wrinkles typical of sun damage. Pharmacies couldn't keep up with the demand, and Retin-A remains the jewel of profit makers for the Ortho Company.

Soon after the craze began, doctors began issuing solemn warnings that Retin-A's benefits were exaggerated, that it doesn't affect the wrinkles of aging and is not a harmless drug. Although true, these turn out to be beside the point because Retin-A appears genuinely useful for skin care in both sexes. Although not FDA approved for anything except acne, that may change by the time you read this.

The action that improves acne, thinning the epidermis with increased shedding, also smooths superficial lines caused by too much sun. Men who value a fine complexion should try Retin-A with the understanding that it comes at a price. Treated skin grows delicate; scaling and flaking may become annoying and require moisturizers. Wearing a sunscreen becomes essential.

I use Retin-A religiously, but not for my complexion (my wife claims she notices an improvement, but I don't). I had a skin cancer ten years ago, and my dermatologist insists that regular application will prevent future skin cancers. Although far from unanimous, a growing consensus exists among dermatologists that Retin-A (and other vitamin A derivatives, including Accutane) eliminate early precancerous skin changes. You'll learn more about this later in this chapter.

Dandruff and Seborrhea: Flaky Situations

Having brushed his teeth, many a man rinses the brush and then proceeds to brush his face to clear away flakes that appear each morning at the side of his nose and around his eyebrows, hairline, sideburns, and sometimes generally over the beard area.

This is the consequence of seborrhea, a harmless but tiresome affliction that probably affects every man sooner or later but begins at puberty for a good number. Prevention is impossible, but suppression works if you keep it up. I mention brushing the face only because so many frustrated men can't resist. Using brushes, fingernails, and other instruments to scrape off unsightly flakes works only for that day and regularly leads to local irritation and minor infections. You can do better.

Why Your Skin Flakes

Although almost everyone with dandruff and flaking believes his skin is dry, the opposite is the case. Normal skin sheds in particles too small to be seen. When the surface becomes oily, skin cells stick together in sheets to make the visible flakes of dandruff and seborrhea.

This disorder owes its name to dermal sebaceous glands, which empty into hair follicles, flow to the surface, and provide protective oils. Areas rich in sebaceous glands enjoy plenty of oil, so they resist dryness but become most susceptible to seborrhea: scalp, beard area, ears, armpits, sternum, groin, and around the belly button. For unclear reasons, epidermal cells in seborrheac skin multiply much more rapidly; this combined with the presence of skin oils produces the seemingly endless supply of flakes. On hairless areas such as the nasolabial folds or upper cheeks, you may not see flakes but only a vivid redness.

Treatment

Modest dandruff is almost universal, but daily washing with ordinary shampoo often removes flakes so well that no special treatment is necessary. Try this first because antidandruff shampoos can cost an impressive amount.

If you're not satisfied, move up to a product containing zinc pyrithionate (Head & Shoulders, X-Seb, DHS Zinc). Give this a month or two before trying a shampoo with selenium sulfide or salicyclic acid such as Selsun, Exsel, Sebulex, or Ionil. Ordinary tar suppresses dandruff best, but it's black and smelly, so manufacturers have worked hard to produce pleasant formulations by dilution and mixing in perfumes. Dilute tar works, but it works better when black and concentrated in shampoos like Sebutone or Pentrax. There's no harm in trying these first, but prepare to pay $10 to $20 for a small bottle.

For stubborn inflammatory (i.e., itchy) dandruff, a doctor can provide dramatic relief with a cortisone lotion or spray. For seborrhea around the face, eyebrows, and ears, rub on 1 percent hydrocortisone cream twice a day. These are available over the counter under a dozen names. The redness or flaking should disappear in a week or two, after which you can reduce applications to daily or stop entirely until the rash returns.

One percent hydrocortisone works so well against seborrhea that a persistent rash is probably something else, so see a doctor. Never use a stronger cortisone cream on this area. Facial skin is so thin that weak creams penetrate completely; stronger cortisone not only suppresses the overactive cells of seborrhea, it suppresses them too much, making facial skin atrophic and delicate. All strong cortisone requires a prescription, and most doctors know their danger, so this is a warning against using prescription creams left over from other skin disorders.

It turns out that the best seborrhea treatment is probably an antifungal antibiotic of the griseofulvin family, discussed in the next section. Not only does the tablet or cream eliminate dandruff and the rash, but relapses occur less often. This means that (although I didn't mention this earlier) fungi may play a role in seborrhea. Then again, they may not. Although studies of antifungals date from the 1980s, experts remain uncertain of how they work against seborrhea. Since other treatments work well, and cortisone creams cost much less, they remain the treatments of choice except for stubborn cases.

Skin Fungi: Why You Itch

Although itchy rashes spring from may sources, a man who itches probably suffers from a fungal infection—provided that he itches in a chronically damp area—between the legs, on the feet and between the toes, and sometimes in the armpit. Fungi grow over every part of the body, but in dry areas they produce mild itching at the most. An intensely itchy rash over the chest, shoulders, or other dry area probably represents local injury from an irritating chemical, and intense generalized itching points to a generalized allergy. Both require medical attention. You can treat many fungal infections yourself, at least at first.

What They Are and Where They Come From

Common skin fungi (ringworm, jock itch, athlete's foot; the medical term is dermatopyte) belong to a distinct class of plants that also include molds, mushrooms, mildew, and rusts. Although they live everywhere and can spread to humans from the soil or animals, most human fungi are unique to humans and cannot survive elsewhere. Infections spread from human to human, but these fungi are so universal that almost everyone harbors a few billion living quietly on his skin along with the resident bacteria. Ill health, poor nutrition, and hot weather impair resistance to these organisms, but a man in good health can suffer when his own fungi decide to multiply for no clear reason.

Harmless organisms, dermatophytes feed on the dead surface of epidermis. Like all fungi, they grow best in warm, damp conditions where they penetrate deeply enough to tickle pain nerves to produce itching (itching is the mildest form of pain). On dry parts of the body, fungi spread with hardly any symptoms.

Jock itch affects men on the upper and inner surfaces of the thighs, occasionally spreading backward toward the anus but rarely involving the scrotum and almost never the penis. It begins as a small, itchy red patch perhaps with a slightly raised border. Scales, crusts, and even small blisters may appear, but the center tends to clear as the rash spreads, a pattern responsible for the term *ringworm.*

Treatment is easy but so rarely effective that it's given self-treatment a bad name. The usual reason for failure of self-treatment is the wrong self-diagnosis, but this is not so with jock itch because, unlike itchy rashes elsewhere on the body, fungi cause the majority of itching between the legs. Treatment of groin infections fails when it stops too soon. Treat jock itch with two months of antifungal cream. Excellent creams, once available only by prescription, were approved for over-the-counter sale in the 1980s. Among them are miconazole (Micatin) or clotrimazole (Lotrimin, Mycelex). Rub a thin coat over the area twice a day; a heavy application doesn't improve the outcome.

Keep this area as cool and dry as possible to discourage reactivation. Wear loose underclothing and pants. Apply an antifungal powder or plain talcum powder liberally after bathing.

Athlete's foot, the most common fungal infection, probably bothers all men sooner or later and smolders on without symptoms between infections. Men quickly seek relief when they experience itching between the toe webs, especially the third and fourth. If relief takes the form of scratching or vigorous scrubbing with a washrag during a bath, the damp, infected skin cracks, replacing itching with painful fissures. Over the rest of the foot, fungi produce a patchy scaling that may coalesce in a moccasin distribution, occasionally with blisters and crusting. Men blame dry skin when they notice diffuse flaking and peeling without discomfort, but they're wrong. However, a rash on top of the foot is probably not a fungus.

Dermatology texts always discuss infections of the hands and feet together, but so many common skin disorders affect the hand that you shouldn't try to diagnose yourself. A peculiar exception is a typical rash affecting both feet but only one hand; that's almost certainly a fungus.

Treatment with several months of cream works well for infections between the toes and small patches elsewhere but poorly for extensive involvement. Furthermore, if toenails are involved no cure lasts. Most men accept their scaly feet as long as itching remains tolerable, but those that don't accept require oral griseofulvin, an antifungal antibiotic that inhibits dermatophytes but not germs or other fungi. You skin surface is dead so the drug can't change its appearance, but new cells growing from below contain griseofulvin, making them impervious to fungi. Since palms and soles contain the thickest epidermis with the longest turnover time, treatment must last three months.

Available since the 1960s, griseofulvin enjoys a good safety record—obviously essential in a drug taken for months to treat a minor infection. A minority of users suffer a headache or stomach upset that may or may not disappear with time. New antifungal antibiotics exist, but like all new drugs they cause more side effects and cost more, so we reserve them for infections that don't respond to griseofulvin.

Nail Infections

As the years pass, many men notice their toenails growing thick and yellow, perhaps even brittle, crumbly, and loose. Although aware, men rarely mention it to the doctor; mostly I bring up the subject when I observe this during an exam for another problem. Men assume that ugly toenails are a sign of aging, but toenails can't age because they're already dead. Thick yellow nails indicate disease, with fungal infection the leading cause.

Topical treatment won't cure an infected nail. Only oral griseofulvin works.

It diffuses into living nail cells under the skin, and as the nail grows out the fungi can't grow backward. Eventually healthy nail reaches the tip. Toenails grow slowly; treatment should last over a year, and you may not notice good nail appearing until after three or four months. Furthermore, a cure isn't guaranteed, but in my experience griseofulvin works over half the time. It worked for me—on the third attempt. I took the drug for about eight months on the first two attempts, and the infection returned in a year or two. After taking it for about fourteen months fifteen years ago, my nails cleared permanently.

Your family doctor may show little enthusiasm for prescribing a powerful drug over an extended time to treat a mere cosmetic problem. Although this is sensible, if you detest your ugly toenails try to persuade your doctor or consult a dermatologist.

Ringworm

Ringworm or fungal infection of nonhairy skin affects adults less often than children. Involvement begins as a pink patch that spreads outward with a raised, scaly border and a clearing center. Typical ringworm itches slightly or not at all. Creams eliminate infection confined to a small area, but extensive ringworm requires at least a month of griseofulvin.

The Universal Fungus: Tinea Versicolor

This may sound like the Latin species name, but it's only medicalese for "fungus that changes color." The organism is *Pityrosporum orbiculare*, another harmless fungus that normally lives on human skin. Although common in hot weather and hot climates, tinea versicolor appears year-round in a large minority of men. As they do with toenail infections, men often pay no attention because the rash doesn't itch or appear on visible areas—face and extremities.

I routinely see men with scattered tan or yellowish patches on the chest, back, abdomen, and shoulders, present for years, perhaps growing more intense with sun exposure and fading in winter. In white men, the patches appear darker than their normal pigment, but dark-skinned men have lighter patches. A mild case consists of a few spots over the sternum, but florid infections cover the trunk from neck to buttocks. Men who bring the rash to my attention complain of slight itching, but I suspect this is because anyone with a skin disease expects to itch.

Harmless and probably not contagious, tinea versicolor doesn't require treatment, and its tendency to recur makes treatment a lifetime proposition. Antifungal creams work fine but become impractical for large areas. Griseofulvin fails, but a short course of a newer antibiotic, ketoconazole (Nizoral) eliminates the infection.

For the average case, practical over-the-counter treatments include selenium sulfide (Selsun or Exsel shampoos) and sodium thiosulfate (ordinary photographic hypo or a commercial product called Tinver). Apply to the entire trunk after a daily shower, leave it on ten minutes, then wash off. Do this daily for two weeks. Treatment kills the fungus, but the spots may persist for months; although not essential, sun exposure speeds up repigmentation. If recurrences become bothersome, treat for two weeks and then once a week for the rest of your life.

Skin Disorders That Never Herald Skin Cancer

Men whose college years are growing distant begin to notice things on their skin that weren't there before. Your life may depend on paying attention to those in the next section, but daily living grows tiresome if you must keep an eye on every blemish and bump, so here are several that you can safely ignore. You may, however, want to take some action for cosmetic reasons.

Too many benign skin disorders exist to discuss in a book like this, so I have chosen the ones that matter most—those that are (1) very common and (2) occur on the face and scalp.

A look around at the beach or locker room reveals that almost every man past thirty-five has a few brown warty patches over his back and chest. Older men may have dozens that spread widely to include the scalp and face. Some on the face appear so ugly that you'll wonder why the men haven't tried to get rid of them. Most likely, a doctor has explained that these are entirely benign and that removal is too much trouble. Often this means too much trouble for the doctor.

Seborrheac Keratoses

After age thirty, small brown spots with a rough surface begin to appear over the back. Since they never cause symptoms, most men don't notice them, but after forty you may see a few on the back of your hands. Not freckles and only distantly related to moles (both of which appear at a much younger age), seborrheac keratoses begin and remain at the top of the epidermis. Called age spots at this early stage, they are easy to eliminate.

Over years, the spots enlarge and grow rougher and often wart-like, but, unlike warts, they never go away. Some grow to an inch or more in diameter and vary from flesh-colored to black. A typical seborrheac keratosis seems stuck onto the skin surface, and many are accidentally torn off or scraped away with a fingernail. This is not always possible, so don't try it.

Treatment. Seborrheac keratoses are entirely benign, and getting rid of a large one takes a modest amount of skill, but I wouldn't want one stuck to my face, and neither would most doctors. Since these are almost universal, you should make plans for dealing with yours early enough to avoid a buildup of these skin barnacles.

When I notice a small keratosis on the face, I dip a Q-tip in a cup of liquid nitrogen and freeze the spot for about five seconds. It sloughs in a few days and heals invisibly. Since almost every man past forty has a few, doctors rarely mention treatment unless a patient brings it up. Keeping liquid nitrogen requires a large thermos and regular refills from the dealer, so many solo doctors don't take the trouble, but every clinic should have it.

Remember that a brown spot appearing on your face after you pass thirty is probably permanent and destined to grow. Doctors will undoubtedly feel that they've done their job when they assure you that it's benign, so you must request that they freeze it for purely cosmetic reasons. You are completely justified, and I'm surprised that doctors (who would quickly treat a wart on the face) have so little concern for early seborrheac keratoses.

Once a keratosis grows large and thick, a doctor can scrape it off with a rake-like instrument called a curette after injecting novocaine. The area should heal without scarring. Unless there's a suspicion of malignancy, surgical excision isn't necessary.

Dermatitis Papulosa Nigra

Black and oriental adults commonly develop dozens of pinhead-size papules over the cheeks. Despite their distinct name, *dermatitis papulosa nigra*, these are identical to seborrheac keratoses. Although the same techniques eliminate them, the end result is often less satisfactory because injury to the skin of nonwhite races tends to heal with a change in pigmentation. Even a minor freezing with liquid nitrogen may leave a small dark or light spot, so any nonwhite who wants something removed from his face should see a dermatologist.

Cherry Angiomas

Almost everyone over thirty has a few small red or purple papules the size of a pinhead on the trunk, chest, or scalp. These are cherry angiomas, clumps of swollen blood vessels in the dermis. No one knows why they occur. Entirely benign, they grow numerous with age but almost never appear on the face. Removing them is impractical, but liquid nitrogen, curettage, and other methods of local destruction work.

Milia

Pearly white cysts a few millimeters in diameter often appear around the eyes and forehead of men over age forty. Called milia, these form when small pieces of growing epidermis become trapped in the dermis just below. Many men choose to ignore them, but a doctor can eliminate each cyst by slicing off the surface with a scalpel and squeezing out some cheesy material.

Freckles

Freckles are irregular tan spots that form on sun-exposed areas of genetically susceptible persons who usually have sandy or red hair. Although harmless, their appearance indicates that the skin is particularly susceptible to the sun. Freckles can be peeled off with acid or liquid nitrogen but tend to recur. Like gray hair, they are better admired than treated.

Liver Spots

Similar to freckles but a consequence of long sun exposure are liver spots (named for the color, not the organ). Favored sites include the forehead and back of the hand, but never the knuckles. Skin with liver spots shows other signs of sun damage such as fragility, depigmented spots, and actinic keratosis (see the next section). Except for their smooth surface, liver spots resemble early seborrheac keratoses, and the same techniques eliminate them.

SKIN DISORDERS THAT MAY OR MAY NOT HERALD SKIN CANCER

Detected early, all skin cancers—including the dreaded melanoma—are cured easily, but in my personal experience curing an easily cured cancer can be remarkably unpleasant. You can reduce your risk by keeping an eye out for benign but ominous skin conditions that are even more easily cured.

Precancerous Skin Conditions

A pink, scaly spot on a sun-exposed area—usually the face or neck—is often an *actinic keratosis*. Men are more likely than women to have them on the rim of the ear. An actinic keratosis may feel rough to the finger but rarely wart-like or raised; usually small, they can spread widely if neglected. Five to 10 percent turn into squamous cell skin cancers, one of the three common types (see page 206).

I treat actinic keratoses (including my own) with liquid nitrogen on a Q-tip, freezing it for about seven seconds. No anesthetic is necessary; the frozen area sloughs in a few days and heals without scarring. In the old days, doctors used an electric spark or scalpel. Some continue to do so, and surgical excision is essential if a doctor suspects malignant change and wants to send the tissue for pathological examination.

For multiple keratoses we can prescribe a cream containing 5-fluorouracial

(Efudex, Fluoreplex). Rubbed twice daily over an area, the cream inflames and then destroys the keratoses—including those formerly invisible. Treatment takes two to four weeks, after which healing takes a few more weeks; angry, red patches cover the area during this time, so patients dislike it.

Actinic keratoses are a snap to treat with liquid nitrogen, a valuable substance useful for destroying many superficial skin disorders. Every family doctor keeps a bottle on hand; if money is no object, there's no harm in seeing a dermatologist, but it isn't necessary.

A thicker, larger red plaque with a heavy scale covering the surface is probably Bowen's disease, a disorder that occurs primarily on sun-exposed areas of older white men. Less common but more vivid than an actinic keratosis, doctors commonly mistake it for psoriasis or eczema, so you may have to remind your doctor that psoriasis rarely occurs in a single patch, and that eczema itches. About 5 percent of Bowen's plaques develop into squamous cell carcinoma.

Harmless and Ominous Moles

Although not in the league of fear of AIDS, fear of moles brings a steady stream of otherwise healthy men to the doctor's office. Everyone knows that a growing or darkening mole can represent the dreaded and often fatal malignant melanoma, so doctors excise many obviously benign moles to relieve a patient's worry. Removing every mole is impossible because the average man has forty.

A mole consists simply of a clump of cells that usually includes melanocytes (skin cells that produce pigment), and its color ranges from gray to tan to dark brown to black, and a black mole is not necessarily ominous. Pigment isn't essential, and many moles are flesh-colored. Shapes vary as much as color: from a flat spot to slightly elevated to an obvious dome; the surface may be rough or smooth. Some grow hair—also not an ominous sign. Although not produced by solar radiation, moles appear more often on exposed areas and rarely on the buttocks, inner arms, and other protected sites.

Newborns possess none or only a few; they begin appearing at six months and continue to increase until the early twenties. Few appear afterward, and existing moles age and fade away with a lifespan of about fifty years. By age eighty, you can expect to be free of moles (but not other colored spots).

Signs of a harmless mole include uniform pigmentation, a smooth border, and unchanging size and color. Use these guidelines for all moles, including those in odd sites such as the inner thigh.

Worrisome signs include enlargement, color changes (including red, white, blue, or black), and any surface changes: crusting, scaling, oozing, bleeding, or thickening. We consider the appearance of pigment spots just beyond the edges especially ominous.

I have never cared for these guidelines because too much overlap occurs, but no better ones exist. Although they tend to grow more slowly, benign moles often enlarge and become bumpy. Furthermore, if you stare at any mole long enough, it begins to look evil. When this happens, see your doctor for an inspection and advice on future visits. You will need a yearly skin exam once you begin worrying about moles.

Skin cancer: a common malignancy

Easily the most common malignancy, skin cancer affects over 600,000 Americans per year, the majority of them men, because men spend more time in the sun. Men also suffer more occupational exposure to coal tar, pitch, radiation, creosote, and arsenic. Smoking induces cancer in areas exposed to smoke—lips and mouth. Finally, like other cancers, a family history increases the risk, and so does a suppressed immune system: AIDS victims have more.

Fair-skinned men of Celtic or Scandinavian ancestry are most susceptible, especially those with red or blonde hair and blue eyes. Black skin protects; whites have twenty-five times more skin cancer and a 15 percent lifetime risk. The incidence doubles with every 265-mile approach to the equator; a Texas resident runs 5.7 times the risk as a person from Minnesota. Living at a high altitude with its greater ultraviolet intensity also raises the risk. Skin cancer incidence is rising steadily.

Know the Three Skin Cancers

The most common and curable, *basal cell carcinoma* attacks about 500,000 Americans per year, the majority male, past forty, and sun exposed. Ninety percent of these carcinoma arise between the hairline and the upper lip. A cancer of the lower lip is usually a squamous cell carcinoma, discussed later.

The usual basal cell appears as a waxy pink pimple with a central ulceration and tiny blood vessels visible around its translucent borders. Medical students learn that the phrase "pink, pearly papule" wins a professor's approval as a description of a basal cell carcinoma. Although not a bad guideline, you're better off seeing a doctor for any new occurrence on your skin that doesn't disappear in a month. As it grows the papule may scab, bleed, or form a temporary crust, but don't depend on appearance or on any behavior except persistence.

Although they almost never spread (metastasize) or kill, a basal cell carcinoma doesn't go away but enlarges slowly, and every dermatology textbook feels obligated to print a photograph of a victim with a hideous gaping hole in his face. Since skin cancers tend to be painless, old people with more pressing medical problems often ignore them, so keep an eye on your elderly relatives.

One tenth as frequent but more serious are *squamous cell carcinomas*. *Squamous* means plate-like; squamous cells cover your epidermis. Their flat, compact shape provides the best protection against injury, but too much irritation from radiation or chemicals will turn them malignant.

To digress slightly, squamous cells appear in areas where they don't belong in response to chronic irritation, most often cigarette smoke. In these locations (mouth, throat, lung, esophagus, bladder), they are always premalignant. Lung and other cigarette-induced cancers are usually malignant squamous cells.

Fortunately (because tobacco-induced cancers spread more readily), smoking plays a minor role in skin cancer, except on the lower lip. A distant second to basal cells over the rest of the face, squamous cells make up almost all cancers on the lower lip, and men suffer over 90 percent of cases (lipstick may provide some protection for women). For unclear reasons, squamous cell carcinomas also occur three times as often as basal cells over the back of the hand. With these exceptions, both appear over identical sun-exposed areas. Unlike basal cells, squamous cell cancers commonly arise from visible premalignant conditions mentioned in the last section (especially actinic keratoses), and less often in areas of obvious injury such as old scars and skin exposed to radiotherapy or cancer-causing chemicals.

An early squamous cell cancer appears as a small crust or bump that expands, ulcerates, crusts, or simply grows into a wart-like nodule. Once again, see a doctor for any skin condition that remains after a month. The doctor will often decide that no treatment is necessary unless it persists. Always ask when you should return if this happens, and then obey.

Panic spread through a medical school class I taught in 1971 after my "Introduction to Medicine" lecture on malignant melanoma. Professors prefer to illustrate with their most vivid cases, and I followed the custom in discussing the third common skin cancer, *malignant melanoma*. A slide of a white woman appeared normal at the time of her diagnosis. A second slide taken a year later, after the cancer had spread, showed only one change: Her skin had turned black. A third slide demonstrated that her urine had also turned black. Further slides showed results of the autopsy after her death. Her liver was black; her brain was black; all her tissues had turned coal black. For weeks afterward, students trooped to the dermatology clinic for an inspection of their moles. It's a tradition that medical students develop symptoms of whatever new disease they study; melanoma remains the overwhelming illustration in my memory.

Although only a rare patient turns black, malignant melanoma deserves some of the concern it inspires. It's the fastest increasing cancer in the United States, doubling every decade and increasing disproportionately in young adults. By the year 2000, a white American will have a 1 percent chance of falling victim over a lifetime (other races suffer much less).

Sunlight plays a role, but cumulative exposure matters less than in other skin cancers. The back, not the face, marks the preferred site in men, although melanoma can appear anywhere on the body, including the eye and inside the mouth. More moles occur on the back, but that's also the site of most sunburn, and studies show that *blistering sunburn during childhood* vastly increases the risk.

Moles and Melanoma

Despite the feared association, only about one melanoma in three grows from a preexisting mole. Most appear from normal skin, so detecting melanoma is little different from detecting other skin cancers. Using guidelines from this and the last section, keep an eye on your moles, but if you're worried or have any risk factor (fair skin, tendency to sunburn, affected relatives), let a doctor inspect your skin.

Treatment

Despite a host of clever new techniques, simple surgery remains the choice for most skin cancers. After injecting novocaine, the doctor cuts away the tumor along with a generous margin of normal skin. A quarter inch is adequate for basal and squamous cell cancers, but not for a melanoma, with its propensity to spread. Doctors keep a half-inch margin for the thinnest, but this may double or triple for thicker melanomas, requiring hospitalization and skin grafting.

For all its disadvantages, the fragile skin of the elderly heals with less scarring, and skin cancers behave less aggressively, so doctors often treat with electrodesiccation and curettage. Under local anesthesia, the doctor scrapes off the tumor with a curette and then scorches the base with a spark and curettes away the burned tissue. For someone who hates the thought of surgery, this also works for small, shallow cancers. Radiotherapy may be best for a large mass or one on the nose or in a tricky area such as the eyelid.

Be careful of treatments such as lasers, freezing, and using chemicals—either smearing them on the cancer or injecting into it. They may sound superscientific, new, or better than brutal surgery or radiation, but they aren't. Freezing has been around for thirty years, and even lasers date from the 1970s. They've never worked as well as their most optimistic advocates claim.

Get the Best Medical Care for Your Skin Cancer

Although there's no reason why a family doctor or surgeon can't cut out the cancer, this rarely happens except in rural areas far from a skin specialist. You're better off with a dermatologist, if only because he or she deals with skin cancer all the time.

Many dermatologists advertise their particular expertise with skin tumors. Pay no attention. All are trained in skin surgery, and all would love your business. Remember that our absurd medical insurance system pays vastly more for a procedure like surgery than for simply examining a patient. For removing the simplest basal cell, a dermatologist could bill over $300 in 1993. Twenty minutes is a reasonable time for the surgery, and he or she would have to see half a dozen ordinary rashes to earn as much.

Although the cure rate with surgery approaches 95 percent, this drops for recurrences, larger skin cancers (over an inch in diameter), those with vague margins, and those around the nose, eyes, and ears. Mohs surgery works far better, but since ordinary surgery works most of the time, that's what you'll probably receive unless you ask.

Mohs Surgery: What You Should Know

A few hundred dermatologists have taken an extra year of training to learn the technique Dr. Mohs developed fifty years ago to deal with difficult skin cancers.

Doctors prefer to cut a wide area of tissue from around a tumor to ensure removal of 100 percent of the malignant cells. This works well over most of the body, but cutting large pieces from the face leaves ugly gaps. Removing less leaves the face looking better, but the smaller the excision, the greater the chance of recurrence.

The Mohs technique takes the guesswork out of determining how much to cut. The surgeon removes a segment around the tumor, marking it to show the orientation. Then he or she prepares it and examines the edges carefully under a microscope. If all margins show only normal cells, the cancer is gone.

If an area shows malignant cells reaching the edge, the surgeon returns to the patient and cuts another small segment from just beyond that spot. It may take many trips from patient to microscope before the surgeon determines that the edges of all segments are free of tumor. Using this technique, a surgeon removes a minimum of skin, and the cure rate approaches 100 percent. However, like all plastic surgery, it's wildly expensive.

When Should You Choose Mohs Surgery? You should choose it for almost any skin cancer on the face, insists at least one expert. It's the only technique that almost guarantees a cure, but it's too expensive, and there are too few Mohs surgeons to handle the traffic. Here are practical guidelines (of course, if you have plenty of money, you don't have to be practical).

1. Mohs surgery is the best for a recurrence. Radiotherapy is also effective; since a recurrence indicates that tumor cells have spread more widely, that seems obvious; repeat surgery doesn't work well.

2. It's the best initial treatment for tumors that may extend deeper or farther than they appear to the naked eye. A dermatologist can tell after an examination and biopsy, and you'll have to trust the decision.

3. It's best where surgery is tricky—around the eyes, ears, and nose. Here the dermatologist does what doctors do all the

time—use judgment. What method is best? Should he or she use ordinary surgery? If so, how much skin should he or she remove? Good doctors have the best judgment, but no one is perfect.

WHAT YOU SHOULD KNOW ABOUT COSMETIC SURGERY

Given a choice between halting aging inside versus outside my body, I'd choose inside, but since my health remains good, the consequences of aging are far more obvious on my exterior. Following my own advice, I apply Retin-A and sunscreen religiously and freeze small keratoses as soon as they appear. Now and then I think about electrolysis to eliminate the hair sprouting from my ears, but that's the limit of my cosmetic efforts.

On the other hand, I don't feel the urge to take more action. As I mention elsewhere, women don't object to the signs of aging in us as much as we do in them, and I don't have features that everyone considers unattractive and which medical science can correct: jowls, sagging eyelids, double chin, deep wrinkles. This is not the case with many men my age. Overwhelmingly, a female preoccupation in the past, cosmetic surgery began to interest more men around 1980, and they now make up a substantial minority of patients.

What to Expect

While I don't perform plastic surgery, I counsel patients who are thinking about it, and here is what I say:

1. It's breathtakingly expensive, rarely covered by insurance, and the surgeon usually expects the fee up front.
2. Surgery will probably make you look better for your age, but don't count on it to make you look younger.
3. Correcting a cosmetic defect often makes a man feel better about himself, and that's a sensible reason for going ahead.

Don't expect it to accomplish any other goal—including making you more popular or improving your sex life.

Naturally, you must choose a reputable surgeon. If your family doctor has personal knowledge of someone accomplished in the procedure you want, that's the best choice. A certified plastic surgeon isn't the only possibility; some head and neck surgeons, ophthalmologists, and dermatologists specialize in certain operations. If you're on your own, choose a surgeon certified by the American Board of Plastic Surgery. Remember the exact name because plenty of organizations exist with "plastic" "cosmetic" surgery in their titles. Only a doctor certified by the American Board of Plastic Surgery has taken the seven-year residency and passed the test. You can obtain a list of specialists in your area by calling 1-800-635-0635.

What's Available?

Here is what to expect of the most popular cosmetic procedures:

Facelifts smooth our sagging, drooping, and heavy wrinkling. To see how you might appear afterwards, look in a mirror, place your palms over your temples and push the skin backwards.

In a typical operation, the surgeon makes a long incision from one ear across the scalp to the other ear. Lifting the skin of the forehead, he or she cuts out frown muscles and others that produce furrows. After extending the incision below the ear to free up the cheek, chin, and neck area, the surgeon separates the skin from the underlying tissue then trims excess skin, pulls it tight, and sews it back. Confined to the hairline, the scar is inconspicuous.

Most surgeons prefer local anesthesia plus heavy sedation because it's safer and doesn't require an endotracheal tube which makes it difficult to visualize the face. Immediately after surgery the face swells and feels tight, but pain is rarely a big problem. Depending on the surgeon's preference, patients go home the same day or in a day or two. Bleeding under the skin produces vivid black-and-blue marks that last about a month, so the patient may want to take time off work.

Like all surgery, healthy patients enjoy the best results. Some surgeons reject smokers because smoking reduces the blood supply to the face. Obese men are not the best candidates because the surgeon can't remove all their underlying fat, so results are hard to predict. Some men, especially those with a dark complexion, are prone to form thick scars, so concealing them may be impossible. Naturally, a man whose hairline recedes will also reveal his scar.

Blepharoplasty removes excess skin from upper and lower eyelids; it is often combined with a facelift. Men look less grim and tired and perhaps younger when this sagging skin disappears. Occasionally a droopy upper lid interferes with vision; more often a lax lower lid leaves the eye unprotected so it burns and tears. If this is the case, your insurance may pay at least part. An ophthalmologist can evaluate this, and he or she may also perform the blepharoplasty.

Under local anesthesia and sedation, the surgeon makes incisions across the creases of the lids and near the eyelashes, trims excess skin and removes underlying fat, then closes the wounds. Since they extend across natural creases, scars are barely visible.

Afterwards, ice packs over the eyes help reduce swelling and bleeding. Most patients go home the same day, but a month may pass before visible bruising fades.

Wrinkle Removal. A facelift improves obvious wrinkles but does little for fine wrinkles around the eyes and mouth. Eliminating these requires removing the surface layer of skin either by scraping with a rotary wheel (dermabrasion) or destroying it with a phenol solution (chemical peel). As a bonus, these can eliminate blemishes as well as shallow scars from acne or chicken pox. Although the surgeon or dermatologist will discuss the pros and cons of either procedure, men tend to prefer dermabrasion because a chemical peel leaves the skin shinier than most men find attractive.

Local anesthesia works for a small area; large areas usually require general anesthesia and hospitalization. The procedure is painful, and the patient must remain immobile during surgery. A crust forms over the treated skin and remains for at least a week. Afterwards, the new skin appears bright pink. This fades to a modest pink in a few weeks, and women can improve this with makeup. Six months may pass before all pinkness vanishes, but the new skin will always look slightly paler.

Plastic surgery with a scalpel is so complex that almost all physicians who perform it have undergone academic training. This is not the case with dermabrasion and chemical peels; the basic procedure is not terribly difficult to learn. A G.P. can charge $200 for a complete physical exam that takes an hour; in contrast, $3000 for an hour's face peeling looks tempting, so plenty of entrepreneurial doctors are tempted. Yet these procedures require as much skill as traditional surgery. Removing slightly too much epidermis leaves scars. Unless the scraping or peeling occurs evenly over the entire face, the end result looks blotchy. Make sure you choose an experienced, qualified specialist. You'd be wise to check out some of his patients.

Rhinoplasty (nose reconstruction). A man who feels his nose is too large, hooked, high, bumpy, or otherwise unsatisfactory can have this corrected. Almost any healthy person is a good candidate although surgery may aggravate an unrelated nasal problem, so doctors discourage men with hay fever and other allergies.

Using drawings and a mirror, the patients spends time in the office choosing the appearance of the transformed nose. During the operation, the surgeon usually makes incisions inside the nostril which avoids visible scars. Correcting a bulbous or overhanging nose requires trimming cartilage without working on the nasal bones themselves, but fixing a large, hooked, or crooked nose demands extensive bone work. Afterwards the surgeon packs the nose to prevent bleeding, and the man wears a dressing for about a week. He goes home the same day or the next and must avoid strenuous exercise for about a month. As with other facial surgery, bruising lasts several weeks.

Liposuction, available in the U.S. only since 1982, has become perhaps the most common cosmetic procedure. Like dermabrasion and chemical peeling, it attracts plenty of doctors eager to share the bonanza, so a man must choose his surgeon with care.

Although it permanently removes fat, liposuction removes only a few pounds, so don't consider it for simple weight loss. It works well for eliminating localized fat deposits. Men are often concerned about bulging breasts or a double chin, but they also choose liposuction to reduce sagging buttocks, thighs, and abdomen. The operation works best in men with skin elastic enough to adjust once fat disappears underneath. If skin quality is poor (or the surgeon unskilled) the surface looks bumpy and irregular afterwards. Obviously, young men are better candidates although many middle-aged men have acceptable skin tone. Older men may benefit from liposuction although the surgeon may have to perform additional plastic surgery to trim redundant skin.

In the usual technique, the surgeon cuts a small incision through which he inserts a metal tube with a sharp tip. Moving the tube around slices fat from other tissue. At intervals a machine connected to the tube suctions out the fat. Over the next several weeks, the cavities that result will shrink, eliminating the undesirable bulge, and this change should be permanent. If the man puts on weight, fat will accumulate everywhere and not reproduce the local defect. The operation causes swelling and bruising which may take two months to disappear.

CHAPTER · 10

WHAT THE SEXUALLY ACTIVE MAN SHOULD KNOW

To many men, a woman's gynecological functions seem a mysterious and perhaps distasteful subject best left unexamined. In past generations, this ignorance inconvenienced the woman, who assumed, not always correctly, that a man gave her whatever gynecological ailment she was suffering. More recently, when the medical profession began taking an interest in contraception, men were happy to discard the condom and allow women to take advantage of the wonders of science.

Today women are less willing to shoulder all responsibility for the unpleasant consequences of intercourse and leave the fun to men, and intelligent men see the justice of this. In any case, sexually transmitted diseases have become both a plague and a perpetual annoyance to our generation. Justice and self-interest demand that a man know something about women: how they handle contraception and what role men play in a host of gynecological disorders.

Sexually transmitted diseases are spread by sex, less often by other affectionate contact such as kissing, and not at all by inanimate objects like toilet seats. In the past, homosexual men had far more venereal disease (VD) than heterosexuals because they tended to be more promiscuous, but their rate is dropping rapidly for reasons everyone knows. The rate for heterosexual men is rising.

When I entered medical practice twenty years ago, I could count the venereal diseases on one hand—literally. There were five. Gonorrhea and syphilis remain with us. Three others are so rare that I've never seen a case, so I don't discuss them, but a host of new ones have appeared. Opening a medical journal today, I expect to read of yet another disease formerly never associated with sex that is now definitely a VD. You may be surprised to know that hepatitis, amebic dysentery, warts, cervical cancer, and probably penile cancer are all sexually transmitted.

UNDERSTANDING CONTRACEPTION

Men should realize that many women resent contraceptive research's overwhelming emphasis on women. Half a dozen new methods for females appeared during the twentieth century, but not one for males. Knowing a woman's choices may help you appreciate your responsibility.

The Pill

You probably never wondered why a pregnant woman never gets pregnant again while carrying her child. Although plenty of room remains in the uterus for the first several months, she can't conceive because the fetus stimulates its mother's hormone output, which suppresses further egg production. Soon after isolating the hormone estrogen in the 1930s, contraceptive researchers gave it to women in an effort to duplicate pregnancy. It turns out that, like male hormones, estrogen performs unreliably. Adding a second hormone, progesterone, produced the breakthrough: a contraceptive essentially 100 percent effective.

The first contraceptive pills imitated pregnancy faithfully, causing as much bloating, weight gain, nausea, fatigue, and breast tenderness as the real thing. Despite this, almost everyone welcomed them as a wonderful medical miracle. An independent woman of the 1960s chose the pill as her contraceptive. It's hard to imagine the sexual revolution without it.

Following our usual behavior toward dramatic advances, doctors appreciated the pill's good features quickly and the bad ones later. After a decade, doctors began noticing a few users suffering blood clots, strokes, heart attacks, gallstones, high blood pressure, and an elevated blood sugar. In retrospect, this should not have surprised us because pregnant women also suffer most of these. When news spread, the media and public turned against the pill with the same passion as they embraced it a decade before.

Compared to 30 years ago, today's oral contraceptives contain a fraction of the hormones and produce fewer side-effects and even some benefits (less menstrual bleeding, milder cramps, much lower risk of uterine and ovarian cancer), so they are regaining popularity. However, many women remain uncomfortable about taking hormones throughout the month.

The IUD

Women throughout history inserted wood, metal, and other materials into their uteruses for contraception as well as abortion. Doctors began inserting their own intrauterine devices (IUDs) after the turn of the century; researchers took an interest only in the 1950s, when population control became popular. The result was a collection of rings, bows, coils, and springs that, lined up on a shelf, look fairly gruesome.

They also behaved gruesomely. Early IUDs functioned as a foreign body, inflaming the uterine lining and making it hostile to a fertilized egg. Larger

IUDs produced more inflammation and better contraception as well as more pain and bleeding. Despite this, a majority of users found the symptoms tolerable and appreciated the convenience of contraception without pills or the bother of inserting creams and jellies into their vagina.

Then disaster struck with the Dalkon Shield. Several years after its appearance in the 1970s, doctors suspected and then confirmed that its design encouraged pelvic infections. The torrent of lawsuits that followed drove the shield as well as all other IUDs off the market. Even today major drug companies refuse to market them in the United States, although several small companies are taking the plunge.

In the rest of the world, including Canada and Europe, IUDs remain more popular than the pill. New ones are much smaller and release tiny amounts of medication locally in the uterus. Because they don't act as a foreign body, side-effects are milder. Many new designs are FDA approved, but they haven't caught on. The risk that an American gynecologist will be sued for malpractice at some time during his or her career is about 100 percent, so gynecologists tend to avoid anything that has caught the attention of lawyers. In addition, women today are less willing to accept objects inside their internal organs when alternatives exist. Given a choice between a solid object inside his penis and something else, most men would not think twice.

The Diaphragm

When pill and IUD use plummeted during the 1970s, sophisticated women led a revival of the diaphragm, a device dating from before World War II that fell out of fashion when easier methods appeared. A flexible ring surrounding a rubber cup, diaphragms come in various sizes; a doctor or nurse must fit a woman with the right size diaphragm for her cervix and teach her how to use it effectively.

Proper technique includes using the right size, filling the cup with spermicide before insertion, and inserting it just before sex. It doesn't work without all these steps. A snug diaphragm seems like a fine barrier, but it isn't; the diaphragm merely acts as a receptacle for spermicide. Women who don't use spermicide get pregnant. Inserting the diaphragm early in the evening also defeats the purpose. The spermicide disperses. Used correctly, the diaphragm works with about 95 percent efficiency.

During the several minutes while his partner fumbles with the diaphragm in the bathroom, a man should give thought to the convenience of a condom. Slipping one on takes five seconds.

Other Barriers

Spermicide without the diaphragm is slightly less effective but quicker and easier. Available without a prescription, it comes as a cream, foam, jelly, suppository, and soaked in a sponge.

The Female Condom

Released in 1993, the female condom is the newest barrier on the market and an ingenious idea. Larger and more expensive than the male condom, it's pushed into the vagina before sex and pulled out afterward.

The Rhythm Method

The rhythm method is not as unreliable as critics maintain and far more inconvenient than enthusiasts admit. Advocates point out that it's a natural method, but a woman who must put a thermometer in her rectum every day of her adult life is not doing what nature intended. However, done properly, rhythm is 95 percent effective—as good as the diaphragm.

To begin, a woman carefully measures her menstrual cycles and time of ovulation for a year. Her temperature drops slightly before ovulation, then rises 0.6 to 1.0 degrees within a day after. This change is often subtle, so she must take her rectal temperature at the same time every day, usually on awakening.

After recording a year's worth of periods (thirteen), she calculates her shortest and longest cycle; this is essential because a woman's period usually varies by at least five days from month to month. Then she calculates her safe time. No magic number exists, but experts agree that the egg survives five or six days after ovulation, and sperm can survive three days after ejaculation. This means that nine days are the shortest possible unsafe period. Most couples must abstain for ten days to two weeks per month. Those who don't want to abstain can use the rhythm method to save money on creams or condoms during safe times.

Unless she is extremely regular, a woman should continue to measure her temperature to detect even greater variations in her cycle. Women with extremely irregular periods can't depend on the rhythm method.

Contraception for Men

Although this section discusses contraception for women, I must include something about contraception for men so I can discuss making a choice later in this chapter. For the average man, contraception means the condom until well into the next century. Research on a male pill continues, but eliminating sperm is proving harder than we predicted. Reducing the sperm count is easy. Giving extra male hormone works (athletes taking steroids produce few sperm), but a reliable male pill must reduce them to zero, and this requires dangerously high doses. Female hormones interfere with a woman's fertility in tolerable doses, so they become popular worldwide when introduced in the 1960s. The first birth control pills turned out to be more dangerous than we thought; today they contain much less hormone.

Coitus Interruptus. An old technique (note the Latin name), this method is not popular in America but is a tradition in France and is largely responsible for the French government's chronic complaint about France's low birth rate.

The man proceeds with sex as usual until ejaculation becomes inevitable, when he withdraws, depositing his semen elsewhere. Aside from waiting too long, the major danger occurs during multiple acts of sex because fluid remaining in the penis may contain sperm. This technique requires self-control as well as a trusting partner, but it works fine. Frenchmen pride themselves on this sort of skill, and perhaps they can teach us something.

The Condom. Although called a "French letter" in England, the condom grew popular through the efforts of an eighteenth-century Italian, Casanova. His were made of lamb intestine, a material still available. The advent of vulcanized rubber in the nineteenth century drove down the cost, making condoms the leading birth control device over most of the world, a position they still hold. Lambskin supporters maintain that they enjoy superior sensitivity. This may be true, and lamb intestine prevents pregnancy as well as rubber, so it's fine if you know your partner. Lamb also screens out germs, but viruses can leak through. Since viruses cause two virulent sexually transmitted diseases, AIDS and hepatitis, anyone having sex with a stranger risks his life by not wearing a rubber condom.

"The condom broke," women often explain during an office visit for an unexpected pregnancy or postsex contraception. I hear this so often that I'm certain it's not the truth but a substitute for a more embarrassing explanation, such as the condom falling off or failure to use any contraception. Condoms are pretty reliable.

Use a condom with a receptacle tip to hold the ejaculate. If yours doesn't have one, leave half an inch of space at the front when you slip it on. A lubricated condom isn't necessary if you have sex with a woman who is aroused, because she will produce plenty of vaginal secretions. If this isn't the case or if you deal with a prostitute, use a lubricated condom. With a prostitute, I suggest wearing two.

Some authorities advise withdrawing immediately after ejaculation, but men prefer to relish the moment. Don't wait more than a few seconds, and hold the condom to prevent it from slipping off. If an accident happens, the woman should immediately use a contraceptive cream. If the accident occurs during the middle of the cycle when pregnancy is a real possibility, a doctor can prescribe the "morning-after-pill," a high dose of hormones for three days. Unreliable if taken more than two days after exposure and often unpleasant for the woman, this is not something you should rely on often.

It's safe to carry condoms in your pocket. Shelf life is several years, and body heat won't damage them. Don't store them in genuinely hot places such as the glove compartment of your car. In poor countries, men wash condoms and reuse them, which is a bad idea. Sperm are amazingly energetic, and it takes only a pinhole to allow them through. Don't keep on the same condom for a second use the same evening.

Choose an Effective Method of Contraception

Although contraception won't be its main purpose, you'll use a condom during sex with anyone outside an exclusive relationship. For a regular partner, deciding on a method should be a subject of discussion.

Almost all couples who come to me for advice insist on safety above contraceptive efficiency and convenience. Despite an ongoing debate, it's not vividly clear which method is safest, and experienced couples gradually learn to value efficiency and convenience. Here's why.

Efficiency. The birth control pill, taken faithfully, prevents pregnancy best. For a woman who knows that she'll forget a pill now and then, an injectable or implantable hormone works best, although the new IUDs also perform well.

Safety. Barrier contraceptives produce no serious side-effects. Although new IUDs and hormonal methods have become very safe, a slight risk remains. To most laypeople the conclusion is obvious: Barriers are safer. But this conclusion is not so obvious if you think more deeply, and it may be wrong. More women using barriers become pregnant, and pregnancy is a slightly risky condition. In fact, a healthy woman is far more likely to die during pregnancy than one taking hormones or using an IUD. Abortions are also safe, but not completely so.

For a couple concerned only about short-term and long-term safety, the best strategy probably requires that the man use a condom while the woman uses one of the barriers, with the understanding that she will see a doctor for the morning-after pill if the condom fails. Condom plus morning-after pill represents a compromise which may or may not be safer than hormonal contraception.

GYNECOLOGICAL DISORDERS THAT A MAN SHOULD KNOW ABOUT

Patient: "My lady friend has an infection, and she wants me to get checked."

Doctor: "Is anything bothering you?"

Patient: "No."

Doctor: "What infection does she have?"

Patient: "I don't know. Can't you do a test?"

Doctor: "There are dozens of tests. I need to know what to look for. Can you tell me her symptoms?"

Patient: "She said she had an irritation."

Doctor: "Could you be more specific? A vaginal discharge? Pain? Trouble urinating?"

Patient: "I'm not sure. Her doctor did a test."

Doctor: "What did he find? Oh, I forgot; you don't know. What did he treat her with?"

Patient: "Pills. Or maybe a cream."

Doctor: "Do you know its name?"

Of course he doesn't. I have this maddening conversation at least once a month. Not only are men ignorant of female problems, they often recoil in disgust and rush to the doctor to make sure that they aren't infected. It turns out that most minor female infections aren't contagious and don't require that you see a doctor, but this is definitely not so for all.

Vaginal Infections

These cause itching, burning, and an abnormal vaginal discharge without generalized illness, fever, or abdominal pain. Like most minor infections, they eventually go away, but medical science has such good treatments that it's foolish to wait.

Yeast Infections A woman with an itch usually makes this diagnosis, because *yeast* is a popular synonym for all vaginal infections. In fact, *Candida* or yeast make up only about 30 percent. Although a different organism, *Candida albicans* resembles the fungus responsible for jock itch in men or athlete's foot in either sex. Of all vaginal infections, yeast causes the most intense itching and sometimes a thick, white discharge that looks like cottage cheese. Treatment is one of many antifungal creams or suppositories.

Like many microorganisms, *Candida* live harmlessly in the vagina unless something encourages them to grow wildly. This may happen if a woman takes antibiotics, which kill germs in the vagina but have no effect on fungi. Diabetes and other disorders that impair the immune system also promote *Candida*, but most cases have no obvious case.

The man's role in yeast infections. There is none. Women catch yeast from themselves. You need not see a doctor or take medicine if your partner has the infection.

The same applies if you're a victim. *Candida* occurs only rarely in men, and you can make the diagnosis yourself. On the penis it causes red bumps that itch mildly or not at all; most often I see it under the foreskin of an uncircumcised man. It can be treated with an over-the-counter cream (Micatin or Lotrimin) twice a day for two months, but you should see a doctor if it doesn't fade within a few weeks. Your partner doesn't need a doctor if she has no complaints.

Trichomonas. Unlike *Candida*, the trichomonad, a one-celled protozoan, doesn't normally live in the vagina and is probably transmitted through sex, although men don't show symptoms. Women notice an unpleasant discharge that usually itches, but not as badly as a yeast infection. Treatment is an antibiotic called metronidazole (Flagyl or Protostat).

The man's role in trichomonas infections. We probably harbor the organism somewhere in our urinary tract, because women with untreated partners suffer repeated infections. After making the diagnosis, I write two prescriptions, and other doctors should do the same. It's a waste of time and money for the man to come to the office, because testing men for trichomonas reveals none, but we always treat. If your partner's doctor sends her away without your prescription, phone and ask him or her to call one to your local pharmacy (use the information prescribed here as an argument). If he or she refuses, call your doctor and explain the situation.

Bacterial Vaginosis. Although responsible for half of all vaginal infections, this condition is not as well understood as the others, so doctors have called it by many names, such as nonspecific vaginitis, gardenerella, or hemophilus vaginitis. We suspect that germs that may or may not normally live in the vagina overgrow, producing a smelly discharge and irritation. Treatment is also metronidazole, but a longer course than for trichomonas.

The man's role in bacterial vaginosis. We're not certain about the man's role. Although sexually active women suffer more, the condition is not unknown in virgins, and no such infection occurs in men. In the past doctors treated partners, but this doesn't reduce recurrences.

Bladder Infections. Although bladder infections are not vaginal infections, symptoms as well as misunderstandings overlap, so you should know about them.

Cystitis, or bladder infections, plague young women. Their short urethras allow germs that normally live just outside to ascend and multiply in the normally sterile bladder. Several extra inches provided by a penis protect young men so bladder infections are rare in them, although men more than make up for this in middle-age, when swelling prostates obstruct the urethra (see Chapter 6).

Infected urine irritates the bladder, so women feel the urge to urinate every few minutes; the urge may be so sudden that they lose control. Since the sensation comes so often, little may trickle out when the woman reaches the toilet, but a short time later the urge reappears. If the infection spreads to the urethra, a woman feels burning as she urinates. Women with vaginal infections experience burning when urinating, but they also feel it continually. Once diagnosed, cystitis responds quickly to antibiotics.

The man's role in bladder infections. A woman's own germs are responsible. Men don't transmit the infection and don't require treatment, yet they exert an influence because the vigorous movements of sex can push a woman's germs into the bladder. Other activity around the genitals, such as bathing and masturbation, do the same. Many women suffer cystitis so regularly after sex that doctors prescribe a single dose of antibiotic to be taken immediately afterward.

Undiagnosed Infections: The Man's Role. On rare occasions, unable to make a diagnosis in a woman with a persistent, annoying irritation, the doctor suggests that the woman's partner "get checked." If you have no symptoms, call that doctor, explain that you feel fine, and ask if he or she still wants you to see a doctor. If the answer is yes, you must go, not because your doctor can solve the problem but out of respect for your partner's misery.

Undiagnosed means an infection in which the doctor says clearly that he or she doesn't know what it is. Matters are different if the woman doesn't know; this happens so often and provokes so many useless office visits that you must know how to deal with it.

Handling the Angry Phone Call

At some point in your adult life, a man who sleeps around receives a call from a present or former lover with the unsettling news that she has VD or an infection along with a hint, suggestion, or angry accusation that he gave it to her. Doctors regularly counsel such men in the office, but as the example on page 220 shows, it's frustrating. Here's how to handle this difficulty.

1. Don't deny it. Not only will it upset her further, but you could be wrong. As this chapter and Chapter 8 reveal, a man who feels fine can transmit infections.
2. Sympathize. Think how you'd feel if your genitals were diseased.
3. Find out more. Absolutely essential is the *name* of her infection. The general terms *VD, vaginal infection,* or *vaginitis* are useless.

Don't see your doctor without a name. If she replies that the doctor didn't tell her, she must phone and ask (her doctor won't tell anyone else). If she's waiting for the results of a test or culture, you must wait, too. If she refuses to call, the name and dosage schedule of her treatment may give your doctor a clue, but this is not certain. A description of her symptoms is usually useless.

4. Use the information in this chapter. If she has a yeast or bladder infection, you can explain that you're not responsible. This doesn't go over well when the doctor has urged that she send her contacts for a checkup. Some doctors routinely urge this on all women with genital infections, and it causes endless inconvenience. To preserve the relationship, you may have to go.

5. Don't act as her proxy. A woman may phone as soon as symptoms appear. Convinced that she's the injured party, she insists that you make the trip to the doctor for a test to determine what you gave her. Gently explain that since you have no symptoms, testing you won't determine if she has a minor infection. If she has a major infection such as gonorrhea, a culture of your urethra might grow the germ, but it takes two days. Waiting two days with gonorrhea could cause her permanent damage; she must begin treatment immediately (doctors treat women without waiting for test results). Use this chapter to back you up.

All this advice is unnecessary if you use a condom, because your chance of transmitting an infection approaches zero. If you don't use one, you should.

WHAT CAUSES A DISCHARGE FROM THE PENIS?

Gonorrhea

Until well after I entered practice in the early 1970s, a man who noticed stinging when he urinated and pus leaking from his penis knew immediately that he had gonorrhea, or he quickly learned after consulting friends. If his infection occurred after the advent of penicillin, one shot cured him like magic.

The oldest traditional VD, gonorrhea is our most common reported communicable disease (chicken pox is next; nongonococcal urethritis is more common but not reportable). Although two million cases per year make it far more common than AIDS, syphilis, or even herpes, gonorrhea has never provoked the same dread. A little dread would be useful, because it can be very destructive, especially in women.

Most infected men develop symptoms within a week of exposure. Before the advent of penicillin after World War II, a man might grit his teeth and wait; most gonorrhea disappeared after a month or so. If he wanted treatment, a doctor inserted a catheter into his urethra and allowed an antiseptic to flow in. Although painful, it probably didn't help. One infection doesn't give immunity, so anyone can catch it again and again. Before the penicillin era, men grumbled about their latest dose of "clap" but secretly looked on it as a sign of virility.

Gonorrhea wasn't considered dangerous, but occasionally men suffered local abscesses, arthritis, or meningitis, and now and then the infection left them sterile. These are rare nowadays because no shame attaches to having a sexually transmitted disease, and victims hurry to a doctor.

Gonorrhea also occurs in the throat and rectum, producing a sore throat or anal pain and discharge. Five to ten percent of men have no symptoms but remain contagious.

In the old days, rectal gonorrhea was a disease of homosexuals (officially, in the old days there were no homosexuals; medical science became aware of them during the 1960s). Today, as a result of AIDS, gays are getting their act together, and their VD rate has been dropping since the mid-1980s. This is not true for heterosexuals. Nowadays when I see someone with any sexually transmitted disease, I never guess at his or her orientation. I've been surprised too many times. I don't assume that anal infection means anal intercourse because too many patients swear indignantly that they never do such things. Experts still teach that anal VD comes from anal intercourse, and I tend to agree, but there's no proof that it can't spread from vaginal contact.

Diagnosis. Diagnosis is easy. Medical students can do it. I diagnosed gonorrhea regularly when I was a student volunteer at a free clinic on New York City's Lower East Side in 1970. A patient squeezed a drop of discharge onto a slide, which I carried into our primitive lab, dipped into a bottle of methylene blue dye, and examined under the microscope.

The gonorrhea discharge is pus: a mixture of white blood cells and the bacteria they are fighting. Gonorrhea germs are tiny dots that stick together in pairs, and they always grow inside a white blood cell, something other germs rarely do. Examining a positive slide, I might see 90, 95, or even 99 percent normal white cells, but sooner or later one appeared packed with tiny pairs of blue dots (because we used methylene blue; other stains produce other colors). It was always exciting to see; it still is. Few serious diseases are so easy to diagnose.

Treatment. Treatment once meant a shot of penicillin. Then it meant a very large shot of penicillin, then two large shots. By the late 1980s, the gonococcus had grown so resistant that our first choice became a different antibiotic: ceftriaxone (Rocephin).

■ DON'T SELF-TREAT WITH ANTIBIOTICS ■

If you kill every germ infecting you, they're dead and don't bother you any more. If you only kill some, *they get stronger!*

This explains why penicillin became useless for gonorrhea. In most parts of the world you can buy antibiotics without a prescription, and people treat themselves for whatever ails them. This is not a good idea. Resistant gonorrhea, malaria, typhoid, tuberculosis, and other infections first appeared in these countries and are gradually spreading everywhere.

It disturbs me when a patient with a sore throat or cough takes a few antibiotics before coming in. This never helps (the chance that he or she made the correct diagnosis and took an adequate dose of the right antibiotic for the proper length of time is zero—especially when you understand that 95 percent of sore throats and coughs don't respond to antibiotics).

When you take antibiotics on your own, you're performing a nasty experiment on yourself: one that researchers perform to produce resistant bacteria.

Scientists add a tiny amount of antibiotic to a culture of bacteria. This kills only the most sensitive germs; the rest multiply. Then they add a slightly larger amount of antibiotic. Again weaker germs die, resistant ones multiply. After many repetitions, all grow happily no matter how much antibiotic is around. Do you really want to do that to yourself?

Never take antibiotics on your own, and if your doctor gives you a prescription, finish the bottle. You want to kill 100 percent of the infecting germs. Killing 99 percent is asking for trouble.

Nongonococcal Urethritis

During the 1970s, doctors became aware that many patients with a discharge weren't cured. These were not cases of penicillin-resistant gonorrhea (which were also appearing) because even massive doses didn't help. We were seeing a new sexually transmitted urethral infection caused by an unrelated microorganism called chlamydia. Penicillin doesn't kill chlamydia.

Called nongonococcal urethritis (NGU) before researchers discovered the cause, we haven't changed the name because a few organisms besides chlamydia may be involved. NGU quickly grew to be the leading urethral infection, becoming so common that up to 45 percent of gonorrhea victims catch chlamydia at the same time. As a result, we always treat a gonorrhea patient for both.

Four million cases per year make NGU a major epidemic, but with so many more frightening diseases raging, it remains in the background. A dangerous infection in women and the leading cause of female sterility, a bout of NGU is mostly an inconvenience in a man.

Overall, NGU produces a milder urethritis than gonorrhea. Incubation takes longer: one to three weeks. The discharge flows less heavily and sometimes hardly at all. Burning may or may not accompany it. Infections without symptoms occur more often than with gonorrhea. A painful infection of the spermatic cord (epididymitis) marks the leading complication. (I discussed this in Chapter 6).

Diagnosis. Despite the differences, doctors who try to distinguish NGU from gonorrhea by symptoms alone regularly guess wrong. A microscopic exam remains essential. If the examiner can't find a white cell packed with dots, the diagnosis is NGU. In the absence of enough discharge, a doctor can swab the urethra and send off a culture for chlamydia.

Treatment. The treatment choice is a week of doxycycline, a convenient form of tetracycline one takes only twice a day. Many alternatives exist, but all forms of penicillin (including amoxicillin and ampicillin) fail.

Prevention. Prevention of urethritis and all forms of VD means wearing a condom. Forget what you've heard about condoms being unreliable. Although not perfect, they're very good. Among hundreds of patients with sexually transmitted diseases, I recall only one or two who swore they used a condom.

Experts with more romantic views urge everyone to stick to a single, monogamous relationship. Who can argue with that? Most people yearn for a single lover, but finding one can be frustrating. Also, monogamy doesn't guarantee safety because many sexually transmitted diseases remain dormant for years. Yet despite these caveats, monogamy remains less risky.

WHAT CAUSES SORES?

The genitals are not an area that men neglect to examine closely, and they should be examined now and then. Do so when you examine your testes. Most abnormalities brought to a doctor's attention are minor and are discussed later in this chapter. Two are more serious—herpes and syphilis.

Herpes

A minor sexually transmitted infection compared to syphilis yet more widely feared, genital herpes causes women great misery. Men suffer less, but the sores are an ugly sight.

A common virus, herpes simplex can attack any organ. It's the leading cause of viral encephalitis, a devastating brain infection; herpes in the eye causes blindness unless promptly treated. As long as the immune system stays healthy, herpes simplex rarely attacks internal organs, but victims of AIDS and other immune deficiencies suffer herpes simplex pneumonia, hepatitis, and esophagitis.

Fortunately, almost all infections occur on the skin, causing fever blisters, canker sores, and small clumps of sores elsewhere on the body. Spread is by direct contact; sex passes it from genital to genital. Skin infections are rarely serious, which is good news because herpes simplex is as universal as its relative, chicken pox (herpes zoster, another virus that causes sores). Most men have had herpes without realizing it.

The Usual Course. The first sign is a vague tingling around the genitals. Nothing is visible for a day or two, and then a few blisters appear. They quickly burst, becoming shallow sores that scab and heal within two weeks. Considerable pain accompanies herpes on sensitive areas like the tip of the penis. On the thigh or shaft of the penis, the discomfort may be hardly noticeable.

Fever and general misery accompany a first attack because the virus is in the blood and spreads throughout the body. Afterward, a victim has antibodies which quickly destroy any virus that reappears in the blood.

Complications. After most viral infections (measles, mumps, polio, hepatitis, yellow fever, smallpox) you are immune forever, but herpes has the peculiar habit of remaining dormant in nerve cells. Although it can never return to the blood, it regularly comes back to life, spreads to the end of a group of nerves, where it kills a patch of skin, and then retreats. Almost everyone suffering one attack of genital herpes will have another.

In case you're curious, nerves supplying your skin also harbor dormant chicken pox virus. Recurrences are less common, but when they happen, you suffer the painful eruption, shingles.

Herpes recurrences occur after local rubbing or injury, a minor illness, sun exposure, or emotional stress, but they often appear out of the blue. A few sufferers relapse every month or two; although maddening, this doesn't last. Recurrences are less severe than initial attacks. They gradually grow less frequent and usually stop within a few years.

Diagnosis. I diagnose herpes by examining the sores and listening to the patient describe his symptoms. If the history sounds typical, and the sores appear typical, I announce that they look like herpes. Some patients accept this, but many want a test. They want 100 percent assurance and believe, like most Americans, that a laboratory test will provide it. Since making patients feel better is a doctor's duty, I often order tests for this purpose alone.

A blood test for herpes antibody exists, but it reveals less than you think. Once you've had herpes, your blood contains the antibody forever, so a positive result indicates an infection sometime during your life. It's positive in 80 percent of prostitutes and 0 to 3 percent of nuns.

A culture gives better information only if herpes turns up. The chances are best if you arrive with a fresh blister. The doctor cuts away the skin covering the blister, rubs the raw surface, and sends the fluid to a lab. Growing the virus takes two to four days. Unfortunately, most patients wait until sores appear. By this time the virus may have disappeared, so a negative culture doesn't prove anything. If a doctor says, "It looks like herpes," that's as accurate as most tests.

Treatment. During the first years of the herpes hysteria in the early 1980s, worthless remedies abounded, and doctors championed many. They ranged from vitamins to lysine to ether to good antiviral drugs such as ioxouridine, which cures herpes of the cornea but nowhere else.

Humans who notice something wrong with their skin—a sore, a rash, an itch—feel an uncontrollable urge to rub cream on it. We have felt this compulsion since the dawn of time, and all healers, witch doctors, and physicians understand it. The advent of scientific medicine didn't change human psychology. Patients are rarely pleased when I explain that their rash will go away after a week or two and that no treatment helps. They look uneasy. Shy patients say nothing; others wonder politely if a cream will help; all are slaves to the deep inner need to rub something on their skin. If my explanation doesn't overcome this urge, I prescribe something. No cream helps herpes, but many victims get Zovirax.

Taken at the first symptom, acyclovir (Zovirax) tablets shorten an attack dramatically. However, acyclovir only suppresses the virus. It does not prevent recurrences, and it's expensive: about $70 for a ten-day course, so treatment isn't necessary if the sores aren't bothersome. Acyclovir is also available as an ointment. Like tablets, it's expensive (about $50 a tube), but unlike them it's useless. Ointment slightly shortens an initial attack but has no effect on a recurrence.

Prevention. Only the first episode of herpes spreads from another person, so prevention must begin at the beginning of your sex life. A victim may or may not shed virus between recurrences, which means that unprotected sex with someone without sores remains risky. Condoms protect against viruses, too.

Syphilis

Called "the white plague" and a major menace for centuries, syphilis is still with us: 50,000 reported cases a year with a large number unreported. It's growing more common in heterosexuals as it diminishes in homosexuals.

Before the antibiotic era, syphilis produced the same panic as AIDS does today, and mean-spirited people announced that victims were paying the penalty of their immoral behavior—another parallel with modern times.

Whatever Happened to Caligula? Historians love to practice medicine, and doctors play at being historians. Both enjoy pinning diseases on famous men, and syphilis wins hands down. Why were Beethoven and painter Francisco Goya deaf? Why were Milton and Bach blind? Why did the composer Schumann, the Roman emperor Caligula, and King George III of England go mad? From syphilis, of course. You can never go wrong with syphilis because late stages take so many forms.

But it's all nonsense. Until well past the middle of the nineteenth century, medical science was too primitive to make sense of complex diseases. Old descriptions of diseased patients make entertaining reading (any large library contains eighteenth- and nineteenth-century medical journals; take a look), but they're gibberish.

Syphilis develops from infection by a corkscrew-shaped bacteria called a spirochete. Like the gonococcus, it prefers the mucus membranes of your genitals, anus, or mouth, but it can penetrate slightly abraded skin, so the first sign of infection may appear on the penis or lips. Unlike the gonococcus, which usually remains localized, the spirochete spreads quickly throughout the body.

The Risk. Tracing sexual contacts, public health workers discover that only half are infected, so the risk from a single sexual exposure is probably lower than one would expect. On the other hand, early syphilis produces less discomfort than early gonorrhea; many victims pass through the early stages unaware.

The Usual Course. Incubation varies from a few days to six weeks, depending on the number of germs acquired. When researchers inject a million spirochetes into a volunteer, visible infection appears within three days. Injecting about sixty people eventually causes syphilis in half.

Traditionally, the first sign is the *chancre*—a painless ulcer on the genitals or anus, occasionally on the lip (a painful sore is more likely herpes or another infection). It persists a few weeks and then quietly heals. At the same time, nearby lymph nodes in the groin swell and shrink, also usually without pain.

Overlooking a chancre is easy. According to one study, only 42 percent of heterosexual men learned their diagnosis at this stage; among homosexual men, only 23 percent; among women, 11 percent.

A chancre marks *primary* syphilis. Almost every victim goes on to *secondary* syphilis one to three months after healing. You can think of this as the stage when the spirochete spreads, although this actually happened much earlier. Blood is infectious even before the chancre appears (transfusions and needle sharing spread syphilis as well as AIDS).

In the old days, a skin specialist was called a dermatologist and syphilologist, because this single disease provided so much of his or her practice. Secondary syphilis typically begins with a spotty pink rash covering most of the body, including the palms and soles. After days or weeks, the rash may progress to bumps or pimples. Five percent of patients suffer patchy hair loss in the scalp, beard, or eyebrows. Ten percent notice wart-like clumps in moist areas between the legs, where pimples have coalesced. One or two warts are probably warts, but a doctor should think of syphilis when he or she sees a large mass. Painless gray patches appear inside the mouth or on the lips or genitals in 15 percent of cases. All these eruptions are painless and not very itchy. Along with a rash, almost everyone notices enlarged lymph nodes on both sides of the groin, armpits, and neck.

To add to our difficulty, many signs of secondary syphilis resemble those of an ordinary virus: sore throat (15 to 30 percent), fever (10 percent), fatigue (25 percent), and headache (10 percent). If you suffer flu symptoms with a rash, flu is probably the diagnosis, but if you have doubts about your sexual partners of the past months, let the doctor know.

Unusual Courses and Complications. Less commonly, secondary syphilis produces hepatitis, colitis, nephritis, gastritis, arthritis, or disease of literally any organ. After recovery, two-thirds of patients never get sick again, although blood tests remain positive and the germ lives on in their body. Untreated, one-third move on to *tertiary* syphilis, in which tissue destruction leads to heart disease, paralysis, insanity, or blindness.

"If you know syphilis, you know medicine," a wise doctor once proclaimed. Thick medical books discussed this single disease. Doctors and hospitals specialized in it. It was the leading diagnosis of inmates in insane asylums. Since the advent of penicillin, advanced syphilis has almost disappeared.

Diagnosis. Men often ask for a "blood test" after a careless night on the town. Unfortunately, no test works so quickly. Your chancre will appear before a blood test for syphilis turns positive.

I also hear this during a routine exam when men want to make sure they're not harboring something ominous. For common sexually transmitted diseases, only AIDS and syphilis blood tests are in general use. You'll read about AIDS later in this chapter.

Several tests exist for syphilis, although I don't order them routinely except on promiscuous men. I want to explain them in detail because many doctors don't see enough syphilis to understand the tests; once or twice a year I see a man needlessly worried by his results.

The test you may know (still required for a marriage license in most states) is the VDRL (Venereal Disease Research Laboratory). Developed before I was born, modern versions are the same in name only, and many go under different names. You should remember only one fact: All are screening tests (i.e., cheap and easy) but less accurate than a diagnostic test.

The VDRL doesn't detect syphilis itself but a collection of antibodies provoked by the interaction of spirochetes with tissue. Produced in large amounts, these are easy to detect, so a negative VDRL is reassuring except during the first weeks after infection. A positive result isn't the last word (remember, it's not a diagnostic test). Many conditions that provoke the immune system lead to a false positive VDRL. Acute infections such as flu and pneumonia can do this for a short time. Long-lasting false positives occur in 25 percent of narcotic addicts, 10 to 20 percent of victims of autoimmune diseases (lupus, rheumatoid arthritis), and in 10 percent of everyone over age seventy. Confronted with a positive VDRL, a laboratory should do the following:

1. Measure the strength of the reaction by repeating the VDRL after diluting your serum. A positive result after a 1:8 dilution makes syphilis a near certainty. The lab will write the dilution on the slip, so your doctor should know it—and tell you.
2. Perform a diagnostic test called the FTA (fluorescent treponemal antibody). If you have a positive VDRL and a negative FTA, you don't have syphilis. False positive FTAs occur, but only rarely.

Although it happens, a doctor should never tell a patient, "Your VDRL is positive, but it doesn't mean anything. Don't worry about it." I'd worry if a doctor told me that. A doctor can give better information; it's probably on the lab slip. You should also remember that if you've had syphilis, your FTA will probably remain positive forever. The VDRL falls slowly after treatment and sometimes remains positive—but only weakly so. If it remains at 1:8 or higher, you need another treatment.

The immune system takes a few weeks to generate antibodies, so neither test is reliable early. Unless you're willing to walk around with a suspicious sore, get a dark-field examination of a scraping from the area. Spirochetes are hard to see with an ordinary microscope, requiring a special lighting attachment plus a doctor or technician trained to use it. Nowadays you'll go to a medical center or public health clinic, but if the scraping is positive, you'll know immediately.

Treatment. One injection of long-acting penicillin treats primary or secondary stages of the disease. We give three injections at weekly intervals for syphilis present longer than a year. Penicillin pills *never* work. We use tetracycline or doxycycline when a patient is allergic to penicillin.

Fortunately the syphilis germ is as sensitive to penicillin today as it was fifty years ago. No other common bacteria has been so cooperative. If you catch syphilis, a few dollars worth of drugs will cure you, a genuine miracle when you realize how much misery and deformity it caused for centuries.

Sexually Transmitted Benign Genital Lumps

Warts

Viruses cause cancer in animals, and researchers are certain that this is true for common human malignancies. Definite proof will be a wonderful advance in the battle against cancer. Evidence is piling up, and I expect a breakthrough at any time, but as I write only the lowly wart virus qualifies.

A wart is a benign tumor. Unlike malignant tumors, pieces won't break off and grow throughout your body. Warts spread because you or someone else rubs virus onto unaffected skin.

The Risk. About one in ten men have warts. Like most highly infectious conditions, they are most common in the young and diminish with age. When a patient over fifty shows me something he thinks is a wart, it's usually something else.

Five percent of adults have anal or genital warts, which are no different from warts elsewhere except that sexual contact spreads them, and they seem even more contagious than warts in dry areas. If your sexual partner is affected, your risk is 64 percent with an incubation period of at least four weeks.

The Usual Course. The wart virus works slowly. After it enters a living cell, a month to a year passes before a pinhead-sized, flesh-colored bump appears. More weeks to months pass as it grows large enough to reveal the typical rough surface. A bump with a smooth surface is probably something else (perhaps a molluscum, discussed later in this chapter). Warts on a moist surface may spread widely, resembling a patch of cauliflower.

Despite popular belief, warts are temporary. One quarter disappear within six months, half within a year, two thirds in two years.

Unusual Courses and Complications.

1. Anal warts in a child are evidence of sexual abuse.
2. Get a test for syphilis if you have anal or genital warts. Most doctors can't tell the difference between warts and the wart-like clumps called condyloma lata that appear during secondary syphilis.

Treatment: *Physical destruction.* Researchers are searching for gentler ways, but results are unimpressive so far. Announcements of a shot that melts away warts appear regularly in the media. Don't believe them. A skilled dermatologist may treat a stubborn infestation with repeated injections of interferon or an anticancer drug. These sometimes work, but they are not gentle.

Current treatments include

1. Burning
2. Freezing
3. Corrosive chemicals
4. Surgery.

This illustrates a law of medicine: If a disorder has many treatments, none are very good. Getting rid of a wart is easy, but maintaining a wart-free body is unrealistic. Don't let this upset you. I spend more time warning patients against wartophobia than attacking their skin. This is essential because warts require a serene Zen detachment for successful treatment. They thrive on attention and flourish in an environment of fear and hatred. If one bothers you, treat it. But never despise your warts.

Although detachment is appropriate for warts in most areas, those on the genitals deserve prompt treatment to avoid infecting a sexual partner.

The Mechanics. For warts on dry skin, try over-the-counter corrosive chemicals such as Compound W, Vergo, WartAway, or Dr. Scholl's. Sometimes effective, they are cheaper than a doctor visit and keep you busy while nature takes its course. Never treat yourself for genital or anal warts.

For those, most doctors use *podophyllum*, a corrosive black liquid extracted from a plant. With a cotton swab the doctor paints each wart, carefully avoiding normal skin. If this is your first treatment, you should wash it off with soap and water after four hours. A few men are too sensitive; they feel burning sooner and must wash it off immediately. Most feel nothing at all and can leave it on longer during later treatments.

Although a field of warts occasionally vanishes, I'm pleased to see a 50 percent shrinkage on the second visit in two weeks. The average infestation requires several trips. If any remain after four visits, the doctor should think about switching to another method after first making sure the podophyllum is not out of date—the most common reason for treatment failure.

Liquid nitrogen is my favorite for warts in most areas. Although it is superior for treating genital warts because it usually works in one treatment, many patients refuse to allow me near such a valuable part of their anatomy with a cup of boiling liquid. Podophyllum is equally destructive but sits quietly in its bottle.

Dipping a cotton swab into the cup of liquid nitrogen, I touch it to the wart for a second, then dip it into the liquid and repeat. The wart quickly turns white as it freezes. A wart the size of a pinhead needs fifteen seconds of freezing; at half an inch it may take forty-five seconds. When the freezing reaches normal skin, you'll feel stinging, but it's tolerable. The penis and even the anus are less sensitive than, say, the fingertips. Everyone grits his teeth when I freeze fingertip warts.

If I've frozen for exactly the right amount of time, the wart withers away over a few weeks. Usually I'm not so lucky, and the freezing kills some normal skin, producing a blister the next day. When the blister heals, the wart should be gone with no scarring.

Prevention. You can't prevent warts on most parts of the body, although it's a bad idea to walk barefoot through public areas such as locker rooms or to use combs, razors, and other instruments that have rubbed against someone else's skin. Condoms prevent genital and anal warts. Wear one for six months after a treatment because warts often lay low for a time.

Handling Other Benign Genital Bumps

Molluscum contagiosum sounds frightening, but a long Latin word merely means that the condition dates from the nineteenth century or earlier, when doctors named everything in a classical language. *Wart* is the popular term for verruca vulgaris; molluscum have never grown popular enough to acquire a simple name, although they're fairly common.

Another viral tumor, molluscum contagiasum grows as a smooth, pinhead-sized dome with a dimple at the top. Often located on the groin or shaft of the penis, molluscum can appear anywhere, but unlike warts you don't often see one alone. Fortunately, the size rarely exceeds an eighth inch.

Direct contact spreads molluscum from person to person, but once infected, a man can acquire more through his own efforts (autoinoculation). The incubation period ranges from two weeks to two months, and an individual molluscum lasts about two months.

A ten-to-fifteen-second application of liquid nitrogen cures the average molluscum; other destructive methods that work for warts also work here.

Pearly penile papules is a name that provokes chuckles except in men who discover them. Always located just behind the head of the penis (glans), they consist of dozens of white warty bumps in a 360-degree ring. Perhaps one man in five notices a few if he looks closely; sometimes they grow in a dense mass but always limited to the circular area behind the glans.

Treatment is reassurance. Not contagious and not a skin disease, pearly penile papules are probably a minor congenital abnormality that grows obvious after puberty—like moles. They are harmless.

Sexually Transmitted Infestations

Infestations are a consequence of poor hygiene throughout most of the world and even in America among the homeless and others not likely to buy this book, but they also strike clean, middle-class individuals. Men recoil with disgust at the sight and appear quickly in the doctor's office.

Fortunately, infestations are easy to treat, and patients are invariably grateful. I reassure them that insects—carriers of plague, typhus, and other deadly diseases throughout history and in poor countries today—represent only an annoyance among the prosperous. Strictly speaking, infestations need not be sexually transmitted; they can spread on clothing and bedding, but this is unlikely among individuals who maintain reasonable hygiene, and impossible during intercourse.

Lice

Unlike bedbugs (which live elsewhere) or scabies (which live concealed under the skin), lice are plainly visible, so a man who sees bugs mostly likely sees lice—and human lice to boot. Although often blamed, pets rarely transmit their own because each animal has a louse species that prefer that animal alone.

Three human varieties exist, each occupying a distinct area of the body. Sucking blood, they exude a saliva that causes a mild allergy; this plus the mechanical puncture produces itching, but some victims are surprisingly tolerant of their lice.

The average man who finds a louse has almost certainly acquired *pubic lice* (crabs, pediculosis pubis). Hearing my diagnosis, a large percentage of male patients denounce the housekeeping practices of hotels, and I nod sympathetically. However, unlike body lice which wander freely, pubic lice cling tightly to the skin, dying in a few days if detached. As a result, close contact between two pubic areas transmits the infestation most efficiently, although clothing and bedding remain a possibility.

Diagnosis. The pubic louse prefer the genitals and lower abdomen. For unclear reasons, it also lives on the eyelashes and rarely in the armpit. Round-bodied unlike its two elongated relatives, three legs projecting from each side produce its crab-like shape.

Almost the color of skin, pubic lice appear as tiny brown or yellow specks, making them hard to identify. I have better luck than patients because I can peer more closely at an infested area, but I find it useful to nudge the specks with a sliver of wood to see if they move. Also visible are the eggs (called nits), tiny white ovals attached to a hair shaft just above the skin. Learning this clue, victims quickly find nits everywhere but they usually point out dandruff, dirt, and nondescript skin flakes. Nits always cling to a hair.

Treatment. Most doctors prescribe the insecticide gamma benzene hexachloride, which gardeners know as lindane but which pharmacists dispense under more colorful names, the most common being Kwell. Using lindane shampoo, patients should lather up, wait five minutes, then wash off. Lindane also comes as a cream, which must remain on the skin eight hours before washing. Hairy individuals must treat themselves from the neck to the knees. Afterward, nits are removed with a fine-toothed comb. You kill lice on the eyelashes by applying a thick coat of vaseline twice a day for eight days.

Many doctors advise a second treatment after ten days to kill any nits that hatch, but this is probably not necessary. Sexual contacts as well as people who share the same bed should receive the same treatment. Laundry or dry cleaning eliminates lice from bedding and clothing; one can also accomplish this by storing the item away from a human body for a week.

A newer cream, permethrin (Elimite) is also effective. Patients tend to prefer a prescription, but anyone can buy a good over-the-counter remedy: A-200, Nix, Rid, Pronto, R&C. Although almost never used, a common oral antibiotic, trimethoprim-sulfamethoxazole (Septra or Bactrim) works well—probably by killing bacteria in the louse intestine.

Dealing With Body Lice and Head Lice

Varieties of the same species, body lice and head lice look identical and can interbreed, but each has different feeding habits. Unlike infestations of pubic lice, these occur more often as a result of poverty and poor hygiene. Spread occurs from clothing and bedding; sharing brushes also spreads head lice. Sex is a less likely source.

Diagnosis. Body lice don't live on the body but in clothing seams, especially where warmth and pressure occur around the collar and beltline. Skin examination reveals tiny pimples and signs of intense scratching, which may produce deep excoriations and infections. Body lice tend to attack the upper back, perhaps because victims find it harder to reach.

Head lice live on the scalp, but they are difficult to find because only a few may be present. Nits are more reliable evidence.

Treatment. The same remedies used for pubic lice work for body and head lice. Once clothing and bedding are cleaned, patients with body lice don't require an insecticide, but most doctors prescribe one anyway.

Scabies

Scabies is infestation by a tiny mite the size of the period following this sentence. The female burrows just beneath the skin, laying a trail of eggs behind her. An allergic reaction to the mite, her eggs, or her feces produces itching, but this may not develop for several weeks.

Personal contact transmits the mite. Although an efficient method, sex isn't required because scabies spreads rapidly through overcrowded institutions, day care centers, and even ordinary families.

Diagnosis. Scabies itches intensely, typically worse at night. The mite may leave a trail of tiny pimples as it burrows, and men often show larger itchy papules over the genitals and penis. Besides the genitals, scabies prefers the buttocks, lower abdomen, forearm, wrists, nipples, belly button, and the skin between the fingers. Textbooks insist that the doctor carefully scrape a burrow with a scalpel and examine the material under the microscope to detect the mite or its eggs. Although the best diagnostic test, it's not as easy as they claim, and few doctors make the attempt.

Unfortunately, while genital papules or a line of pimples make the diagnosis more certain, both are often absent, so the doctor sees only small scattered pimples and scratch marks. In the end, we frequently use a trial of therapy to make the diagnosis (i.e., if it works, the patient had scabies; if not, we keep looking).

Treatment. Permethrin is probably best, although lindane also works. Apply the cream from the neck down (scabies doesn't affect the head), leave on for eight hours, then wash off. Launder clothing or store for ten days. Treatment must include everyone who shares the residence as well as sexual contacts.

Bedbugs

Although they live in beds, bedbugs are unlikely to inhabit the one in which most Americans sleep regularly, so associating them with sex is not unreasonable.

Diagnosis. Larger than a louse and easily visible, a bedbug is a flat, oval brown bug about one-quarter-inch long. Remember this because unless you produce one for the doctor to identify, the chance of accurate diagnosis is low as the bite shows no feature to distinguish it from any insect bite.

Bedbugs hide in crevices during the day, leaving at night to bite a few times before returning. The bite is painless at first, and some victims never notice it. Others awake with a few itchy pimples; sensitive individuals suffer severe itching with a generalized rash. Occasionally the bites bleed, so anyone who sees spots of blood on the skin or bedclothes should suspect bedbugs.

Treatment. The bites disappear in a few days; treatment doesn't speed healing, but soothing lotions or cortisone creams relieve itching. If you plan to use this bed again, spray it as well as nearby furniture, floor, and walls with insecticide. Use a professional exterminator.

Considering AIDS

I thought a long time before deciding what to include in this section. Preventing AIDS is relatively easy; I can cover that in a few sentences. The dozens of complications and their treatments would take up an entire book. Furthermore, although the media cover the subject regularly and almost everyone knows someone affected, AIDS represents a small risk to most readers of this book. You are unlikely to inject drugs or have frequent sex with someone who does. Now that blood banks test blood for HIV, your chance of infection from a transfusion approaches zero. Homosexual readers have long since learned what they must do.

I decided to take a cue from my practice, which includes mostly middle-class and working people. I doubt if I see one new AIDS patient per year, but many are already positive HIV or taking medication for AIDS. Far more numerous are patients who ask for an AIDS test. Except for a few homosexuals worried about past indiscretions, most don't need it. Perhaps they had intercourse with a woman whose hygiene seemed suspicious or broke up with a lover who may not have been faithful. When I explain that they are not at risk and that the test isn't necessary, they listen politely.

In the past I assumed this meant that they accepted my explanation and we could discuss other things, but I am wiser now. Although the test will undoubtedly be negative, I explain, I'll order one if they still want it. Invariably, they want it. My success rate where I predict a negative HIV test is 100 percent.

This chapter reviews what you should know about AIDS and explains why most of you need not worry. It also explains why AIDS is the worst plague in history, with no end in sight.

The HIV Virus

The disease begins with infection by HIV-1 (human immunodeficiency virus type 1). An HIV-2 exists; closely related, it's rare except in Africa and less virulent. Despite the common belief, HIV-1 is not mysterious or obscure. It's a retrovirus, a family known since the beginning of the century and responsible for many animal infections. The first human retrovirus disease was not AIDS but a rare leukemia.

A Primer on Viruses. A thousand times smaller than a germ, a virus is simply a chromosome (a long, coiled molecule containing information for making that virus) inside a protein coat. Completely inert outside a cell, a virus doesn't breathe, eat, move, or reproduce, and scientists debate whether to call it a living organism. Only when a virus touches the right cell does something happen. The protein clings to the surface and injects its chromosome into the cell. Traveling to the nucleus, the viral chromosome disappears into the cell's own chromosomes. For a time (hours to years) nothing happens. Then the cell stops normal activity and begins manufacturing viruses inside itself. After filling up, the cell dies and disintegrates, releasing viruses to begin the cycle again.

Their extraordinary simplicity make viruses difficult to destroy. Boiling and strong acids work, but these are not practical treatments for human disease. Safer methods such as antibiotics, which poison bacteria by interfering with their activity, fail to harm viruses, which have no activity at all. Only when an infected cell is making new viruses can a drug interfere, but the cell, not the virus, is doing the work, so an antiviral drug must interfere with a cell's activity. Doing so without poisoning the cell is a tricky business, and current antiviral drugs are much more toxic than antibiotics. But researchers have had 60 years to refine their techniques with antibiotics, so we should do better with time.

Transmitting the Virus

HIV spreads through blood, semen, and breast milk, not through saliva, sweat, tears, nasal mucus, urine, or feces. Even spread by semen is inefficient; a woman infected by a man has had a great deal of sex with him as wife or lover. A single episode of sex has a low probability of transmitting AIDS—much less than its chance of spreading hepatitis, gonorrhea, syphilis, or warts.

One explanation for the appearance of AIDS first among homosexuals in the United States is that many were more promiscuous than the average heterosexual man. Now that they are getting their act together, their incidence of new infections has dropped dramatically. The greatest increase is now among drug users who share needles. Although heterosexual sex produces only about 5 percent of AIDS, this category is also increasing, with women making up the great majority. Drug addicts are mostly men, so it's their wives and lovers that suffer.

Sex with an HIV-positive woman can infect a man, probably because she often has some blood in her vagina, but this is less common than transmission from a man to a woman. Prostitutes suffer AIDS mostly because they use drugs, not because of sex.

Clinical Course

Most victims feel fine after infection, although a minority develop a flu-like illness three to six weeks later. Symptoms, include fever, body aches, headache, a generalized rash, and diarrhea that resolves itself after a few weeks. It's identical to other viral illnesses, so almost no one suspects AIDS—and most men who think they have the flu have the flu. The HIV blood test doesn't become positive until two or three months after infection. Ninety-five percent of patients become positive after five months, although this may take years in a rare case. Researchers are developing tests to detect infection earlier, and these may be available by the time you read this.

For years after infection, the patient remains healthy. Even tests of immune function remain normal, but after three years these begin to decline in almost everyone. Most commonly, doctors measure a key blood cell called the T4 lymphocyte, normally present at greater than 800 per cubic millimeter. (Although recommendations change, when the level drops below 500 doctors consider beginning drugs such as zidovudine—ZDV or AZT—to slow this decline. Below 200, immunity is so impaired that doctors often prescribe drugs to prevent certain infections that occur commonly, such as pneumocystis pneumonia.)

During this decline patients may feel fine. Some notice generalized enlarged lymph nodes, which may represent an attempt (unfortunately ineffective) to fight the infection. Men who have read this grow frightened when they feel an enlarged node, so read on and remember. Experts define the generalized enlarged lymph nodes of HIV infection as palpable nodes in two or more parts of the body that persist more than three months—and *nodes in the groin don't count*! An isolated lump under your jaw or in the armpit doesn't qualify.

Seven years after infection, symptoms have appeared in 75 percent of individuals. Often a specific infection or tumor, it's also frequently a poorly understood illness called AIDS-related complex (ARC), consisting of persistent fever, weight loss, fatigue, diarrhea, or skin rash. Once again, you must maintain a sense of proportion. Several days of fever and fatigue, perhaps with diarrhea, makes me think of a routine viral infection. Don't worry about HIV until a month has passed.

Fullblown AIDS (acquired immunodeficiency syndrome) is not a specific disease but the consequence of severe immune deficiency. Before AIDS, immune deficiencies were rare and usually the result of a genetic defect in the immune system or its suppression by drugs or disease. The average physician never saw a case, which was just as well because victims suffered complex illnesses that were difficult to treat.

Typically a person with inadequate immunity grows susceptible to opportunistic infections—infections with organisms that are relatively feeble and easily suppressed in someone with normal resistance. Easily the most common is pneumonia caused by *Pneumocystis carinii*, a fungus which attacks perhaps 80 percent of AIDS victims at some time. Like most opportunistic organisms, *Pneumocystis* exists widely in the environment, and most of us have a few living quietly in our lungs. Other opportunists include formerly obscure organisms with names like *cryptosporidium, cryptococcus, toxoplasma,* and atypical *mycobacteria.*

Closely related to opportunists are infections like herpes, warts, and yeast, which produce annoying conditions in most of us but widespread infection where immunity is weak.

Finally, most people wonder why AIDS victims suffer obscure infections and seem to escape the common virulent ones that can overwhelm even a vigorous immune system such as strep, staph, tuberculosis, etc. Partly, the answer is that once a person has antibodies to an infection, AIDS won't eliminate them. Thus most adults have had their immunizations; also they are no longer susceptible to bacterial infectious so common in children, such as strep throat and ear infections. Partly, we have good treatments for common bacterial infections—even in AIDS patients. Treatments for opportunistic infections have been bad because these were so rare that few researchers paid attention to them. This is being remedied.

Finally, AIDS victims *are* susceptible to virulent infections. Tuberculosis in the United States had been declining for the past hundred years, but since 1985 the rate has climbed steadily because of AIDS. Furthermore, the tuberculosis spreading among AIDS patients has turned particularly nasty, often resisting the usual antibiotics. You should understand the ominous implications. If you don't have HIV now, it's easy to make sure that you'll never have it. Your intact immune system makes it unlikely that you'll catch *Pneumocystis, cryptococcus*, or other opportunists, but healthy humans are quite susceptible to tuberculosis, salmonella, many bacterial pneumonias, and a host of other virulent infections. As these spread in the AIDS population, they'll spread to us.

Although less well publicized, HIV virus infects the brain as well as the immune system. Half of its victims suffer neurological disease, most commonly a diffuse brain deterioration called AIDS dementia complex that begins with apathy, weakness, and unsteadiness and progresses (provided that the patient doesn't die of another complication) to severe senility and paralysis. This vaguely resembles Alzheimer's disease in the elderly, another poorly understood disease which some experts also blame on a virus. Experts are uncertain why AIDS victims suffer a high rate of several malignancies: tumors of lymphoid tissue (lymphomas) and a formerly rare tumor called Kaposi's sarcoma.

What Treatments Exist?

No disease better illustrates the superiority of prevention to treatment. By 1985, we knew how to prevent AIDS with essentially 100 percent success and at trivial cost. Despite impressive advances in treatment, as of 1993 AIDS remains a 100 percent fatal illness, and the expense of treatment is straining the finances of the wealthiest countries.

Drugs to cure infections are one of the great triumphs of twentieth-century medicine. Opportunistic infections should accumulate better treatments over the next decades; the first ten years of research has already produced impressive progress. Unfortunately, in the absence of a healthy immune system, a patient cured of one infection remains susceptible to that as well as all the others. Many opportunistic infections recur so predictably that a patient must continue treatment for life.

Obviously a limit exists on the number of prophylactic drugs a person can take. It is far better to begin treatment earlier to slow the decline of the immune system. The development of zidovudine (AZT, ZDV) in the mid-1980s was a significant advance. Subsequent drugs with names like DDI, DDE, and D4T complement ziduvudine without improving on it, but I predict better drugs as time goes on. Somewhat toxic and wildly expensive, antiretroviral drugs slow the drop in T4 cells and seem to provide more normal life before the inevitable. In the absence of a breakthrough, these are the best we can offer, and they may be the best for a long time.

Vaccines offer a chance to reduce AIDS to the same level as polio or tetanus today. Trials of several are in progress and laboratories are developing others. Unfortunately, we don't understand how the body fights retroviruses, and (a good rule) until scientists understand a problem, they have a hard time solving it. Traditional vaccines, like those for polio or tetanus, give the body a slight taste of a disease. In response, the immune system produces a line of cells that quickly pour out antibodies whenever those disease organisms appear again. The antibodies quickly destroy them.

The difficulty with retroviruses is that antibodies against them seem ineffective. A blood test revealing antibodies against, say, measles or polio means that the person has successfully fought off the infection. A positive HIV test (which measures antibodies) means exactly the opposite.

Current vaccines employ the usual strategy—injecting either harmless retroviruses or pieces of the AIDS virus in an effort to provoke a protective reaction. Experts regularly make hopeful announcements about their vaccine—but scientists are human; they always love their latest project. Although I'm sticking my neck out since you'll be reading this at least two years after it's written, I don't see a vaccine against AIDS in the near future.

Popular articles and media documentaries on AIDS give the impression that a vaccine is on the horizon, but that's misleading. You won't read a downbeat article on any health subject in a popular magazine. If I submit an article to a magazine (and I've written hundreds), the editor quickly returns it for revision if I haven't given readers enough good news or optimistic predictions. If I can't comply, the article doesn't appear. For this reason, I've never written an article about AIDS. There's not much good news.

Prevention

Everyone knows about condoms. As I mentioned earlier, the chance of catching AIDS from an single sexual contact with a woman is low but not zero. If you decide to take a chance, I guarantee that you'll start to worry.

It is commonly agreed that sexual activities can be categorized according to their HIV risk status. Examples would be:

Unsafe Sex Practices

1. Anal intercourse without the use of a condom
2. Vaginal intercourse without the use of a condom
3. Swallowing semen
4. Swallowing menstrual blood
5. Swallowing vaginal fluids
6. Nonprotected oral-anal contact
7. Nonprotected manual-vaginal contact

Somewhat Risky Sex Practices

1. Fellatio without ejaculation
2. French kissing
3. Stimulation to orgasm between the thighs or buttocks
4. Contact with urine
5. Anal intercourse with condom
6. Digital-anal sex without barrier
7. Fellatio with ejaculation into a condom

Safe Sex Practices

1. Dry kissing
2. Taking a bath together
3. Masturbation
4. Licking healthy, clean skin
5. Hugging
6. Massage
7. Stimulation to orgasm on any external body part

A few other minor tips. If you travel to a country outside of Europe or Japan, don't accept any blood products. That includes vaccines and gamma globulin as well as transfusions. Don't even accept an injection unless you know that the needle is being used for the first time. This means that you must receive all your shots before traveling. Otherwise a country may insist on immunizing you at the airport before allowing you in.

The future: What we can learn from Africa. I'm not convinced that AIDS in Africa offers a cautionary lesson for the United States, but plenty of experts have drawn one, so you should know about it.

AIDS has devastated black Africa. Beginning in the late 1970s, about the same time as the U.S. epidemic, the virus has spread much more quickly and now affects 10 to 50 percent of the population—twenty or more times the rate in the United States. Unlike the pattern in advanced countries, AIDS in Subsaharan Africa (and other poor nations) behaves as a typical heterosexually transmitted disease, striking men and women equally. Experts aren't certain why AIDS spreads so rapidly in these nations, but most believe that poverty and the presence of other sexually transmitted diseases on the genitals make exchange of blood during sex more likely.

By the late 1980s, AIDS was established in Thailand, India, and other nations of Asia and spreading rapidly. There is no reason to doubt that the 1990s will see the poor nations of Asia afflicted as badly as those of Africa.

The future in America. In 1991 the number of HIV-positive persons in the United States passed a million. AIDS cases total over 250,000. Both numbers are rising steadily.

America spent 1 percent of its entire public and private medical care budget to treat HIV infections in 1992. This will rise to 2 percent within three years. Much of this frightening increase is not the result of more cases but of scientific progress. New treatments for an AIDS infection are invariably expensive. Treating one healthy HIV-positive case costs $6,000 per year.

If a perfect vaccine appeared now, and everyone received it, costs would continue rising for another ten to fifteen years while all current infections ran their course—and you should know that no good vaccine exists for malaria, leprosy, tuberculosis, or even ordinary strep throat despite 100 years of research.

The safe sex campaign among the general population is having a good effect; the effort in public schools is making progress despite some opposition to passing out condoms. Although an important public health measure, the campaign directed at heterosexuals will have little effect on AIDS. Those who should practice safe sex (addicts and prostitutes) have more important priorities. The AIDS risk among other heterosexuals is slight, but safe sex will protect them from the unpublicized but raging epidemic of other sexually transmitted diseases—hepatitis, genital warts, herpes, vaginal infections, lice, cervical cancer, as well as the tranditional venereal diseases. I see a hundred of these for every AIDS case.

One unexpected effect of the AIDS crisis has been breaking the barrier to good sex education in the schools. Until the 1980s, sex education, if taught at all, consisted of innocuous instruction on hormones and biology. Any attempt to teach something useful, such as contraception, provoked violent opposition in the community. European schools teach about sex routinely, but an unpleasant puritanical streak runs through America to a greater extent than any other advanced country. Many otherwise decent people believe that educating teen-agers about sex encourages them to engage in it. Although reasonable, this turns out to be wrong. Forty percent of American teenagers become pregnant before leaving high school, the highest rate among wealthy countries—and that includes nations that teach children about sex.

CHAPTER · 11

COMMON SEXUAL PROBLEMS AND THEIR SOLUTIONS

During most of this century, polls revealed that money led the list of stresses in marriage. Money led because researchers didn't ask about sex, and subjects didn't volunteer the information. When researchers began asking, sex rivaled money. Among happily married couples, half of men report some sexual difficulties (women show even less satisfaction; over three quarters complain).

Although some men find this hard to believe, intercourse is not essential to anyone's health. Ascetics who abstain for philosophical or religious reasons suffer no ill health, just as no harm results from forgoing tasty food and other physical comforts. On the other hand, as one of life's pleasures, satisfying sex contributes to the emotional well-being of those who achieve it. Sexual problems cause a great deal of unnecessary misery because good treatments exist.

WHAT YOU SHOULD KNOW ABOUT IMPOTENCE

Thirty years ago, experts agreed that 90 percent of impotent men suffered emotional problems. Older general practitioners gave testosterone shots, which probably didn't work. Newer, better trained physicians looked down on this mumbo-jumbo. They sent men for psychotherapy, which also didn't work.

Twenty years ago, doctors began finding more physical causes, and by ten years ago the tide had turned. We now believe that organic (i.e., not psychological) disorders lead to most impotence. Today a family doctor treats some of these patients; a urologist handles most of the remainder.

What Happens During Normal Intercourse

1. The Anatomy. Although the penis feels like a tube, it's actually three separate tubes with a fleshy cap at the end called the glans. Most of its length consists of two side-by-side tubes called the corpora cavernosa (cavernous bodies). Running underneath, a smaller tube called the corpus spongiosum (spongy body) carries the urethra down its middle. Pressing firmly, you can feel all three.

Cavernous and *spongy* accurately describe these tubes because they're interlaced with large veins that remain empty except during erection. A thin cylinder of muscle, the bulbocavernosus, envelops all three. Its contraction allows you to expel the last few drops of urine, but it doesn't play a major role in erection. Paired ischiocavernosus muscles originate on the pelvis and attach to the base of the penis. Contracting, they sustain an erection by preventing blood from leaving the penis. However, muscles can't produce an erection; it occurs when the penis fills with blood. This requires healthy blood vessels as well as nerves.

2. Nerves. Nerves controlling erection originate in centers low in the spinal cord. Although impulses from the brain (thoughts, pleasant sensations) can travel down the cord and produce an erection, they aren't essential.

Experts identify three forms of erection.

1. Reflex erections occur from genital stimulation. Like another reflex, the knee jerk, the reflex erection occurs when a nerve impulse travels to the spinal cord and provokes the return of another impulse that leads to the response. A paraplegic with a spinal injury can produce this form of erection.

2. Psychogenic erections result from daydreaming or any sort of sensory stimulation, such as sound or pictures. This requires intact nerves because only a few patients with damage in the low spinal cord can achieve them.

3. All men from early childhood on experience nocturnal erections during sleep or on awakening. Although still not well understood, these provide evidence that the basic mechanism works properly. Patients impotent from psychological problems or lack of male hormone continue to have erections during sleep. Their absence points to a physical disorder.

3. Hormones. Essential for sexual maturity, male hormones (testosterone and dihydrotestosterone) enhance erections, but they aren't indispensable. Men with a deficiency lose interest in sex, and their ejaculate diminishes slightly, but they continue to have all forms of erection. Giving extra hormone to a man with a normal level increases sexual desire but makes him more irritable and increases his blood cholesterol without correcting whatever prevents his erection.

4. The Mechanics of Intercourse. Erection begins with a rise in blood flow into the penis, filling the network of empty veins in the corpora cavernosa and corpus spongiosum. The penis grows thicker and longer until it can hold no more. At this point the ischiocavernosus muscle contracts, compressing the base of the penis, preventing blood from entering or leaving and producing a rigid erection. Urination is difficult, and almost no blood flows into the penis. Gangrene would eventually result, but fortunately this phase doesn't last long enough.

Ejaculation occurs when muscle contractions along the epididymus, spermatic cord, and prostate transport semen into the urethra. The bladder neck contracts to prevent backward flow; penile muscles contract to expel the 2 to 5 cubic centimeters of ejaculate. We take great pleasure in the rhythmic muscle contractions that produce ejaculation and call them an orgasm.

Afterward, penile muscles relax, blood leaves faster than it enters, the erection subsides, the man loses interest in intercourse, and erection and ejaculation become impossible for a time. This refractory period may last only a few minutes but it varies greatly with health, motivation, and habit. Age lengthens the refractory period as it does all phases of sex, but impotence is never normal.

Meaning "no strength," the term *impotence* can include any disorder that interferes with sex, but laypeople take it literally to mean lack of strength in the penis. A man whose penis softens too quickly or who loses the ability to become erect considers himself impotent, a humiliating affliction that men have feared throughout history. Even during the most prudish years of the Victorian era when no mention of sex appeared in popular literature, advertisements for physicians, tonics, and quack remedies boasted of their ability to restore a man's vigor. Everyone knew what that meant.

The most common male sexual disorder, men find impotence so embarrassing that they never speak the word. They may casually ask for a shot to increase their energy, complain wryly about trouble "keeping it up," or request a complete physical exam while insisting that nothing in particular bothers them. In twenty years of practice, no man has called himself "impotent," and I suspect that many never mention the subject. They should realize that medical science doesn't do badly in this area.

Failure of Erection—Causes

Starting with the simplest cause, every man fails now and then. Worry, fatigue, a bad cold, a quarrel with the partner, and other stresses can defeat an erection despite the best efforts. Unless this occurs regularly, we don't call it impotence.

Drugs. Medical references include an enormous list of offenders, including dozens that I prescribe regularly without a problem, but some drugs interfere predictably with sex. Although a leading cause, they don't present much difficulty because their action is transient. A few men insist that an ongoing problem dates from an old prescription, but drugs don't cause permanent impotence.

Several classes of antihypertensives produce impotence often enough that some doctors issue a warning at the time they hand over the prescription. The warning alone may or may not cause impotence, but it definitely increases the number of men who thank the doctor, leave the office, and never fill the prescription. Since untreated high blood pressure leads to catastrophes, I always explain that

1. These drugs affect only a minority of men. The majority feel fine.
2. Some classes of antihypertensives never cause impotence, so a doctor can always control blood pressure without this difficulty. These drugs tend to be more expensive, so I urge men to try the cheaper treatment first.

Alcohol and marijuana as well as sedatives, tranquilizers, antidepressants, and other drugs that affect the brain (antihistamines, seizure and nausea medications) make up the other large group of offenders. Stopping restores potency, and switching to another class of drug sometimes helps.

Circulatory Insufficiency. Without adequate blood supply, the penis swells slowly or not all. Just as cholesterol buildup reduces blood flow to the heart, it does the same to the penis, and the incidence of both impotence and coronary artery disease rise in parallel as men grow older. Since cholesterol buildup (atherosclerosis) is the leading disease among American men, it also causes the most impotence.

Just as the low-cholesterol diet discussed in Chapter 2 prevents atherosclerosis, it eliminates the risk of this form of impotence. Once a man falls victim, I encourage him to think about diet as a general health measure but not as a quick solution to achieving an erection. That may require the artificial means discussed later, although X-ray studies sometimes reveal a local blockage in a penile artery that surgery can correct.

Disorders of Nerves. Any central nervous system disorder from a brain tumor to a slipped disk can interfere with sexual function, although (as

I mentioned earlier) erections remain possible in many men with severe damage.

Disorders that injure peripheral nerves produce more victims. Chronic alcoholics tend to be impotent. Diabetics blame an elevated blood sugar, but damage to peripheral nerves is usually responsible; this is a poorly understood consequence of long-term diabetes that eventually affects half of cases. Severe vitamin deficiency leads to impotence, but doctors in the United States rarely see this. Surgeons have grown skilled in avoiding injury to penile nerves during bladder, prostate, and rectal operations, but it remains a risk.

Hormone Disorders. Although men immediately think of testosterone, diabetes causes perhaps 90 percent of hormonal impotence. Doctors theorize (i.e., evidence exists but it's not overwhelming) that keeping blood sugar normal prevents this as well as the other complications of diabetes: eye and kidney damage. Strict control requires a rigorous diet, maintaining a normal weight, and (if necessary) many insulin injections during the day. Once present, complications aren't reversible, so every man should make the effort from the time he hears the diagnosis.

Other hormone disorders (testosterone deficiency, naturally, but also thyroid and pituitary disease) interfere with erections but do more harm by suppressing sexual desire.

Other Causes. Many exist, but they aren't common. Kidney failure causes impotence, but it must be severe. Half of men on dialysis are affected; most recover after successful kidney transplantation.

Generating an erection requires some degree of healthy body function, so victims of severe, chronic diseases such as cirrhosis of the liver or cancer have difficulty. Traditionally, men have difficulty after a heart attack, but this results from drugs or anxiety, not heart disease. Men with high blood pressure worry, but hypertension doesn't cause impotence.

Psychogenic Causes. Severe depression or anxiety produces a major fraction of impotence. Victims of depression lose the ability to feel pleasure, a big barrier to making an erection. They lose hope and self-esteem, rejecting advice to cheer up on the grounds that they deserve their misery and, in any case, are incapable of changing. Victims of other serious mental illnesses such as schizophrenia or mania behave in ways that amuse onlookers and interest doctors, but not depressives. They are boring, but nothing is accomplished by pointing this out because they will agree. A painful and often life-threatening disorder, depression leads to suicide.

Depression seems a perfect example of a strictly emotional problem (i.e., caused by a stressful life, treated by kindness and psychotherapy, not drugs). Like so many commonsense impressions, this is wrong. Evidence is growing that severe mental illness is brain disease, and nowhere is this more clear than in depression. Traditional psychotherapy works poorly. Medical treatment with drugs and electroshock works well, better than for many strictly physical diseases.

Now that doctors aggressively search out physical causes, we no longer conclude that every impotent man who feels anxious can blame his problem on anxiety. Impotence is upsetting. Yet some men remain in whom anxiety is the correct diagnosis; convincing them isn't difficult because of their intense level of suffering. Every man under stress becomes impotent now and then, but it requires experiences like losing a job or a severe marital conflict to do this regularly.

Those who lack conviction that sex is fun risk trouble, so we find impotence among men with intense religious feelings, those who have been abused sexually, and men with unrealistic expectations about their performance. Men exist who have little sexual interest, but absence of intercourse isn't a disease unless someone suffers because of it. Finally, a man may need a nontraditional sexual situation. Some homosexuals are impotent with women. Paraphelia (i.e., voyerism, transvestitism) sometimes reveals itself as impotence in the absence of the required stimulation.

Diagnosing the Problem

Although impractical to demonstrate in the office, a doctor must discover whether or not impotence is absolute before launching into complex and expensive studies. An erection requires so much coordinated activity from nerves and blood vessels that a man who succeeds even 1 percent of the time probably suffers psychogenic impotence.

A man who experiences only nocturnal erections is physically intact, so a doctor must know if these occur. A urologist may send a patient home with a strain gauge attached to a recorder, but you can test yourself by wrapping a strip of postage stamps around your penis when you go to bed. If they remain unbroken in the morning for a week, you've proved the absence of nocturnal erections. If you're too thrifty to waste stamps, try plumber's tape; it stretches but doesn't contract.

Every man concerned with impotence deserves a thorough physical exam. The doctor will measure the testes. A length of less than 3.5 centimeters (1.4 inches) points to lack of male hormone, as does an abnormal pattern of hair such as none in the pubic area. The doctor will check pulses for signs of arterial blockage and test muscle strength, reflexes, pain, and light touch to detect subtle neurological defects. After checking the knee and ankle jerks, the doctor should test an unfamiliar reflex often absent in neurological impotence. You can test the bulbocavernosus reflex at home. Squeezing the tip of the penis makes the anus contract.

Of all blood tests, glucose turns up the most abnormalities because even early diabetes can produce impotence. Only rarely does another test make the diagnosis, but everyone receives the usual battery as well as several hormone assays including the obligatory testosterone. Occasionally a hormone deficiency prompts the doctor to order a CAT scan to search for a pituitary tumor.

Any family doctor or internist can perform the investigation to this point. If the diagnosis remains obscure, further tests grow more technical, so almost every patient sees a urologist if not doing so already.

Until the 1980s, checking penile circulation required arteriography—injecting dye into the penile artery and tracing its progress with X-rays. Although highly accurate, arteriography is complex, expensive, and slightly risky, so we'd rather not perform it without a strong suspicion that something correctable will turn up. Fortunately, newer and simpler screening tests allow us to be selective.

Urologists now check circulation by injecting papaverine or phentolamine, drugs that dilate blood vessels, directly into the penis. A normal erection within fifteen minutes almost certainly indicates good arterial and venous flow. Because a nervous patient may not develop an erection, an abnormal result isn't as revealing.

Another simple test measures blood pressure in the penis (using a baby's cuff). Normally this is at least 90 percent of traditional arm blood pressure. A reading of 75 percent or less suggests a problem; less than 60 percent points to serious circulatory blockage. Experts praise a host of other noninvasive tests, mostly using ultrasound, that pose no risk and reveal interesting information about circulation but rarely discover a solvable problem.

Treating the Problem

An impotent man suffering depression, uncontrolled diabetes, or an infected prostate can expect no relief while these persist, so our first step is to control whatever disease is controllable. Although quitting smoking and drinking only occasionally restores potency, not quitting maintains a man in a state of ill health, a poor environment for an erection. Finally, drugs like aspirin or vitamins have no record of interfering with sex, yet stopping them is so simple that it's worth trying before proceeding on.

Testosterone treats testosterone deficiency. Pills are absorbed irregularly and sometimes cause liver damage, so doctors prefer injections, one every two to three weeks. Skin patches will be more convenient when they appear; rumors of FDA approval have been circulating for years.

Not essential for life or even health (eunuchs live longer), male hormone is a convenience that produces significant side-effects. Taking extra stimulates benign and malignant prostate tumors so efficiently that patients should have a rectal exam every six months. By suppressing certain pituitary hormones, testosterone diminishes fertility. At the same time it increases sexual desire, a distressing side-effect if impotence persists.

Like testosterone, other drugs occasionally cure impotence, but mostly they don't. Although experts shake their heads at this vast overprescribing, men find the alternatives daunting. Faced with surgery, implants, or a Rube Goldberg device to pump up his penis, anyone prefers to try drugs first, and doctors are right to go along.

Drugs That Help Impotence Problems. Yohimbine (Yocon, Yohimex) possesses a widespread underground reputation because it's not a product of Western pharmaceutical research but derived from a Chinese herb. Although a segment of our population believes in the superior qualities of alternative remedies, there is less here than meets the eye. Although possessing a rich culture, the Chinese lack our passion for gadgets and clever technology (see the discussion of penile implants later in this chapter). Yet historically Chinese men have been perhaps more obsessed with sexual potency than we in the West. Their solutions have their own cultural bias, which is more environmentally destructive than ours. Every wildlife poacher knows that a rhinoceros horn or tiger penis brings $20,000 in China for use as an aphrodisiac. In China itself, more people search for fossils than in the rest of the world combined. When found, they are sold to pharmacists who grind them up for medicines.

Although evidence from studies is not overwhelming, yohimbine may help impotence, perhaps by slowing venous outflow from the penis. The dose is 5.4 milligrams three times a day.

Zinc. Although our diet contains a reasonable amount of zinc, certain groups are at risk of zinc deficiency: those on dialysis, diabetics, and anyone taking diuretics. A blood test can make the diagnosis. The result of the test is usually normal, but it's hard to resist a trial of therapy. Try 220 milligrams of zinc sulfate or 420 milligrams of zinc gluconate daily for two months.

Bromocriptine (Parlodel) counteracts overproduction of prolactin, a pituitary hormone. Tumors as well as many drugs provoke this overproduction, and it may occur during kidney failure, thyroid disease, or after surgery.

Isoxsuprine (Vasodilan, Voxsuprine), 10 to 20 milligrams three times a day, and *pentoxifylline* (Trental), 400 milligrams three times a day, are drugs given for senility on the grounds that they increase blood flow to the brain. They may do the same to the penis.

Nitroglycerin increases blood flow to the heart. Taken orally or under the tongue, it has little effect on potency, but reports occasionally appear of good results from a paste applied directly to the penis.

Injecting *papaverine* or *phentolamine* into the penis, useful for diagnosis, has become a popular treatment, effective in all types of impotence: arterial, neurological, and psychogenic. Not to be undertaken lightly, a man should consider such drugs if surgery is the only alternative. Before sending a patient home with vials and syringes, a urologist will teach the technique after a careful explanation of the side-effects (scarring after long use; an occasional erection that won't subside) and alternatives; he or she will also require the man to sign a detailed consent form that stresses our uncertainty about the long-term complications of repeated injections.

External Devices You Might Try. In an article written in 1988, I mentioned an apparatus, worn like a condom, that produced an erection through a simple suction action. For months afterward, the magazine forwarded letters from readers asking how to buy one. None of my other hundred magazine articles produced a comparable response. Clearly a huge market exists for a good machine to make an erection. The half dozen available today are not ideal, but a surprising number are sold (men tend not to discuss the subject). Urologists, sex therapists, and some family doctors know about them and teach their use.

The condom device is a double-walled silicone sheath that fits over the penis. A syringe or mouth suction evacuates air from the sheath, drawing the penis inside. Tubing wrapped around the base maintains the vacuum. Other devices consist of a hollow plastic cylinder connected to a pump. Placing the cylinder over his penis, the man operates a hand-held pump to remove the air, drawing blood into the penis. When pumping is complete, he slips a rubber band off the base of the cylinder onto the base of the penis to trap the blood.

Types of Surgical Implants. Although it seems drastic to slice open a penis to insert a rod, urologists have been doing just that since the 1970s with increasingly good results. If all else fails, an implant provides an acceptable erection.

Three types exist. In order of complexity they are semirigid, intermediate, and inflatable. As you'd expect, simple implants are more reliable, complex ones are more convenient. Urologists have their favorites, but the man should make the final decision.

Semirigid devices are often simple enough to be implanted under local anesthesia. Typically they maintain stiffness when straight but bend for concealment. With no moving parts, these rarely fail, but they don't increase length or girth of the penis and are difficult to conceal.

Intermediate types are also contained entirely within the penis, but much of their length consists of a flexible cylinder. Repeatedly compressing the tip of the device inflates the cylinder. Bending the erect penis in half deflates it. These lengthen the penis more than semirigid implants and are easier to conceal when not in use.

Completely inflatable prostheses provide the most natural erection by increasing both length and girth of the penis as well as allowing it to shrink to normal size. In one device, tubes connect the implant to a fluid reservoir in the scrotum. Squeezing the scrotum fills and empties the implant.

Great profits lie in a device to make a better erection, so a great deal of engineering energy is devoted to the search, and improvements occur steadily.

WHAT TO DO ABOUT PREMATURE EJACULATION

We define this as ejaculation sooner than the man or his partner desire. Everyone agrees that ejaculation is premature when it occurs before the penis enters; some experts assign thirty seconds to two minutes after entrance as the upper time limit. No consensus exists, but this is a disorder where the patient makes the diagnosis. If a man or his partner believe that premature ejaculation occurs, they're probably right.

Timing Normal Intercourse

Studies on the average sexual encounter reveal that three minutes elapse from the time a man begins thinking about intercourse, achieves an erection, and obtains enough stimulation to ejaculate. For a woman, time from arousal to orgasm averages *thirteen minutes.* Although not directed at premature ejaculation, these studies show that it occurs so routinely that one could classify it as normal male behavior.

In a zoological sense, this is true. Animals spend a long time in courtship and display, but coitus takes a few seconds. Humans invented the idea of intercourse as a prolonged and pleasurable activity, but since it's not instinctive, men and women must learn how to accomplish it.

How a Woman gets to Orgasm

Women achieve orgasm slowly, although the mechanics are similar to those for men. During arousal, vaginal blood flow increases, producing swelling of her external genitals and clitoris (the female equivalent to the penis). At the same time, small glands pour out secretions to lubricate the vagina. You can easily detect a well-lubricated vagina; women rarely enjoy intercourse before this takes place.

Afterward they are more amenable, so men tend to plunge ahead, a risky step because lubrication appears at an early stage in a woman's sexual cycle, perhaps ten minutes before the possibility of an orgasm.

Rhythmic contractions of her vaginal wall provide an orgasm similar to a man's, but her refractory period passes quickly, so she can experience orgasms rapidly after her first. In Polynesian cultures a man did not feel manly unless he gave his partner multiple orgasms. This has never caught on here; in fact, only 20 to 30 percent of American women experience even one per encounter.

Why You May Ejaculate Too Soon

Unlike the case with impotence, physical disorders are almost never responsible. Doctors have long blamed anxiety or conflicts in a relationship. This is hard to contradict because stress interferes with any pleasant activity, but my philosophy on stress teaches that it makes everything worse but doesn't cause anything. Some premature men wonder if they are too sensitive to erotic stimuli; doctors wonder, too, and have long prescribed circumcision, which renders the penis less sensitive. Since most American men are already circumcised, excessive sensitivity can't be a major cause, but it's on the right track.

Men ejaculation too soon not because they feel too much pleasure but because they haven't learned to control the sensations that lead up to ejaculation and make it inevitable. In nature, as I mentioned, male animals ejaculate as quickly as they can. Adolescents in America experience their first erotic stimulation through masturbating, where no motive exists for delaying. When early sex occurs with prostitutes or in anxiety-producing situations such as the back seat of a car, the same urgency applies. In societies where adolescents of both sexes experiment freely, girls quickly teach boys that hasty ejaculation is not a good idea.

Treatment

No drug reliably retards ejaculation, but the unreliable ones are safe enough to try first. Antidepressants and antipsychotic medications may help, probably through their ability to delay nerve transmission. A doctor begins with 25 milligrams of an antidepressant such as amitriptyline (Elavil, Endep) or the antipsychotic thioridazine (Mellaril) three hours before sex. If necessary, the doctor raises the dose until results are good or side-effects (dry mouth, drowsiness, dizziness) become too unpleasant.

Scattered reports describe good results from phenoxybenzamine and the tranquilizer lorazepam (Ativan), so they're worth a try.

Good techniques exist for retarding ejaculation, but they involve a major commitment from a man and his partner. Several simple methods work, although they sacrifice some of the man's pleasure.

The old complaint that condoms reduce sensation works to advantage here. Use two or three if one isn't adequate.

Prematurity puts a damper on the evening, so men rarely get a second chance. Yet many discover that they can maintain their second erection much longer and the third longer still. Some men routinely excuse themselves at the beginning of a romantic evening, masturbate in the bathroom, and then return to continue the overtures. Underused and unmentioned in manuals, the second ejaculation method forms a mainstay for men unwilling to try sex therapy.

A rare internist, a few family doctors and urologists, and all sex therapists teach techniques that require practice but enable a man to hold back ejaculation voluntarily. Sex therapists produce good results but at a great expense that's probably not covered by insurance. This is also a field full of charlatans, so choose one recommended by your doctor or associated with a medical school.

Having a good teacher improves the results, but there's no harm in trying without one.

The Squeeze Technique The woman takes the active role, providing foreplay while the man relaxes. If he has been hypersensitive in the past, she caresses his genitals lightly until he feels the earliest sensation that ejaculation is on the way. As soon as he announces this, she grasps his penis behind the glans, thumb at the bottom, first and second fingers at the top, squeezing firmly until his sensation disappears. He may or may not lose the erection. Then she resumes as he tries to lengthen the period of her caresses. Experts advise the man to proceed to ejaculation after the third or fourth squeeze and to repeat the session several times over a week, but this seems optimistic. In my experience it takes weeks of practice, and there's no harm in half a dozen or more squeezes per night.

Both partners must practice. The man must not concentrate so hard on suppressing ejaculation that he delays signaling for the squeeze. At first men wait too long, but the quickly discover the pain of ejaculating into a squeezed penis. A woman must learn to squeeze quickly and firmly; the man should find it unpleasant.

Eventually he learns to maintain an erection until both partners grow bored. At this point the woman moves on to more intense stimulation. Applying a lubricant (Vaseline or K-Y jelly) to one hand, she rubs his penis with an up-and-down motion, applying the squeeze with the other hand when he signals. A man who delays ejaculation for several minutes under this stimulation has made real progress.

Finally the woman sits astride the man, inserting his penis into her vagina then sitting motionless until his signal, when she quickly dismounts and applies the squeeze. When he can hold his erection inside for several minutes, she begins moving her pelvis slowly, again squeezing when he feels ejaculation approaching. After a few dozen sessions, most men learn to delay ejaculation long enough so that both partners enjoy intercourse.

Studies show that premature ejaculation tends to recur, so a man must continue to concentrate if he wants to avoid backsliding. When this happens, another course of squeeze therapy helps. I also suggest that a man practice on his own—masturbating and then applying the squeeze himself. In my experience most men don't do well at this—they enjoy it so much that they wait until it's too late.

The Stop-Start Maneuver Because the woman plays a central role in the squeeze, a man who wants to succeed by himself chooses the stop-start maneuver. More difficult, it may have a better long-term cure rate. This simply repeats every step in the squeeze technique without the squeeze. The man tells the woman to stop whenever he feels ejaculation coming on, breathes deeply, focuses on relaxing, and rests until the desire fades. Again, a man can practice the early steps while masturbating.

INFERTILITY PROBLEMS

A growing problem, infertility affects perhaps 15 percent of couples compared to 10 percent when I began practice in 1973. Two factors are responsible: the sexual revolution and its resulting increase in infections plus the growing custom of delaying pregnancy. Older couples are less fertile.

Eighty percent of fertile couples conceive after a year of trying, so doctors should not begin testing until this period has passed. Because half the remainder conceive during the next year, we get much undeserved credit, but it's reasonable to take action after a year.

Women received the lion's share of medical attention during past generations, but today an infertility investigation involves both sexes. Men produce once third of cases, women another third, and both share the blame for the rest. Not only must the man accompany his partner to the doctor, his examination comes first because male screening tests are quick and cheap.

Are You Doing it Right?

To maximize the chance of conception, experts advise couples to have intercourse every other night from day ten to eighteen of the menstrual cycle, a woman's most fertile period (day one is the first day of menstruation). One ejaculation every other day keeps sperm concentration at its highest. The couple must avoid lubricants, and the women shouldn't douche afterward. Position probably has no influence, but this doesn't prevent experts from recommending the missionary position, adding that the woman should remain on her back with legs drawn up and knees bent for twenty minutes after ejaculation.

A Quick Review of Fertility

Girls generally begin menstruating between ages eleven and fifteen, and boys produce their first sperm between twelve and fifteen. Both sexes remain relatively infertile for about a year as their glands mature. Maximum fertility occurs around age twenty-five and declines significantly in women after thirty-five. Menopause occurs between forty-five and fifty-two. Although male fertility also declines with age, it probably never reaches zero in the absence of disease.

Primitive cells inside the testes divide several times to produce a mature sperm, taking seventy-four days to accomplish this—a period worth remembering. Far tinier than a human egg, sperm exist in enormous quantities. A woman releases a few hundred eggs during her reproductive years (girls are born with all their eggs present in the ovary). A man produces 50,000 sperm *per minute* during his peak years.

Each sperm contains twenty-three chromosomes, half that of other body cells, a necessity because the egg contains the other half. About half of sperm contain a Y chromosome, the only chromosome absent in women (all eggs contain an X); eggs fertilized by a Y sperm become males (i.e., they are XY). The remaining sperm contain an X chromosome and produce females (all women are XX). In humans and other mammals, sperm determine the sex of the offspring, but this is purely a chance of evolution. In birds, the female's egg contains the deciding chromosome.

A mature sperm in the testes is simply a special cell with no power of movement or ability to fertilize an egg. It acquires these capacities after spending several days moving through the epididymus, a tightly coiled tube that nestles behind each testes. From the epididymus the fully capable sperm enters the foot-long spermatic duct (vas deferens—the tube cut during a vasectomy) that extends from the epidiymus up into the abdomen and then coils back to empty into the urethra near the prostate. At any given time, the epididymus and vas store about 500,000,000 sperm.

What Causes Infertility?

Congenital Causes. Men invariably worry that they were born with a subtle physical defect, but usually they weren't. While a host of congenital disorders cause infertility, they are not terribly common and are almost always accompanied by obvious signs such as chronic illness (cystic fibrosis, sickle cell anemia) or underdeveloped genitals (chromosome abnormalities, hormone deficiencies). A man in good health who undergoes a relatively normal puberty and appears masculine probably acquired his infertility later in life. An exception: the few percent of infertile men with congenital absence of the spermatic duct.

Undescended testes, present in 1 percent of newborns, make up another congenital cause. Sperm can't survive at body temperature; even if they could, undescended testes function poorly in ways we don't understand. Although surgical correction in infancy improves fertility, they still tend to produce inadequate amounts of sperm after puberty. This remains true for both testes, even when only one began life undescended.

Hormone Disorders. Overlapping with congenital disorders, these cause a modest fraction of infertility: 5 to 10 percent. A man may pass through a form of male menopause called testicular failure but more often suffers injury or disease near the pituitary (tumors, cysts, infections, congenital hormone excess or deficit). Rarely subtle, men who acquire these after puberty may notice only a lack of sexual desire, but more likely they show other signs such as testicular atrophy, headaches, or swelling of the breasts. When present during childhood, sex hormone abnormalities lead to premature puberty or none at all.

Drugs and the Environment. Drugs, excessive heat, chemicals (lead, vinyl chloride, benzene), and radiation can suppress fertility. Tracking down these offenders is rarely difficult, but in stubborn cases a doctor must investigate a patient's occupational or environmental exposure. Narcotics, cocaine, and marijuana as well as heavy smoking and alcohol abuse lower fertility, most likely a consequence of general ill health. Among prescription drugs, cancer chemotherapy often permanently impairs fertility. A few other drugs do so temporarily; stopping them corrects it.

Anabolic steroids are probably the leading offender—more so because athletes and body builders consume them surreptitiously and fail to reveal this even when infertility brings them to the doctor. Furthermore, because it's reasonable to assume that male hormone enhances fertility, men are surprised to learn that the opposite occurs. I explain that pituitary hormones, not testosterone, stimulate sperm production. As the master gland, the pituitary also regulates testosterone production from the testes. When a man takes extra male hormone, the pituitary detects this and compensates by inhibiting the testes. As a result, they grow inactive and shrink.

Infections. Any severe illness or infection or even a bad attack of the flu suppresses sperm production, but this should return to normal within three months (remember that a sperm takes seventy-four days to develop). Permanent sterility after illness occurs less often than men believe. Mumps strikes terror into a male who catches it, but his chance of sterility is low (for a discussion of mumps orchitis, see Chapter 6). Among other infections, syphilis, leprosy, and tuberculosis occasionally destroy the testes. More commonly, gonorrhea and chlamydia leave behind scarred and blocked spermatic ducts.

Antibodies to Sperm. These occur in 3 to 7 percent of infertile men. Although rarely leading to complete sterility, they don't help. Our immune system attacks invading organisms with specialized blood cells and sticky proteins called antibodies. Naturally it doesn't attack our own cells (except in autoimmune diseases like rheumatoid arthritis or lupus). We are protected from attack in the womb because our developing immune system is exposed to the rest of our developing tissues and learns to recognize them as self. Thereafter it ignores them but springs to life when anything unfamiliar appears.

We are born without sperm, so the immune system considers them unfamiliar. Fortunately they develop in the testes, isolated from the bloodstream.

where watchdog immune cells circulate. When blood contacts sperm after an injury, surgery, or repeated infections, antibodies appear and attack them. Sperm with antibody attached swim more slowly and may clump together, but this isn't inevitable. Many men with antibodies remain fertile.

The Varicocele. Early in any investigation, the doctor will search for a varicocele and probably find one. Ten to 15 percent of men are affected; this percentage doubles in men evaluated for infertility, so a connection may exist. Urologists blame varicoceles for infertility more often than nonurologists, and their role remains controversial.

A varicocele is a varicose (i.e., a stretched and flabby) vein draining a testis. Separate vessels drain the left and right, but 90 percent of varicoceles affect the left testis because that vein travels high into the abdomen before reaching its outlet. The right testicular vein travels only a short distance. Like varicose veins in the legs and anus (hemorrhoids), varicoceles occur when high pressure of the blood exceeds the strength of their thin walls.

You can diagnose yourself by feeling above your testicles. If you detect an area that resembles a clump of worms, you've found one. Performing a Valsalva maneuver (holding your breath and bearing down) increases venous pressure and makes the veins stand out. Many men with a varicocele remain fertile; others have some impairment, perhaps because sluggish blood flow leads to higher temperature in the testes.

Retrograde Ejaculation. Ten percent of men with no sperm in their semen ejaculate backward. A common result of prostate surgery (see Chapter 6), this can occur from any disorder that damages nerves around the bladder neck—most often diabetes. Normally the wide bladder sphincter shuts during orgasm, forcing semen forward down the narrow urethra. When this doesn't occur, the ejaculate takes the path of least resistance, ending up in the bladder. Every man with a zero sperm count or a small volume of semen should have a urinalysis to look for sperm.

Examination and Tests

Every man worried about fertility deserves a complete medical history and physical exam. The doctor should learn about past medical problems, surgery, and bad habits. The physical exam pays special attention to body proportions and hair pattern (for evidence of hormone deficiencies or chromosome abnormalities) and genitals. If his arm span measures 2 inches or more than his height, the man is eunuchoid: He hasn't passed through puberty. The testes must measure more than 3.5 centimeters across the long axis. A careful search should turn up the spermatic cord, epididymus, and seminal vesicles; rarely are they congenitally absent.

The doctor may order simple tests such as a blood count and urinalysis, but complex ones await the results of a semen analysis. Every infertile man must have one, and it should precede the more demanding tests that a woman must undergo.

The Semen Analysis

After two or three days' abstinence, the man masturbates into a sterile glass kept at body temperature. He can do this at home, but analysis must take place within two hours, preferably one. Results are too important to rely on a single specimen, so the doctor must order at least two.

The laboratory records the following:

1. Volume should vary from 1.5 to 5 cubic centimeters (5 cubic centimeters is a teaspoon). Variation within these limits makes little difference. Each day of abstinence increases volume about 0.4 cubic centimeters, but it plateaus at one week and shouldn't pass 5 cubic centimeters. Since over 95 percent of semen represents fluid from the prostate and seminal vesicles, presence or absence of sperm has little effect on semen volume. This is why men notice no change after vasectomy. Low semen volume points to blocked or absent seminal vesicles; an infected prostate may produce excess fluid.

2. Appearance is pearly and opaque, like egg white. Normal semen quickly coagulates and then liquefies within half an hour. Once this happens, it will pour, drop by drop. Slow or absent liquefaction prevents sperm from moving easily.

3. Sperm count in a normal ejaculation ranges from 20 to 150 million per cubic centimeter. Although simple to measure, sheer number seems less important than we once believed. As a result, the lower limit of normal has drifted downward over the past decade, although some experts still prefer 50 to 60 million. Men with counts under 20 million aren't necessarily sterile since we have techniques to collect and concentrate sperm for artificial insemination.

4. The most important single gauge of semen quality, good motility can compensate for a low count. The technician records two elements:
   a. The number of moving sperm, normally over 50 percent
   b. The quality of motility: how rapidly and straight they swim. To avoid depending on individual impressions, laboratories now use computers, lasers, video cameras, and specialized counters.

5. Sperm morphology: Over 60 percent should appear normal.

Sperm come in an amazing variety of size and shape, including some with multiple heads and tails. To be classified as normal, the sperm must have an oval headpiece with a normal midpiece and active tail.

6. Fructose: When volume or sperm count is low, the laboratory should test for this sugar, which is produced in the seminal vesicles. Its absence points to a blocked duct.

7. Cultures: Although infections cause sterility, they are usually long gone by the time the man sees a doctor. Ongoing infections are uncommon, but if the semen exam shows suspicious cells or clumped sperm, the doctor will order a culture to search for a disease-causing organism. As a safety measure, a doctor always cultures semen before performing artificial insemination.

8. Antibodies: Most infertile men with sperm immunity have a normal semen analysis; a minority show clumped sperm or obviously abnormal swimming movements. Because clues are so often absent (and also because immunology is an exciting field with many interested researchers), more and more experts order antibodies during an infertility workup; some do so routinely.

The Best Test: Postcoital. Isolated tests have their limits; in the end, pregnancy is the only irrefutable proof that sperm can do their job. Although possible, watching sperm trying to fertilize a human egg remains a research tool. Substituting hamster eggs gives valuable information, but this is complex and expensive. The postcoital test remains the best easily available evidence of a man's fertility.

A couple has sex near the time of the woman's ovulation. That same day, the doctor extracts a sample of the woman's cervical mucus for examination under the microscope. Finding five or more active sperm per field under high power provides better evidence for male fertility than any semen test alone. An abnormal result is not so revealing because problems in the woman can contribute.

Hormone Evaluation

Since endocrine abnormalities contribute only modestly to infertility, doctors don't search for them unless small testes or other areas of the physical exam raise suspicions, unless sperm density is very low, or unless routine tests reveal nothing, so both doctor and patient are growing frustrated.

Besides measuring testosterone, the doctor orders blood tests for the two pituitary hormones that control testicular function: follicle-stimulating hormone (FSH), and luteinizing hormone (LH). Abnormal results follow three patterns:

1. Low testosterone and high pituitary hormones point to a testicular defect. Reacting to low testosterone, the pituitary secretes excess FSH and LH in a futile effort to stimulate the testes.

2. Low testosterone, LH, and FSH indicate disease in or around the pituitary. Testosterone is low despite normal testes because of inadequate pituitary stimulation. Although rare, these central nervous system disorders are among the easiest to treat.

3. Normal or elevated testosterone with elevated pituitary hormones is a sign of androgen resistance: Hormones are adequate, but the sex cells refuse to respond.

Excess production of another pituitary hormone, prolactin, whose function in men is unclear, is rare. Rare tumors of the pituitary as well as drugs and other obscure disorders can lead to this. Since excess prolactin suppresses other hormones, doctors may measure it.

Just as women produce small amounts of male hormone, men secrete estradiol, a female hormone. Men with androgen resistance produce excess estradiol; rare tumors of the testes or adrenal gland do the same, but liver disease is the leading culprit. The normal liver breaks down estradiol; a diseased liver works more slowly, so the level rises. Alcoholics with cirrhosis have a high estradiol along with small testes, large breasts, and infertility.

More Sophisticated Tests

Chromosome Analysis. One male in 500 is born with an extra X chromosome: XXY instead of XY, called Klinefelter's syndrome. Otherwise healthy, he may or may not look feminized but always has small testes and infertility. To diagnose this as well as other rarer abnormalities, a laboratory grows his cells in a tissue culture, then treats them to make the chromosomes visible for counting (humans have forty-six pairs) and examination under the microscope. At a cost of perhaps $1,000, abnormalities occasionally turn up in men with small testes or a low sperm count. The yield is much lower in physically normal men.

Treatment may improve the appearance and potency of a man with a chromosome abnormality, but infertility remains.

Testicular Biopsy. This is a simple office procedure in which the doctor cuts a small piece and submits it to a pathologist for microscopic exam. Unlike its high priority in a search for cancer, a biopsy is well down the list as a test for infertility. When a patient's ejaculate shows a reasonable quantity of normal sperm, the odds of something wrong in the testes are very low. When we see few or abnormal sperm and the testes feel wrong, we assume that they aren't making sperm; we can't do much about that.

When a man with normal testes produces a good volume of semen containing few sperm, the doctor will consider a biopsy. When the microscope reveals no sign of sperm production, the man was probably born with this isolated defect. Provided that his hormone levels are normal, no treatment helps.

If the microscope reveals normal sperm, an obstruction exists somewhere along the spermatic duct.

Checking for Blockage: the Vasogram. Similar to an angiogram of the coronary arteries, in the vasogram a doctor injects dye into the spermatic tube through a small incision in the scrotum and follows its progress with X-rays, searching for an obstruction. Although simple in principle, a vasogram requires skill to outline the tiny ducts without damaging the delicate walls. A trained surgeon performs the procedure with instruments and an operating microscope nearby, so that he or she can quickly repair an obstruction as well as any damage caused by the vasogram.

Before considering a vasogram, some experts search for a blockage by making a tiny opening in the vas to extract samples of fluid. The presence of sperm proves that the block lies further on. The doctor may also inject saline into the vas; if it flows out the end, the tube is open. If not, the doctor may pass a hair-thin catheter to probe for the site of blockage. When these don't provide a clear answer, the vasogram comes next.

When Every Test Is Negative, Try the Hamster Assay

When semen appears normal, and the remainder of the couple's evaluation is unrevealing, doctors wonder if the sperm harbor hidden defects. Although observing sperm penetrate a human egg has become routine at in vitro fertilization clinics, doctors don't like to harvest a woman's eggs for a purely diagnostic test. Hamster eggs provide a practical substitute.

Intact hamster eggs accept only hamster sperm. To circumvent this, technicians treat the eggs with enzymes that dissolve the outer coating, the zona pellucida. A zona pellucida surrounds all human and other mammal eggs to prevent fertilization by other species; it also prevents more than one sperm from penetrating an egg. After mixing hamster eggs and human sperm, a technician records the percentage of eggs successfully penetrated as well as the number of sperm penetrating each egg.

This is a complex test, so experts at different laboratories use different guidelines for a successful result, but general agreement exists that infertile sperm penetrate less than 10 percent of zona-free hamster eggs. Passing the test is a good sign, although some men remain infertile for obscure reasons. Although discouraging, an abnormal result doesn't prove that sperm can't function. Five to 10 percent of these men father a child with assisted technology such as sperm concentration or in vitro fertilization.

After All Tests. Despite steady advances in our diagnostic skills, we find the source of infertility in just 60 percent of men. We'll do better as time passes, but the prognosis isn't hopeless for the remaining 40 percent. If they keep trying, one quarter father children.

Surgical Treatment

Varicocelectomy. The most common surgical treatment for infertile men, tying off a varicocele improves sperm quality in over two thirds; about half of these father a child over the following few years.

Compared to varicose vein surgery in the leg, fixing a varicocele demands more skill. Urologists choose among several techniques.

1. *Traditional.* Through an incision in the groin, the surgeon exposes the spermatic cord. Carefully avoiding the artery, nerves, lymphatic ducts, and vas deferens, he or she ties off the swollen veins. Most urologist prefer this method; some use local or spinal anesthesia (always preferable to general anesthesia), and the man spends a few days in the hospital.

   Taking about half an hour, this is a safe operation; damage to other structures in the spermatic cord occurs, but not often. As with all varicose vein surgery, recurrences make up the leading complication. Occurring after 10 to 20 percent of traditional varicocelectomies, they are not serious but may require a repeat operation.

2. *Microsurgery.* Although performed through a smaller incision, a surgeon using an operating microscope enjoys a much closer view of the spermatic cord, so he or she can identify and cut smaller veins without risking harm to other structures. As a result, complications and recurrences happen less often. Less traumatic than traditional varicocelectomy, microsurgery can be an outpatient procedure, with the patient sent home the same day.

3. *Balloon Occlusion.* Even more benign than microsurgery, this involves no cutting around the cord. The surgeon makes a half-inch incision in the groin to reach a large thigh vein and then threads a catheter (a long flexible tube) upward, guiding it into the kidney vein and then down the testicular vein. Checking with

X-rays, he or she makes sure the catheter is in position and then inflates a balloon in the tip, blocking the vein. Withdrawing the catheter, he or she leaves the balloon permanently in place.

Requiring only local anesthesia and an office visit, this is worth considering if you hate the thought of surgery and the doctor has learned the procedure or knows someone who performs it regularly. Positioning the catheter may take an hour or two, much longer than traditional surgery, and the end results are similar. Recurrences occur at a similar rate, perhaps 10 percent. Now and then the balloon breaks loose, floats into the heart and then out to the lung, where it lodges. Although rare, this resembles a pulmonary embolism or blood clot in the lung, a serious complication.

Clearing Obstructed Ducts. Using an operating microscope, a urologist can remove or bypass a blockage along the epididymus and vas deferens.

An impressive technological feat, unblocking a duct allows sperm to exit but doesn't guarantee fertility. For example, scarring from a sexually transmitted disease often blocks the epididymus. Surgery relieves the blockage, but he epididymus has usually sustained other damage from the infection—and sperm must spend time in a healthy epididymus in order to mature. As a result, only 15 to 20 percent of men who have suffered an infection become fertile after surgery.

A better outcome occurs when ducts are otherwise healthy despite the obstruction. Damaged ducts result accidentally after hernia surgery and deliberately from vasectomy. In both cases, careful microsurgery restores fertility most of the time.

Drug Treatment

Men and women produce the same male and female sex hormones; only the proportions differ. It follows that we treat infertile men and women with the same hormones, although women respond better. A distinct glandular defect occasionally makes a woman infertile, but more often she suffers a change in the elaborate rise and fall of hormones that must occur for her to ovulate. Correcting this is not terribly difficult. Hormonal defects in men are rarely as simple.

Treatment of Hypogonadotropic Hypogonadism. Although a mouthful, this condition responds best of all hormonal deficiencies. Hypogonadism means simply "too little gonad function," a cause of many forms of infertility. Gonads are sex glands: testes in men, ovaries in women. *Hypogonadotropic* reveals the cause of this particular infertility. *Gonadotropic* means "stimulating the gonads"; pituitary hormones, LH and FSH, accomplish that. Hormone tests revealing the second pattern mentioned earlier (low FSH, LH, and testosterone) point to hypogonadotropic hypogonadism.

These men have underdeveloped testes. To correct this, a man receives hCG (human chorionic gonadotropin) injections three times a week. Ideally he should receive human LH, but extraction—from pituitaries or the urine of postmenopausal women—has proven difficult. Genetic engineers have developed bacteria that secrete LH, so we should have a dependable source in the near future. For now, doctors use hCG, secreted in large amounts by pregnant women and similar to LH.

Six or more months must pass before the testes appear normal. At this point the doctor adds FSH to the injections to encourage sperm production. More months may pass before the count rises to an acceptable level: 2 to 5 million. Although this is a low count that rarely rises higher, sperm quality is high, and about half of men become fertile.

Clomiphene (Clomid). Often successful in women, this drug probably leads the list of drugs given infertile men, although with less success. Clomiphene stimulates LH and FSH production; after several months almost all men show a rise in sperm count and testosterone level. Although very satisfying and responsible for its persistent popularity, this improvement doesn't seem to translate into an improved pregnancy rate.

Bromocriptine. When the blood prolactin level is high, bromocriptine lowers it, restoring fertility and potency when these are impaired. Results are poor in the absence of elevated prolactin.

Testosterone. Male hormones don't improve sperm production; they suppress it, but men occasionally receive a course to provoke "testosterone rebound." After three months of suppression, therapy stops in the hope that sperm output will rebound to a higher level. As with many ingenious treatments, those who originated it published studies with excellent results. Others had less success, but giving testosterone seems so reasonable that it is still used after many decades, although less and less often.

Vitamins, Minerals, Zinc, Nutritional Supplements, Exercises, etc. These alternative remedies have their enthusiasts. Frustrated men give them a try; no evidence exists that they help, but unlike other drugs mentioned, they're cheap and harmless.

Treating Retrograde Ejaculation Ordinary decongestants (Sudafed, Ornade, Teldrin) stimulate nerves that shrink swollen nasal tissues. The same family of nerves tightens the bladder neck, so a course of cold remedies sometimes helps. Other experts prefer a low dose of antidepressant such as Tofranil, 50 milligrams per day.

When drugs fail, doctors can retrieve sperm from the bladder. Sperm die in the usual acidity of urine; to alkalinize it, the man takes a large amount of sodium bicarbonate beforehand. After recovery, sperm are washed, concentrated, and artificially inseminated.

Semen Processing

Over the past decade, specialists have developed clever ways to improve semen quality either by extracting and concentrating healthy sperm or by eliminating harmful elements in seminal fluid. Among them are the following.

Sperm Enhancement. A technician places semen at the bottom of a test tube. The more energetic sperm swim to the top to be recovered for artificial insemination, leaving the slower swimmers behind. Depending on the preference of that fertility clinic, the sperm swim through layers of fiber filters, silica powder, or a mixture of proteins designed to improve motility.

Sperm Washing. Semen added to a special fluid spins in a centrifuge, forcing sperm to concentrate in a pellet at the bottom. After discarding the fluid, a technician resuspends the sperm in a solution designed for artificial insemination. Clinics may wash semen several times to remove chemicals, dead sperm, blood cells, and other debris.

Eliminating Antibodies. Because they stick to sperm, antibodies remain after enhancement and vigorous washing. If sperm appear otherwise healthy, the doctor may proceed with artificial insemination. If a doctor feels that it's important to reduce antibodies, a man must take a course of cortisone to suppress his immune system before producing the semen sample.

CHAPTER ▪ 12
A MAN AND HIS
DOCTOR

Next to immediate family and close friends, a family doctor plays the most important role in your life—certainly in its later years. Choosing one should require some effort, but much of the advice I read in popular writing misses the point. Writers as well as laypeople tend to place competence first among the qualities of a physician. The fact is that sheer medical knowledge matters most if you suffer a rare or complicated disease. Certainly competence is an essential quality in a family doctor, but it's not in short supply, so I advise against making it the basis of your search.

To choose properly, you should know what a doctor actually does and what a doctor enjoys about being a doctor.

How to Choose a Doctor

The Wrong Way. Since young women require extensive gynecological up-keep as well as obstetrics, and since they suffer more from sexually related disorders, they know the value of a sympathetic doctor. Young men mostly require medical attention for injuries, skin disease, and job-related exams: occasions that aren't particularly intimate or upsetting. A lucky man can reach advanced age comfortable in the belief that a good doctor provides efficient maintenance for his body just as a mechanic cares for his car. Asked about the most desired quality in a doctor, he would agree on the importance of a warm beside manner—but mostly for a few neurotic relatives, hypochondriacs who need endless patience and hand holding. For himself, he wants a smart doctor with finely honed skills who can keep him running smoothly.

A Doctor Who Takes Care of Things

The term *bedside manner* has a warm, cuddly sound that many men don't value until they need it and don't get it. I avoid the term because it doesn't explain how a really good doctor behaves. A good doctor obviously wants to help. If you're worried, the doctor knows. If you're in pain, the doctor feels a little pain, too. The question of competence never arises because the doctor is clearly doing everything that has to be done. In the worst case, the doctor will always be there. Abandonment and uncontrolled pain, the most frightening elements of serious illness, are never part of the picture. A really good doctor takes care of things.

This sounds wonderful, but how often will you require this wonderfulness? Ninety percent of a family doctor's appointments involve colds, minor ailments or injuries, and other routine conditions that don't worry the patient or require more than a friendly manner and simple techniques from the doctor. From a strictly mechanical aspect, a bright high school student could handle them. Two or three times a day we see someone who requires either deep thought or deep understanding. When the time comes that you're among that number, you'll appreciate a good bedside manner, but you'll benefit on every visit. If you want someone who returns your calls, talks long and hard about preventive medicine, or fits you into a crowded schedule when you feel bad, you also want a humanitarian. Most patients don't require heavy problem solving or major fixes, but everyone requires care.

Terrific doctors aren't rare. Perhaps 10 percent of us are genuine humanitarians with a generous supply of problem-solving and fixing ability. Filling in the other 90 percent, I estimate that 10 percent are bad, mostly because of personality defects or personal problems such as alcoholism. Sheer incompetence exists, but not as often as you'd think (I discuss malpractice later in this chapter). The remaining 80 percent range from good to barely adequate, so taking pot luck will get you a reasonable doctor most of the time. But you can do better.

Do Your Research

Besides this chapter, you'll find advice on choosing a doctor in at least one entire book. Magazine articles also cover the subject regularly, invariably featuring it prominently on the cover. Slavishly obeying the rules of marketing, no writer discusses how to find a good doctor. They tell you how to find "the best." Written by laypersons, all fail to avoid two pitfalls:

1. They're dazzled by scientific glitter and reputation. This is not terribly off base, because doctors highly regarded within the profession are usually good. However, doctors acquire national reputations by advancing medical science or occupying impor-

tant positions at a medical school—not by taking care of people like you. Many see few or no private patients, and you probably won't learn that from the writer.

2. They give reasonable but impractical advice. Writers who tear themselves away from medical superstars and do their homework can come up with genuinely useful characteristics of a potential doctor. Many make up a checklist that includes information about training, office routine, charges, and perhaps some questions on how the doctor would handle certain situations—his or her approach to testing, prescribing, referring, etc. Then ask these questions of a selection of potential doctors. But I realize that most of you lead busy lives and would not take the time to do this. Long experience has taught me that it's not fruitful to give patients advice that they won't follow. There's usually a better approach.

Feel free to consult the media, but do the following five things.

1. Ask around.

A doctor practicing a highly technical subspecialty may conceal brilliance behind an unpleasant personality, but this never happens in primary care and rarely in the common specialties. If a doctor is terrific, his or her patients know it and will be happy to pass on the news.

Don't stop after one enthusiastic endorsement. People show an amazing range of tastes, so even the worst doctor has fiercely loyal patients. Two testimonials should give you pause, and three or more indicate a serious candidate. Don't be cynical here; naturally laypeople are mostly impressed with a friendly, caring doctor, so they overestimate the competence of someone they like. My patients often give me credit for curing ailments which run their course unaffected by medical science. I enjoy the acclaim, but patients also benefit. A good doctor cures few patients but makes everyone feel better, and even effective therapy works better when the patient believes that his or her doctor is the best.

2. Ask other doctors.

This includes those you know socially. You might think that doctors know the absolute best in their fields, but don't count on it. Doctors know their friends, colleagues, and some to whom they refer patients, but beyond these they are influenced by the same credentials as magazine writers. Although asked regularly by readers, I have no idea who's good outside of my local area—the only exception being an outstanding dermatologist in Orlando, Florida, who was my best friend in medical school.

I know perhaps a dozen whom I'd consider excellent. They combine a high level of competence (I've discussed medicine with them or heard them lecture and been impressed) with a warm personality: Patients whom I have referred have praised them. But I don't know everything about everybody; several doctors to whom I refer seem OK. Nothing bad has happened to my patients, and no one has complained. But I don't know these doctors personally; some I have never seen.

Expect this level of help from most doctors you query. They know some dirt that's not general knowledge, and they know more about a doctor's competence or technical skills. But even doctors have their limits, and you shouldn't trust one good report. Doctors have their own quirks; they're are partial to their friends as laypeople are and often make referrals out of habit or to doctors who do them favors in return. But pay attention if several speak enthusiastically about a colleague.

3. Make sure of their training.

For your family doctor, choose either a family practitioner or general internist. Historically, internal medicine encompasses adult medicine—not adult surgery, psychiatry, urology, etc. A newer specialty, family practice includes training that doesn't concern you, such as pediatrics and obstetrics, but includes minor surgery and other areas traditionally skipped by internists. In reality, general internists pick up skills outside their specialty, so they usually do fine. In the past, internal medicine training focused on serious diseases while a family practice residency, being newer, brought in more routine care and preventive medicine. Lately, feeling the competition, internal medicine residencies are coming around.

If you decide on an internist, make sure he or she is a generalist by training. Plenty of internal medicine specialists (cardiologists, gastroenterologists, endocrinologists, etc.) practice general medicine and most perform adequately, but I see no reason to prefer one. During training, specialists spend two or three years exclusively in their specialty, after which they cram to pass a difficult test. In the end they know a great deal about one field of medicine; presumably they enjoy this field or they wouldn't have spent so much effort to learn it. Starting out, many accept all patients until they build up a practice in their specialty. Most remember enough general medicine to handle it, but, as a patient, I'd feel uneasy if my problem didn't belong to the area that that doctor enjoyed. Some specialists decide that they prefer the variety that comes with general medicine; in that case their training has been skewed.

4. Keep a sense of proportion about impressive institutions.

I wouldn't go to the Mayo Clinic for routine care even if I lived in Rochester, Minnesota. I wouldn't travel there unless my doctor knew of a particular subspecialty that my disease required—and that would be unlikely if I lived outside the area or even in Minneapolis, a city with fine medical facilities. The Mayo is an excellent institution, but in hiring doctors its standards are not higher than those of other good clinics.

Lay writers overstress the virtues of large medical centers, especially those affiliated with a medical school. Doctors who teach students and residents must give out the best information, these writers explain, so they keep on the cutting edge of science. There is some truth in this, but much of it doesn't matter to you unless you suffer a rare or complex disease. On the other hand, teaching, like medicine, is a noble profession, so anyone who enjoys both has superior instincts. During my training, I couldn't fault the competence of most of my instructors, although some had unacceptable personalities, and when pure researchers came out of the lab to take their turn teaching, it was usually obvious that they didn't know what they were talking about.

You must also realize that the world has changed since the era when a medical school was a shining ivory tower. Throughout this century and peaking during a the golden years of the 1960s, medical schools made little effort to attract paying patients. The richest schools paid professors a salary and forbade them from practicing. Others held their nose and permitted it because their teachers needed the money, but the more private patients a professor saw, the lower his or her status.

Medical students, interns, and residents positively disliked paying patients unless they suffered interesting diseases. We preferred poor people who had no private doctor to outrank us. Good teachers used their practice solely for income and admitted their middle-class patients to private hospitals elsewhere. But others couldn't resist the temptation. In a teaching hospital, a resident would perform the admitting physical exam and paperwork and handle the routine work as well as wee-hour phone calls from the nurse, but the private doctor still collected the fee. Naturally the doctor was supposed to teach us in exchange for this work, and a few remained in the background, allowing us to make all the decisions (would you have liked that?). But most zipped in and out, ignoring us unless they needed an errand.

Then the world began changing. Throughout most of history, a day in the hospital cost less than a day in a hotel. By the 1940s, rates were about the same; today a hospital day costs twenty times more. Although doctors in training continue to prefer poor people, by the 1970s their superiors found it more and more painful to contemplate a bed that didn't pay its way.

Generous government grants for training disappeared (if you recall, the United States was supposed to have a physician shortage in the 1950s and 1960s). Research grants (which also paid salaries) declined, so many doctors found that they had to earn a living. Medical schools reversed themselves and became positively eager to care for patients with private insurance. Twisting arms, medical schools set up faculty practice clinics, in which professors saw private patients but the school collected part of the fee.

Forced to hustle even more, schools borrowed from banks to construct the massive medical office buildings that surround university hospitals today. Although near enough to share the medical school aura, the sole qualification for practicing in these offices is ability to pay the rent. Their tenants are mostly a cross section of ordinary doctors, but the medical school hopes that patients notice the convenient hospital next door, a hope generally fulfilled to the bitter complaints of outlying hospitals.

So don't head for the nearest big medical center if you're serious about researching a family doctor. On the other hand, if you don't want to work at all, you can't go wrong choosing a doctor at the Division of Family Practice at a medical school. Don't worry about being handed over to a resident. This is only likely if you're not paying or are covered by Medicaid (which, as of 1994, pays a fraction of what your care costs). As a patient who pays your way, you'll get someone who's completed training, and since medical schools rarely take on duds, he or she will be at least average. The best of these are on the university staff who spend part of their time deciding what to teach the residents and then teaching it. You can find them by asking, but their titles give them away. Look for the titles *professor, associate professor,* and *assistant professor.* The other side of the coin is that doctors who teach a great deal don't practice full time. If they're truly brilliant, the school will promote them, so they'll have even less time for you.

Any title preceded by *clinical* (i.e., clinical associate professor) is strictly honorary: payment in lieu of money for helping out. The doctor may spend one afternoon per month chatting with colleagues in the teaching clinic while residents see patients and occasionally ask his or her advice. Although not the mark of a true academic, you should consider such volunteer work a plus. Furthermore, these doctors practice full time and won't move up the academic ladder, so you can count on them over the long haul.

5. You can search for skeletons if you're aggressive.

If you write your state medical board (*not* medical society), most will tell you of complaints against a doctor that were upheld and any actions the board took against that doctor (don't expect information on complaints that it didn't pursue). Malpractice suits don't involve a state board, so it probably won't help you there.

A few years ago, the federal government set up a database for every successful malpractice claim, whether settled in or out of court. Its purpose was to allow clinics, hospitals, and other institutions to check the background of doctors they were hiring, so this data isn't available to anyone else. However, trial lawyers would love to get their hands on it, and many consumer groups feel that the public should have access. Past efforts to pry restricted information from government agencies have often succeeded, so soon you may be able to learn how many times your doctor has been sued. What should you do with this information? Do you want a doctor who's lost even one suit?

Even without checking, if you want to minimize your chance of seeing a doctor who's been sued, choose one as young as possible. The older the doctor, the more likely that he or she has been sued. For some specialities such as orthopedics and neurosurgery, this encompasses the majority of older doctors. In the case of obstetrics, the odds approach 100 percent. All obstetricians are sued sooner or later.

What is Malpractice?

Some doctors are sued for malpractice because they commit malpractice, but in the litigation explosion of the past generation, malpractice (faulty and injurious medical treatment) has become only one of many reasons that patients file suit and probably not the major one.

An English patient saw a doctor and learned that he had cancer. Naturally the man was devastated. Months later, after many ordeals, he learned that the diagnosis was wrong. There was no cancer. Halfway through the trial that followed, the English judge stopped the proceedings and said, "The doctor in this case made a serious mistake, but no one has accused him of incompetence or dishonesty. Everyone makes mistakes; a mistake is not malpractice. Case dismissed."

American doctors chuckle at this story. I tell it to illustrate that things are different over most of the world. In legal theory, the statement, "a mistake is not malpractice" holds true everywhere, but in reality a mistake wins in a U.S. court.

Americans sue when something dreadful happens to them, whether the reason is malpractice, a mistake, or simply a bad result. *Bad result* is a euphemistic term meaning "the doctor did everything right, but something terrible happened anyway." Surgery is risky; patients of even the most brilliant surgeon occasionally suffer a heart attack, stroke, hemorrhage, or infection. Now and then a doctor prescribes a popular, safe drug, and the patient has a violent reaction. One percent of babies are born with serious defects, an awful blow to the parents. They often ask whose fault it is.

Having learned all this, would you choose a doctor who's been sued once or twice? You might hesitate. I'd feel uneasy, too. In case you're interested, I don't know the malpractice history of any doctor to whom I refer unless the news appeared in the paper. I don't know this about my physician friends or even my brother. Doctors freely discuss their mistakes as well as triumphs with other doctors, but malpractice suits rarely come up; the subject is painful.

If I could easily look up this information, would I? Perhaps for a doctor about whom I already had doubts, but not otherwise. It would be like inquiring into someone's sex life—information that was none of my business and that shouldn't affect our professional relationship.

WHAT TO DO ONCE YOU'VE DECIDED

Make an appointment—not for a physical but for whatever the doctor does with a new patient. Not every doctor performs an extensive exam on the first visit, especially with a young patient, but all gather information. You should be asked your medical and family history (make sure you know it). You'll almost certainly receive more lab work than I recommend, but doctors as well as patients enjoy tests.

This is your chance to evaluate your doctor, so relax and observe. Ask whatever medically related questions you want, but I have no additional ones. I can't think of any that will enable you to assess the doctor's judgment and knowledge, and the interview itself will provide information on his or her personality. Although it's traditional to poo-poo first impressions, they are reliable.

It's all right to dismiss some impressions. Don't pay great attention to the office decor. Give the personnel only passing notice (despite the white uniforms, they're probably not nurses). In a large clinic, the doctor doesn't hire or fire the help. Even in a small practice, good office personnel are hard to find and keep, and it's difficult to evaluate them unless you're ill and need sympathy or something upsets their routine (e.g., your appointment wasn't recorded).

"Go Into That Room and Take Your Clothes Off"

When the time arrives to see the doctor, if the aide conducts you to an examining room and then asks you to undress and put on a gown, my advice is to walk out. You've discovered a very bad quality, no sensitive doctor conducts an interview with a naked patient. If you're more assertive, disobey the aide and remain clothed. A doctor who proceeds without insisting that you undress gains a few points. However, the initial meeting between you and a quality doctor should take place in his or her office. In fact, except in an emergency, a good doctor always talks to you while you're clothed before getting down to business.

What to Expect and What You Don't Need

Friends and relatives regularly consult me about medical problems. Now and then a problem requires serious attention, but the majority don't. I provide reassurance and simple advice; I almost never perform an exam or write a prescription. Naturally my wife consults me frequently, and when her problem is clearly minor she often grows irritated at the speed of my diagnosis.

"Someday you're going to say 'it's probably nothing' when it's something," she complains. I agree that this is possible while pointing out that it hasn't happened in fifteen years. My wife is not a hypochondriac, and her complaint is reasonable. She's uneasy because I'm not behaving like a doctor.

But I can't behave like a doctor twenty-four hours a day. Most of the time I'm an ordinary person except that my brain is full of medical knowledge. People are welcome to tap into that knowledge, but knowledge is all they get. For minor ailments in people I know well, I don't do those things that make patients feel that I am a wise and powerful healer. Most doctors do the same in social situations, but they know better than to behave this way on the job.

Perhaps one half of patients who consult a doctor suffer an upper respiratory infection, flu, upset stomach, or other common, self-limited ailment. The diagnosis is obvious as soon as the patient explains why he or she came. Doctors beginning practice often announce it immediately, but they quickly learn that laypeople are less impressed than other physicians with an instant diagnosis. Some patients feel ashamed at the implication that the problem was so simple, perhaps too simple to bother the doctor with. Others become suspicious. Why is the doctor so sure so quickly, they wonder. He or she didn't ask questions or do an exam or any tests. Maybe this doctor is lazy or sloppy or in a hurry.

So an experienced doctor takes even routine ailments very seriously. He or she asks questions (more than necessary), performs an exam (even when unnecessary; putting hands on the patient is part of the therapeutic encounter), and then announces the diagnosis and plan of treatment. For disorders such as viral infections and many minor injuries, a doctor who says "it'll go away soon; you don't need any treatment" has spoken the literal truth. Many patients feel relieved at this news; perhaps you are among them, but this places you in the minority.

Mumbo-Jumbo versus Ritual

Doctors save lives, cure disease, relieve suffering, teach, and perform other noble functions, but they also engage in a great deal of what cynical doctors call mumbo-jumbo. I prefer to call it ritual. By this I mean behavior which does not help diagnose or treat an illness but which makes the patient feel that we are proper doctors.

Most humans who feel bad enough to see a physician expect the physician to "do" something. Young doctors believe that they have performed an excellent service when they provide an accurate diagnosis and explain what will happen, so they grow puzzled when so many patients merely thank them politely before leaving. Despite our high income and status, doctors enjoy gratitude and we're very sensitive to a patient's behavior at the end of the encounter. An obviously pleased patient gives us pleasure. Since few laypeople are willing to show anger at their physician, a polite thank you is usually the only evidence of profound disappointment.

Disappointed patients depress us. Although doctors come out of training convinced that reassurance and education form an essential part of care, they quickly learn that patients don't value this as much as professors of medicine, especially for minor ailments. They value medication, and as a result doctors vastly overprescribe. Critics, including me, denounce the profession for this avalanche of unnecessary drugs, but to a certain extent this must continue. Doctors in Western culture give drugs. American physicians prescribe 1.1 medications per visit.

If you go to an acupuncturist, you'll get acupuncture; a nutritionist will provide nutrition; a witch doctor will do whatever a witch doctor does. Healers in all societies are expected to heal, so traditional physicians never tell you that you'll feel sick for a while, then you'll feel better, and nothing they do will make a difference. Being in a scientific discipline, medical doctors shouldn't feel obligated to act when no action helps, but this is hard to resist. To a patient with a nasty cough, an ugly rash, or a red eye, the news that nothing helps seems completely wrong.

Time and again, I've heard myself explaining to patients about their illness—why they got it, how long they'll have it, reassurance, home remedies, etc. At the same time, observing their reaction, I've thought to myself, "It's not working . . . he's not buying it . . . he wants a prescription . . . should I give it to him?" Sometimes I do. Invariably the patient looks relieved and rewards me with a dose of gratitude before leaving. But I witness more than my share of disappointment because I am not as generous as most physicians with certain important drugs—antibiotics, for example.

Most antibiotics given to outpatients function as placebos. Doctors prescribe them for colds, the flu, and other viral coughs and sore throat for which they are entirely useless. Hearing this statement, laypeople look skeptical and assume that I'm expressing my opinion. In fact, it's not controversial. Giving antibiotics for viral infections is so routine that you can't use it to measure competence. Even good doctors do it.

Dealing with Overprescribing

As with many problems, doing nothing is a reasonable tactic. If you like your doctor, everything he or she does seems right, so my statements on overprescribing won't seem to apply. Furthermore, although I'm an expert on drugs and prescribing (my last book covered the subject), you might simply assume I'm wrong in your particular case. If I see a patient with a miserable sore throat which his or her previous doctor invariably treated with amoxicillin (the most popular prescription drug in the United States), my lecture on the uselessness of antibiotics for viral infections will go in one ear and out the other.

If you still want to avoid getting an unnecessary drug, you must let the doctor know that you're unlike the average patient. The doctor will soon forget, so you'll have to remind him or her on each encounter for a while. Let him or her know early in the visit. As you explain your illness, say something like "I've had this cough for a week, and it's beginning to get me down. I'd like to know if it's anything to worry about and what I should do. If it'll go away on its own,

I don't need an antibiotic." If this sounds like you're dropping hints on how the doctor should do his or her job properly, you're right.

Make a habit of asking "Do I really need this?" Aspirin takes the edge off pain for a few hours. Cough medicine never cured a cough. Antihistamines don't cure allergies. Cortisone makes everything feel better, but it doesn't cure anything. Relieving symptoms is a legitimate medical function, so giving a symptomatic remedy isn't necessarily overprescribing, but doctors lean over backward to provide relief. If your symptoms are tolerable, let the doctor know, but don't decide on your own whether or not to take a drug.

DOCTORS AND ALL THOSE TESTS

For most of this century, when a laboratory received a tube of blood from a doctor, a technician sitting at a bench surrounded by chemicals, a scale, and a few simple machines performed whatever analysis the doctor ordered. This might take five or ten minutes. Doing tests one at a time was not cheap, so doctors ordered modest numbers.

The 1960s brought wonderful contraptions with names like Coulter Counter or multiphasic analyzer, which accepted a quantity of blood at one end, sped it through any number of chemical, electronic, or colorimetric processes, and then disgorged a printout containing a half a dozen to thirty or more test results. The process became so cheap (provided that the machine ran constantly) that when a doctor ordered a single test, the technician might simply use the analyzer, throw out nineteen results, and send back the one the doctor ordered. Naturally, doctors quickly learned that they could get twenty for the price of one.

The avalanche of testing became overwhelming. A doctor whose patient suffered liver disease once wrote the names of one or two tests on his lab slip; now he or she could check off "liver panel" and see the results of ten. It's too cynical to claim that these duplicated each other; some liver tests look at different aspects of liver function, but most patients don't require such subtlety. Laboratories now offered "kidney panels," "arthritis panels," "lipid panels," and collections of tests limited only by the laboratory director's imagination.

Although individual panels were cheap, the machines cost a fortune, so they had to keep busy. Quickly the word went out that screening panels were available for healthy people. In the old days, a man underdoing a physical received a chest X-ray, a urinalysis, and perhaps a blood count and blood sugar. Now his doctor routinely ordered twelve or twenty tests. By paying extra the patient could opt for an "executive panel" of thirty. Bypassing the doctor, laypeople could buy tests at a health fair or through entrepreneurs who offered them through businesses, unions, churches, etc. Customers received an impressive printout; the abnormal results were flagged with alarming warnings to consult

A Typical Multiphasic Screening Panel

Test	Value	Description
Albumin N=3.0-5.5	5.0 gl/dl	A blood protein. Reduced in severe malnutrition.
Inorganic Phosphorus N=2.5-4.5	3.6 mg/dl	Reduced in severe malnutrition. Elevated in advanced kidney disease.
Alkaline Phosphatase N=30-115	85 U/l	Liver test. Slightly elevated, but the patient has no evidence of liver disease, so nothing further will be done.
LDH N=100-225	223 U/l	Liver test. Also elevated in heart disease, lung disease, kidney disease, and blood disease.
Total Bilirubin N=0.2-1.2	1.9 mg/dl	Abnormal in several rare glandular diseases. Elevated in some cases of advanced cancer.
Potassium N=3.5-5.0	4.7 meq/l	Reduced in patients taking diuretics. Elevated in advanced kidney failure.
Calcium N=8.5-10.5	10.1 mg/dl	
Total Protein N=6.0-8.5	8.1 g/dl	Reduced in severe malnutrition.
Carbon Dioxide N=24-32	31 meq/l	Elevated in severe emphysema. Low in very poorly controlled diabetes.
ALT N=0-41	35 U/l	
Chloride N=96-106	101 meq/l	Abnormal in severe vomiting & diarrhea
SGPT AST N=6-53	30 U/l	Abnormal in severe vomiting & diarrhea.
Cholesterol N=150-300	210 mg/dl	A useful test.
Sodium N=136-145	139 meq/l	
CPK N=0-225	105 U/l	Elevated during a heart attack (but not before).
Urea Nitrogen N=10-26	18 mg/dl	
Creatinine N=0.7-1.5	1.2 mg/dl	Kidney test. Does not become abnormal until at least 50% of kidney function is lost.
Uric Acid N=2.5-8.0	7.6 mg/dl	Elevated in severe kidney failure and some types of cancer. Sometimes elevated in gout.
Glucose N=65-115	136 mg/dl	Elevated, but patient ate shortly before the test.
Triglycerides N=30-175	155 mg/dl	
A/G		
Globulin N=2.0-3.9	3.1	A blood protein. Elevated in some long-standing diseases such as chronic hepatitis or rheumatoid arthritis.

a doctor. Most of these screenings were dotted with abnormal results because (as I explained in Chapter 5) 5 percent of all tests performed on a healthy person are out of the normal range. Every so often a worried patient would arrive in the office with his or her printout, and I would review it and reassure him or her as follows:

"Your BUN is a bit low, but a low BUN has no significance."

"Your white count is a little low, but that's not important. An ordinary cold can do that. But we'll repeat it."

"Your boy's alkaline phosphatase is very high, but that's normal for a child. Growing bones produce lots of alkaline phosphatase."

"Your LDH is high, but that's not a good test. No one pays much attention to it. But we'll repeat it."

"Your wife's thyroid hormone level is elevated because she's on birth control pills. Estrogens make the test seem higher than it really is."

"Your blood sugar is below what that lab considers normal, but it's OK by other standards, including mine."

"Your phosphate is low. In a healthy person with a normal calcium, it probably doesn't mean anything, but we'll repeat it."

As the decades passed, doctors realized that these tests caused more problems than they solved. We spent a great deal of time explaining trivial abnormalities and repeating tests but discovered little significant disease. A buzz word during the 1970s, multiphasic testing has fallen out of fashion but still occurs often enough to be a bother.

Why Tests Have Appeal

It's easy to understand why laypeople take tests so seriously. First, they involve expensive and complicated machinery. Most Americans believe that information produced by advanced technology must have value. Second, the workings of a doctor's mind and hands are mysterious, so it's hard to speculate on what they mean. But a test seems easy to understand. Doesn't a blood sugar reveal if you have diabetes? Doesn't an electrocardiogram detect heart disease? The answer to both questions is sometimes. No test measures everything. A stomach X-ray doesn't tell everything there is to know about the stomach. A urinalysis reveals something about kidney function, but one can have kidney disease and a normal urine.

Despite limitations and gross overuse, tests have important uses. Here is what's worth knowing about the common ones.

Understand the Complete Blood Count (CBC). Being "complete" it measures too many things, but'the machine churns them out so easily that we no longer order a simple hemoglobin or white count. In fact, electronic blood counters represent a major advance. In the old days, a blood count was literally that: A technician sat with a microscope and counted. The machine not only saves money and tedium, it's more accurate.

A blood count measures formed elements in the blood (i.e., everything visible). Formed elements include red cells, half a dozen types of white cells, platelets, and—rarely in the United States and a source of great excitement when they turn up—parasites.

Red cells carry oxygen from lungs to tissues and then pick up carbon dioxide from tissues and return it to the lungs. Men normally have about 5 million red cells per cubic millimeter (4.5 to 5.7 million). The blood count also measures hemoglobin, the protein in red cells that carries gases back and forth. Fourteen to 17 grams per 100 milliliters is normal for a man. Another number the hematocrit, measures the precise volume of red cells in a quantity of blood: 41 to 50 percent for a normal man.

It sounds like the red cell count, hemoglobin, and hematocrit measure the same thing, but knowing all three allows some clever calculations. For example, dividing the total volume of cells (hematocrit) by the red cell count gives the volume of a single cell. Some diseases such as iron deficiency produce abnormally small red cells; others such as vitamin B_{12} deficiency lead to excessively large cells, so mean corpuscular volume is another useful number.

Anemia occurs when the red count (hemoglobin, etc.) falls below normal. Anemia is merely a description of the laboratory results, not a useful diagnosis. A thousand disorders can produce anemia, and a doctor is obligated to find the one that applies to each patient. Some anemias are inherited, untreatable, and harmless. Others are a sign of serious diseases such as cancer. Stress and overwork never cause anemia; diet almost never causes it in the United States.

Anemia is not healthy, but neither is its opposite: polycythemia. Too many red cells make blood sluggish and prone to clot. Polycythemia occurs in a few uncommon blood diseases as well as in any condition where tissues have trouble getting enough oxygen, such as living at high altitude or in severe lung or heart disease. Most often, when I see a hematocrit of, say, 54, the patient turns out to be a heavy smoker.

White cells take part in immune reactions. Half a dozen white cell types normally appear in the blood with names like lymphocyte, monocyte, neutrophil, eosinophil, etc. Much less numerous than red cells, white cells should range from 4,000 to 10,000 per milliliter. During an infection this may double or triple, but sometimes it drops into the 3,000's, either because the infection has suppressed white cell production in the bone marrow or because the cells have left the circulation and concentrated in the site of infection. Very low white counts occur in immune disorders; this usually happens when infections, malignancies, or drugs damage the bone marrow, where all blood cells are born.

Although some doctors believe a high white count points to a bacterial infection and a low count to a viral infection, they are wrong (not entirely wrong, but too many exceptions occur to rely on). A white count interests me if I'm uncertain whether or not an infection is present, but I don't often encounter this problem. An abnormal count in someone obviously suffering an infection doesn't provide more information or help me in treatment, so there's no reason to know it.

The Differential. Although machines are getting better, counting the various white cell types remain a job for a technician with a microscope. Mostly this duplicates information in the white count, but occasionally a differential helps. A very high eosinophil count provides good evidence for a severe allergic reaction or parasitic infection. When the white count remains normal but the percent of young (immature) white cells rises, we know the body is struggling to fight an infection. When the technician sees peculiar looking (atypical) lymphocytes, the patient often has infectious mononucleosis. Once again, however, the doctor must rely more on his or her brain than the lab test. Mono typically produces a great many atypical lymphocytes, but other viral infections do the same.

The differential often hints at other diseases but only rarely makes a distinct diagnosis.

Why You Should Not Have a Lab Test Without a Good Reason. During my residency twenty years ago, a young man came to our clinic with a minor injury. Although the injury didn't require it, his resident ordered a few blood tests, including a CBC. All that came back were normal except the blood count, which shocked everyone. The man had leukemia.

Primitive cells in the bone marrow that generate red cells and white cells normally don't circulate in the blood. During leukemia they multiply wildly and often escape, so a technician can observe them when performing a differential. Leukemic cells can appear in the blood months or years before a patient feels ill. This man felt fine.

Was he lucky that we detected his disease so early? No. Drugs cure some forms of leukemia, but no good treatment existed for his. It was a death sentence. Naturally, no one wanted to break the news: the resident, the chief resident, even the attending physician in charge. After much agonizing, they informed the man that something peculiar had turned up on his blood test and gave him an appointment to the hematology clinic. I never heard what happened.

Platelets are small cell fragments that clump around blood vessel injuries to begin clot formation. Since clotting disorders are uncommon, the machine ignores platelets unless programmed to do otherwise. During the differential the technician scans the slide and writes a comment—usually "platelets adequate."

Blood Lipids: Cholesterol, Trigylcerides, High- Versus Low-Density Cholesterol.

The most useful blood tests for a healthy person, lipids predict susceptibility to atherosclerosis and its consequences.

Triglycerides is a medical term for fat. Everyone has a certain amount of fat circulating in the blood; the level rises after a meal, so you must fast overnight before giving blood. Twenty years ago, we considered you at high risk when triglycerides exceeded 150 to 175 milligrams per 100 cubic centimeters. Unlike cholesterol, whose "normal" range has dropped, doctors have grown more liberal with triglycerides, and now we feel comfortable until the level reaches 250 milligrams.

Medical opinion changes. Twenty years ago we considered triglycerides as important as cholesterol as a risk factor for atherosclerosis, but today we're not so certain. Studies provide some evidence, but it's not as overwhelming as that for cholesterol. Although neither doctors nor popular health writers spend much time denouncing triglycerides, you're better off keeping your level below 100. Achieving a low triglyceride is simpler (although not necessarily easier) than reducing cholesterol. A low-fat diet accomplishes this. It turns out that most men with an elevated triglyceride are overweight, and the best treatment is weight loss.

Cholesterol makes up the actual material deposited on blood vessel walls in atherosclerosis. Animal (not plant) tissue contains cholesterol, but your body also manufactures it as an essential ingredient in synthesis of cortisone and sex hormones. Dietary cholesterol plays a less important role in atherosclerosis than your natural production, and eating doesn't change your level significantly, so a fast isn't necessary before drawing blood. A doctor should order a cholesterol on your first visit. If it's in a healthy range (below 200; see Chapter 2 for more information), a repeat every five years or so is fine.

High-density and Low-density Cholesterol. If you've read about cholesterol, you've heard about subtypes: high-density lipoprotein cholesterol (HDL—a good cholesterol; higher is better) and low-density lipoprotein cholesterol (LDL—bad cholesterol; lower is better). Measuring subtypes helps in borderline situations. For example, if your total cholesterol is 220 (not so good) but your HDL is high, you're not as badly off. Perhaps you have the risk of a person with a level of 200. However, once you drop below 180 your risks are too low for subtypes to matter.

Glucose (Blood Sugar)

A normal fasting glucose ranges from 60 to 100 milligrams per 100 cubic centimeters. Dropping a little below probably has no significance. Fasting means no eating for eight hours, but even after days of fasting blood glucose remains normal because this is the level needed to nourish tissues. In the absence of food, the body breaks down muscle and fat to produce glucose. After eating, the level rises modestly but returns to normal within three hours.

The hormone insulin permits glucose to enter cells from the blood. When there's too little insulin, tissues have difficulty taking in glucose, so its level rises higher after a meal and takes longer to return to normal. When diabetes worsens, the fasting level rises above normal (fortunately, the brain and heart don't require insulin, so they remain well nourished even in severe diabetes). No symptoms occur in mild diabetes, but as blood sugar rises the kidneys work to get rid of the excess, so the victim notices that he or she is urinating a great deal. Provided that the kidneys are healthy, sugar doesn't appear in the urine until the blood level rises over 200. Extra urination requires extra water, so the brain produces thirst to encourage the necessary drinking. Finally, when tissues can't take in enough sugar to nourish themselves, they starve, so the person loses weight.

Diagnosing and Overdiagnosing Diabetes. The most common hormonal disease, diabetes affects 1 to 2 percent of the population; the risk increases with age. Establishing its presence is easy when symptoms occur. A single random glucose over 200 in the presence of thirst, excessive urination, and weight loss makes the diagnosis.

Matters are not so simple when the person feels well, and doctors often forget that they must not diagnose a serious disease with a single lab test in the absence of other evidence. Diabetes in a person without symptoms requires two fasting glucoses above 140. If results don't reach this level but remain above 110, the doctor can order a glucose tolerance test. After an overnight fast, the person drinks a sweet solution containing 75 grams of glucose, and then a technician draws blood every half hour for two hours. A glucose over 200 at two hours and on at least one earlier sample makes the diagnosis.

Anything less but still above normal defines something called impaired glucose tolerance. This is not mild diabetes or early diabetes or borderline diabetes—all ominous diagnoses that oppress too many patients. Three quarters of those with impaired glucose tolerance never develop diabetes, and almost everyone that progresses is overweight. Being overweight itself increases the risk of diabetes as well as plenty of other disorders, and weight loss is the treatment of impaired glucose tolerance. Losing only 10 or 20 pounds often returns the glucose level to normal.

Uses of the Blood Glucose. Naturally we check blood glucose to follow treatment of someone with diabetes. Since diabetes can begin without symptoms, it seems reasonable to include a glucose in the periodic exam, and doctors commonly order one. However, preventive medicine guidelines discourage this, except that footnotes mention exceptions if the risk of diabetes is very high: in someone who is grossly obese or whose two parents have diabetes. Almost every adult with diabetes is overweight. Naturally, overweight men should lose weight. When they develop diabetes, the best treatment is not drugs or insulin but weight loss, so ordering a lab test doesn't change the treatment.

The Urinalysis

Like *blood test, urinalysis* means nothing specific. If he or she wished, the doctor could check for a hundred substances, but a routine urinalysis tests for half a dozen. Mostly we do this with a clever tool called a test strip, a plastic strip containing a row of paper squares impregnated with chemicals that change color when dipped in urine. I carry test strips in my bag.

Drug companies sell them in bottles of 100, and, depending on the number of test squares (from two to ten), each strip costs from 20 to 60 cents. Performing the test takes a minute. In the office, an aide reads the color changes from a picture on the side of the bottle and records them on a lab slip. For this service, you or your insurance pay $15 or $20.

Quick and simple, this is probably the most overused test performed during a periodic exam. Despite this simplicity, a routine urinalysis is not considered worth the trouble except in patients with a high risk of kidney disease: diabetics and pregnant women.

Here are the usual elements we check on the test strip.

Protein. The healthy kidney filters so efficiently that almost no large molecules like proteins appear in the urine. While any positive finding is abnormal, it's not necessarily ominous because protein can appear during a viral infection such as the flu, during a high fever, and after vigorous exercise. Like all findings on the test strip, readings are crude. In the case of protein, color changes indicate only trace, small, medium, and large amounts. Doctors often ignore trace and even small. If the doctor decides to take the test seriously, the next step is to collect a patient's urine for twenty-four hours to measure the exact amount excreted and determine the type of protein.

Glucose. This is a traditional test but surprisingly useless. As I mentioned, glucose doesn't spill into the urine until the blood level approaches 200, so the strip can't detect early diabetes. In the past, diabetics tested their urine to monitor treatment; this turns out to be wildly inaccurate; no diabetic should rely on this today. Home blood tests are far more dependable. One useful function of the strip is to confirm quickly a new case of diabetes when a patient comes in with symptoms.

Blood. Blood sometimes (but not always) appears in the urine during a kidney, bladder, or prostate infection, an injury (such as that from a kidney stone), or malignancy of the urinary tract. Since urinary tract cancers grow more common with age, some experts encourage this urine test in older patients.

Checking for blood in the urine helps me most when I wonder if a patient with back or flank pain is suffering a kidney stone. It helps less in an infection because symptoms are usually obvious.

Nitrite, Leukocyte Esterase. These substances may appear in infected urine; then again, they may not. Both are among many tests that help only if they're positive. I carry strips on housecalls, and when a test indicates an infection, I treat. When the test is negative but I believe the patient has an infection, I treat anyway.

Ketones. Ketones appear in urine when tissues break down fat to produce energy. Although this typically happens when diabetes goes out of control, I see it mostly in patients with flu or gastroenteritis who haven't eaten. After less than a day of fasting, the body runs out of stored carbohydrate and begins burning fat.

Bilirubin (Bile). The spleen removes aged red cells from the blood, breaks them down, recycles the iron, and then converts the hemoglobin to bilirubin, which reenters the blood. The liver takes up this bilirubin and uses it to make bile, which is secreted into the small intestine to help digest fats. A diseased liver has difficulty taking up bilirubin, so the blood level rises, and bilirubin spills over into the urine. Urine containing bile looks brown, so I usually know beforehand that the strip will turn positive, but this is a good quick test for hepatitis.

pH and Urobilinogen. Included on all but the most limited test strips, both are almost entirely useless. pH measures the acidity or alkalinity of the urine. This changes with diet and many diseases, but I can't remember the last time knowing a pH helped me.

I confess that I've looked up urobilinogen a dozen times during my life to remind myself what it means. As I write this chapter I must admit I've forgotten again, so I'll have to look it up. Colon bacteria break down some bile to form urobilinogen, which is then reabsorbed into the blood and either taken up again by the liver or excreted into the urine. Various liver and blood diseases increase urinary urobilinogen.

Specific Gravity. Urine is slightly denser than water, and a test strip can easily measure this density. If you drink a great deal of water, specific gravity drops; dehydration increases it. Diseases can do one or the other, but this information is rarely helpful.

The Sediment or "Microscopic." Although only useful if the doctor suspects urinary tract disease, this is usually included with all urinalysis. The technician pours urine into a test tube, spins it in a centrifuge, and then discards the liquid and examines the sediment under the microscope. More than a few white blood cells raise the suspicion of an infection or inflammatory disorder. More than a few red cells shows bleeding even if the test strip doesn't. A diseased kidney sheds cells and other debris detectable after centrifugation.

The microscope also reveals bacteria, but we don't pay much attention because routine urinalysis are often contaminated. Usually a doctor treats if the patient has symptoms of an infection and the sediment reveals white cells. Proof of infection requires a culture, which takes a few days. If the urine was contaminated, the culture reveals either a mixture of bacteria or a bacteria that normally doesn't cause urinary infections.

What the Electrocardiogram Shows

Of all office tests, the electrocardiogram (ECG) provides most patients their first experience with the wonders of technology. No pain or radiation is involved. The patient rests comfortably on a table while wires connect his or her wrists, ankles, and chest to a compact machine that whirrs, clicks, and spews out yards of paper tape covered with jiggly lines. To many laypeople, this tape records all the secrets of the heart.

An ECG records some secrets, but like all tests it can't measure everything. In order of accuracy, here are three aspects of cardiac function that doctors examine.

Most Accurate: The Heart Beat (Electrical Activity, or Rhythm). If your heart beats irregularly, skips beats, or becomes too irritable or the opposite, an ECG reveals what's going on in precise detail. A doctor can determine the source of the abnormal electrical signal, its path across the heart, the seriousness of each particular abnormal rhythm (hundreds exist; some are deadly, some trivial), and the effect of treatment on the rhythm.

The electrocardiogram measures electrical activity superbly because that's what it measures. The wire leads detect tiny electrical signals from the heart, and the machine amplifies them. The blips and lines on the paper don't measure muscle activity or pumping but simply the path of electricity across the heart. A nonbeating heart can still produce a regular tracing.

Health Care for the Healthy Man

Here is the consensus on the following tests that doctors routinely perform during a routine physical exam.

Generally considered essential	Generally considered of little use	Controversial
Taking blood pressure	The blood count	Stool exam for blood
Blood cholesterol	Blood sugar	Blood triglyceride
Sigmoidoscopy	Chest x-ray	Urinalysis (except after 65)
Dental checkups	Electrocardiogram	
Digital rectal exam	Treadmill test	Prostate specific antigen
Testicular exam	Multiphasic blood tests	
Initial head-to-toe physical exam	Regular complete exams in young men	Regular complete exams after fifty
Glaucoma check by an ophthalmologist	Glaucoma check by a family doctor	

This teaches an important rule that doctors as well as laypeople often forget: *The best way to test for something is to test for it.*

No matter how clever, a test that tries to detect something by detecting something else doesn't work as well. As you learned, for example, the best way to diagnose a bacterial urine infection is to observe the bacteria with a culture. Observing white cells, which are presumably fighting the bacteria, is easier but less accurate. Easiest and least accurate of all is dipping a test strip into the urine to look for suspicious chemicals.

Remembering this should give you a sense of proportion on the information an electrocardiogram provides in the two following areas.

Less Accurate: The Heart Muscle. Injured, dying, and dead tissue usually affects the electricity traveling across it. I can easily identify a pattern typical of ischemia (lack of blood) and tell a patient that he or she is probably having a heart attack. I can even determine the location of the injured muscle. A patch of dead scar tissue changes the electrocardiogram in a different way, so I can also tell a patient that he or she has probably had a heart attack in the past (some heart attacks don't produce symptoms).

But remember the rule: The best way to test for diseased heart muscle is to test for diseased heart muscle. Such tests exist using radioactive tracers that concentrate in either diseased or healthy heart muscle. A scanning camera than produces an image of the heart outlining the bad areas. Unfortunately, these take too long to be practical.

Examining the flow of electricity across the heart is fast, ingenious, and often useful, but it's indirect. Time and again current flows happily past a seriously damaged area with hardly a pause, producing an entirely normal tracing or perhaps one with vague nondiagnostic abnormalities. A doctor who sees a normal ECG on a person he or she suspects is having a heart attack must admit that person until repeated ECGs and blood tests (which detect chemicals released by dying heart cells—another indirect test but fairly accurate) confirm or rule out the diagnosis.

Least Accurate: The Health of Your Heart. Although doctors order it routinely, no expert recommends an electrocardiogram for this purpose. It doesn't detect early coronary atherosclerosis. In fact, it doesn't detect moderate and rarely detects advanced disease unless symptoms are also present. Piles of plaque might nearly choke your coronary arteries, but as long as barely enough blood trickles through, the ECG remains normal.

A tracing taken during vigorous exercise can reveal the ischemic changes mentioned earlier if the narrowed arteries don't supply enough extra blood. Some exerts recommend a regular exercise ECG for people at high risk such as hypertensives, smokers, and those with a high cholesterol, as well as anyone whose heart disease would endanger the public (such as airline pilots).

For the average man approaching middle age, the exercise ECG begins to look interesting, and fee-for-service doctors order it generously, but this is terribly risky. A positive test will come as devastating news to a man who thought he was healthy—rather like an abnormal mammogram affects a woman of the same age. But the woman with breast cancer enjoys a big advantage because doctors know how to treat a woman with an abnormal mammogram. We're much less certain how to handle a man who feels fine but has an abnormal exercise ECG. (I discussed this in the "Health Priorities for Men in their Fifties" section in Chapter 3.)

What X-Rays Are All About. Many men confuse X-rays with Superman's X-ray vision, believing that the rays can peer deeply into the area that's bothering them and find what's wrong. If they have a headache, they think they need skull X-rays; a backache requires back X-rays. Yet these are surprisingly unrevealing. Although a valuable tool, the X-ray helps only in certain situations.

An X-ray is not a photographic image. Unlike light rays which a lens can focus, X-rays travel in a straight line through the body to the film. Denser parts (such as bone) stop more of the rays than less dense parts (such as muscle). Lung, which is mostly air, stops hardly any. The result is a collection of light and dark shadows that vaguely resemble body parts.

Using a chest film as an example, here's what an X-ray can and can't reveal.

Shadows Where They Don't Belong. A tumor or infected fluid from pneumonia shows up clearly in the lung because malignant tissue and fluid are much denser than lung. A tumor in the heart or bowel would probably be invisible because tumor, heart, and bowel have the same density.

Irregular Shadows That Should Be Smooth. A fractured rib appears distinctly, especially if the ends are slightly separated, but a fine crack may be undetectable. An X-ray is unreliable at identifying anything smaller than half an inch in diameter.

Abnormally Large or Small Shadows. An X-ray can identify a grossly enlarged heart or collapsed lung. A heart attack doesn't change the appearance of the heart, nor does an asthma attack alter the lungs, so a chest X-ray appears normal although the patient may be desperately ill.

Generalized Disease. A normal chest X-ray often reassures smokers. Occasionally one promises to quit the instant his or her film reveals the first sign of emphysema. During emphysema lung tissue simply disappears, so the lung fields appear abnormally dark, but an X-ray is too crude to show darkening until most of the lung is gone. The first sign of emphysema on a chest X-ray means advanced disease. Similarly, osteoporotic bone appears lighter, but at least half the bone must vanish before anyone can detect this change, so a diagnosis of osteoporosis on an X-ray is evidence of severe disease.

When tuberculosis was common, a regular chest X-ray worked well at detecting early cases. Today, when TB occurs rarely except among immigrants and those who are HIV positive, the skin test has replaced it. Using the analogy with TB, doctors once X-rayed smokers to detect their lung cancer at an early stage. They succeeded, but unfortunately lung cancer is particularly virulent, and patients diagnosed on a routine X-ray died as often as those whose disease turned up after symptoms appeared. Despite this, practicing doctors feel uneasy allowing a smoker to leave the office un-X-rayed, so they continue the practice although experts no longer recommend it.

Once a traditional feature of the periodic exam and preemployment physical, the X-ray no longer serves a useful purpose, and you should refuse one if offered. Other screening tests offer little more. Despite all the miracles wrought by medical science, only a few reveal hidden, treatable disease in people who feel well: the blood pressure check, cholesterol, stool for occult blood, and perhaps the prostate specific antigen and glaucoma test.

To investigate an illness or accident, X-rays and other tests help a great deal, but by themselves these produce only numbers, pictures, or wavy lines, and they form a subordinate part of what doctors do. Doctors gather information, and then they think. Their greatest source of information is your description of what's happening to you. After considering this, the doctor can gather more information through an examination and tests, and the best diagnosticians order the fewest tests. Once you've chosen a good doctor and explained your problem, you've provided most of what's necessary to get the best medical care.

Dealing with your doctor

Two people take part in every doctor-patient relationship. During the past few decades, it's become fashionable to assert that the patient is an equal partner, and I even read this in editorials in my medical journals. This represents a misguided holdover from the 1960s, when my generation discovered that people in authority were receiving more respect than they deserved. The exhilarating battles that followed produced less than total victory but succeeded in curbing some major abuses.

In the process, however, many battlers stretched the meaning of *authority* into areas where victory was impossible. When you or I suspect that a police officer, a government official, or our boss is doing a bad job, we're usually right. Matters become more complicated with, say, a plumber or dentist. They have technical expertise which most of us don't share, so employing them involves a certain amount of blind faith. Faith plays a central role in our relations with a doctor, not necessarily because medicine is so technical (most of the time what we do is quite simple) but because so many visits involve fear. The saddest patients I see are those who are frightened but who, for various reasons, have no faith in the doctor.

I encourage everyone to learn as much science and medicine as possible from books like this and to ask plenty of questions about whatever a doctor is doing. We never explain enough; our thousandth what-to-do-about-your-hemorrhoids discussion is almost certainly shorter than our first. But, in the end, you have to trust that the doctor will take care of things. An earlier section in this chapter gave advice on picking a doctor worth trusting. This section explains your role.

What Your Role Should Be As a Patient

Proud of his strength, a man performs well at tasks that require suffering—*provided that he remains in control.* As a result, men do better than women at losing weight and quitting smoking. But they do worse at anything that involves giving up control: taking pills, keeping appointments, admitting that an illness is too much for them. Like all generalizations, it doesn't apply to everyone, but read on even if you think you're an exception.

Patient comes from an old French word meaning "to suffer," and the derivation continues to make sense. Since the dawn of history, no one thought of seeing a doctor unless he or she felt sick, and this remains true over most of the world today. The idea that a doctor could help someone who feels fine originated well into the twentieth century in a few industrialized Western countries and hasn't spread widely.

Paradoxically, the better you feel when you see the doctor, the greater your responsibility. If you have a broken leg, the doctor has little trouble making the diagnosis. For chest pain, you'll have to answer a few easy questions. If you feel only vaguely under the weather, the doctor conducts a more extensive interview, and if you're in perfect health and getting a physical exam he or she needs a large volume of information that only your lips can provide. You'll not only avoid blank spaces and question marks in your chart, you'll impress the doctor as sensible and well organized if you do some research. Do it before the first visit.

1. Talk to your mother.

An unrivaled source of information about the early years of my patients, mothers also provide fanciful and inaccurate diagnoses that stay with their sons throughout life.

Ask about early illnesses, especially those that required hospitalization. Try to learn facts rather than her opinion; an essential question is "What did the doctor say?"

Most important, if she has always insisted that you're allergic to something, find out how she knows. Mothers tend to be overly generous in diagnosing allergies, some of which can become a major burden to their offspring. For example, 90 percent of adults who say they're allergic to penicillin are wrong (proving they're wrong with skin tests is tricky and not routinely done). Besides its lifesaving qualities, penicillin has few side-effects and costs pennies a pill. Substitutes have more side-effects and may cost dollars a pill, so if you have an infection that penicillin cures, you're better off with penicillin.

You can't be allergic unless you suffer an allergic reaction (and diarrhea doesn't count). So you're home free if your mother decided that you were allergic because

- Your father was violently allergic.
- You had asthma and the doctor mentioned that he or she pre-
  ferred to avoid certain drugs.
- You had too much of that particular drug as a child.
- It gave you diarrhea.

Many rashes blamed on penicillin are actually part of the illness, but this is a decision that the doctor on the spot must make. Ask your mother what the doctor said at the time.

I stress getting the facts from your mother because you must not expect the doctor to take responsibility. (Let's say that, in answer to a routine question about allergies, you make the sort of statement I hear regularly: "I might be allergic to penicillin. My mother once said so. . . . No, I don't remember any problem, and I think other doctors have given me penicillin since she told me. Probably she was wrong.''). Thirty years ago the doctor might have agreed and prescribed penicillin when you needed it. If you suffered a reaction, he or she would apologize (most such reactions aren't serious).

Hearing this same statement in the 1990s, a reasonable doctor would slap a large red "allergic to penicillin" sticker on your chart. Once a patient barely hints that he or she might be allergic to a drug, any reaction that occurs if the doctor ignores the hint is the doctor's fault—and in the 1990s an apology might not be enough. While not major malpractice, in legal terms the reaction is a sure winner—rather like being rear-ended in your car. The patient who contacts a lawyer will collect a few thousand dollars, the doctor will have a loss on his or her record, perhaps a boost in his or her malpractice insurance, and he or she will have to explain the settlement on every future job application.

2. Find out about your relatives.

Doctors learn to take an elaborate family history in medical school, but as they gain experience this history gets shorter and shorter. Doctors are only human, and they gradually stop asking routine questions that patients can almost never answer.

Your chart probably contains a form for family history. Most doctors ask the appropriate questions during their introductory exam, but it's unlikely that they'll return to it, so any blanks that remain after the visit will stay blank. You can avoid this by doing some research.

Know the ages of your siblings, parents, and grandparents, or their age at death. This information about uncles and aunts is a bonus; cousins are less important unless a hereditary disease runs in the family.

Try to learn their significant medical problems. Don't theorize and don't allow your source to theorize. For example, if your father said his father died of a heart attack, ask how he knows. If your grandfather collapsed and died at home, a heart attack is only one of a dozen possibilities (unless an autopsy confirmed this). "Died suddenly at home" is all you can say. Suicide, alcoholism, and severe mental illness are all important parts of your family history as well as ongoing abnormalities such as high cholesterol.

3. Find out about yourself.

During the nineteenth century, tetanus and diphtheria were diseases of children, and they remain so in poor nations. In the United States today, tetanus and diphtheria are diseases of older adults who have neglected their immunization or never received them. Do you know when you had yours? Several, including tetanus and diphtheria, require periodic boosters. Your parents probably didn't discard your childhood shot record; find it and keep it current. Once again, don't theorize ("I broke my arm five years ago; I think I got something then"). If there's any doubt, ask the doctor to repeat your immunizations.

4. Communicate.

Despite the miracles of modern technology, 90 percent of our knowledge about our patients' problems comes from what they tell us. "Talk to your patients," professors of medicine teach students. "They'll tell you their diagnoses."

But sometimes they don't. Sometimes extracting information is so frustrating that the doctor ends up feeling worse than the patient. Here's an example from a man complaining that his stomach was bothering him.

> *Doctor:* "Bothering you in what way?"
> *Patient:* "It's been acting up since I moved to Chicago."
> *Doctor:* "A couple months?"
> *Patient:* "Three years. I saw a specialist when it began."
> *Doctor:* "What happened?"
> *Patient:* "He did tests."
> *Doctor:* "And what were the results?"
> *Patient:* "He gave me a prescription that helped. Could you give me a renewal?"
> *Doctor:* "What was the prescription for?"
> *Patient:* "Little white pills."
> *Doctor:* "Do you remember the name?"
> *Patient:* "No, but they were little white pills. For stomach trouble."

This obviously represents a communication problem. Don't assume it's entirely the patient's fault. The patient may have been a victim of poor communication from the previous doctor.

Since your information is so valuable, your doctor will work hard to get it out of you. You can make the job easier by following a few commonsense guidelines.

Be Specific. You wouldn't say to a mechanic: "My car hasn't been working right . . . it hasn't been itself . . . it's a little out of sorts." Faced with a patient who says he or she isn't feeling well, a doctor will probe for the facts. Why make the doctor work so hard?

What's wrong with this dialogue?

> *Patient:* "I've had this cold since last week."
> *Doctor:* "Last week . . . you mean seven days?"
> *Patient:* "Well, three days."
> *Doctor:* "A cold . . . you mean a runny nose and sore throat?"
> *Patient:* "No. A cough and sinus."
> *Doctor:* "Sinus . . . you mean pain over your cheeks?"
> *Patient:* "No. My nose is plugged."

The average doctor may say "you mean" a hundred times a day. Minimize this by telling exactly what's bothering you.

> Say "My ear hurts," not "My ear is infected."
> Say "I have an itchy rash," not "I'm allergic to something."
> Say "I hurt all over" only if your hair hurts along with everything else.

Don't assume the doctor can read between the lines.

> *Bad:* "My stomach kept me up all night." (How did it do this? Practicing its trombone?)
> *Good:* "The nausea (or pain or bloating) kept me up."

Don't give your diagnosis.

> *Bad:* "I think I'm having a nervous breakdown."

I know what *frightened* and *anxious* means, but when a patient tells me he or she is worried about a nervous breakdown, I'm mystified. That's a popular term that means different things to different people. Ditto for *pinkeye, tonsillitis, infection,* and *indigestion.*

Good: "I've been so depressed that I can't concentrate at work."
"My eye itches and there was a crust over it this morning."
"My throat hurts."
"I get stomach cramps and gas about an hour after I eat."

If you feel terrible, say so, and describe your feelings. Don't use a medical term to mean "serious." A bad headache is not necessarily migraine. A bad cough is usually not bronchitis. A bad sore throat is rarely strep.

Know Your Medical History. Don't assume "it's in the chart." That impressive folder on the doctor's desk may look like an organized, fact-filled record, but in my experience it could be illegible jumble of incomplete data. Remember, it's your body. The best place for the basic facts about it is in your head.

"I see you were hospitalized in 1973? What for?"
Useless: "For tests."
Not much better: "For my back."
Fair: "My back went out and stayed out."
Pretty good: "My back hurt worse than usual, and I felt it down my leg. The doctor thought it might be a slipped disk."
Ideal: "The doctor ordered tests. One showed a slipped disk. I felt better after a few days, so he said surgery wasn't necessary unless it kept bothering me."

Don't assume the doctor can "send for the records." He or she can, but it takes time, and sometimes they never arrive.

Very bad: "I don't remember . . . it's a long word."

I hear this several times a day when I ask the name of a drug or a medical condition. Frankly, it's hard to believe. People remember what's important to them. How many inhabitants of Indianapolis or Guadalajara would say, "Sorry, I don't remember where I live. It's such a big word"?

Encourage the Doctor to Communicate With You. If you're the sixth headache that the doctor has seen that day, his or her discussion may be shorter than it was for the first. It's the doctor's fault if you don't understand, but the only one to suffer will be you. Make sure you have answers to the following questions before leaving the office.

What Is My Problem? Don't accept meaningless descriptions such as "weak back," "nervous stomach," or "poor circulation." Would you pay a mechanic who told you that your car had "engine trouble?"

The problem should have a name. If it's a big scientific term, you should know what it means. Many impressive words are useless—they are simply a fancy name for your symptoms. Examples are dermatitis (rash), gastroenteritis (upset stomach), or arthritis (inflamed joints).

It should have a cause. A dermatitis may result from a germ, fungus, chemical, or allergy. Viruses cause most gastroenteritis, but bacteria or spoiled food are possibilities. Dozens of conditions produce arthritis. Never assume you know the cause. In my experience, you'll be wrong. Perhaps once a week a patient tells me that she (usually a she) has anemia. When I ask why (there are a hundred possibilities), she is usually surprised at the question. Don't you get anemia from a poor diet? Yes—in Bangladesh. In America it's rare.

The problem should have a treatment. If there's none, you should be told. Many doctors use a disease as a substitute for "no one is perfect," or "when you're under stress this is how your body responds." Some people prefer a medical problem to one of the proceeding statements. If you don't, make sure you know exactly what the treatment is and how long it should last. An important clue: No significant disease is treated by tranquilizers or multivitamins.

Do I Really Need This? Besides saving time and money, this lets the doctor know that you are a particularly sensible and self-reliant patient.

Most doctor visits are for minor problems that medical science cannot cure. Coughs, colds, viral infections, and upset stomachs last as long as they last no matter what the treatment. Minor injuries heal in their own time. Doctors vastly overtreat these conditions because experience has taught that most patients feel better if they receive something from the doctor: a shot, a prescription, a bandage—anything.

When I give a cough medicine for a cold or a cortisone cream for an itchy rash, I explain that it will help but it won't make the problem go away more quickly. Only rarely will a patient say, "If it's not essential, I'll skip it." So if temporary relief is not important, ask this question (but don't decide on your own whether the medicine is necessary).

A good relationship with a doctor involves more than handing over your body at regular intervals. Communication is indispensable. A physician can learn some things by examining you and a few others by ordering lab tests. But the greatest source of information is what you tell him or her. The most useful thing you can do in the doctor's presence is talk—and hope that he or she talks back.

INDEX